HANDBOOK OF FRACTURES

SECOND EDITION

D0168887

HANDBOOK OF FRACTURES

SECOND EDITION

Kenneth J. Koval, M.D.
Chief, Fracture Service
Department of Orthopaedic Surgery
New York University Hospital for Joint Diseases
New York, New York

Joseph D. Zuckerman, M.D.
Professor and Chairman
Department of Orthopaedic Surgery
New York University Hospital for Joint Diseases
New York, New York

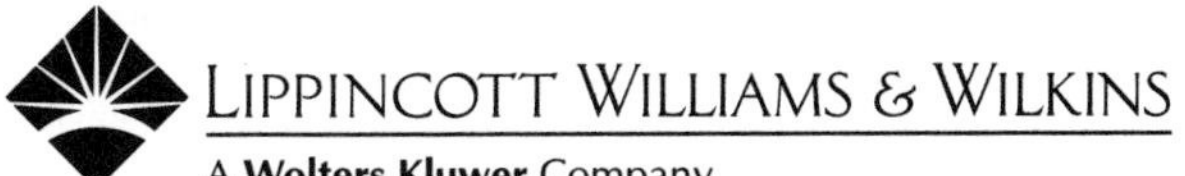

Philadelphia • Baltimore • New York • London
Buenos Aires • Hong Kong • Sydney • Tokyo

Acquisitions Editor: Robert Hurley
Developmental Editors: Brian Brown and Jenny Kim
Production Editor: Christiana Sahl
Manufacturing Manager: Benjamin Rivera
Cover Designer: Jeane Norton
Compositor: Circle Graphics
Printer: R.R. Donnelley/Crawfordsville

© 2002 by LIPPINCOTT WILLIAMS & WILKINS
530 Walnut Street
Philadelphia, PA 19106 USA
LWW.com

All rights reserved. This book is protected by copyright. No part of this book may be reproduced in any form or by any means, including photocopying, or utilized by any information storage and retrieval system without written permission from the copyright owner, except for brief quotations embodied in critical articles and reviews. Materials appearing in this book prepared by individuals as part of their official duties as U.S. government employees are not covered by the above-mentioned copyright.

Printed in the USA

Library of Congress Cataloging-in-Publication Data

Koval, Kenneth J.
Handbook of fractures.—2nd ed. / Kenneth J. Koval, Joseph D. Zuckerman.
p. ; cm.
Rev. ed. of: Fractures and dislocations / Scott W. Alpert . . . [et al.]. 1994.
Includes bibliographical references and index.
ISBN 0-7817-3141-0
1. Fractures—Handbooks, manuals, etc. 2. Dislocations—Handbooks, manuals, etc. I. Title: Handbook of fractures. II. Zuckerman, Joseph D. (Joseph David), 1952-III. Rockwood, Charles A., 1936-IV. Fracures and dislocations V. Title.
[DNLM: 1. Fractures—Handbooks. 2. Dislocations—Handbooks. WE 39 K867r 2001] RD101 .K685 2001
617.1′5—dc21 2001029666

Care has been taken to confirm the accuracy of the information presented and to describe generally accepted practices. However, the authors and publisher are not responsible for errors or omissions or for any consequences from application of the information in this book and make no warranty, expressed or implied, with respect to the currency, completeness, or accuracy of the contents of the publication. Application of this information in a particular situation remains the professional responsibility of the practitioner.

The authors and publisher have exerted every effort to ensure that drug selection and dosage set forth in this text are in accordance with current recommendations and practice at the time of publication. However, in view of ongoing research, changes in government regulations, and the constant flow of information relating to drug therapy and drug reactions, the reader is urged to check the package insert for each drug for any change in indications and dosage and for added warnings and precautions. This is particularly important when the recommended agent is a new or infrequently employed drug.

Some drugs and medical devices presented in this publication have Food and Drug administration (FDA) clearance for limited use in restricted research settings. It is the responsibility of the health care provider to ascertain the FDA status of each drug or device planned for use in their clinical practice.

10 9 8 7 6 5 4 3 2

This book is dedicated
to my understanding and patient wife, Mary,
and to my fantastic children, Courtney, Michael, and Lauren
—the loves of my life.

Kenneth J. Koval

To my wonderful wife, Janet,
and to my outstanding sons, Scott and Mathew,
for teaching me important lessons
about life and family.

Joseph D. Zuckerman

CONTENTS

IV. LOWER EXTREMITY FRACTURES AND DISLOCATIONS

V. PEDIATRIC FRACTURES AND DISLOCATIONS

PREFACE

This book represents the work of many physicians who trained at the Hospital for Joint Diseases. Starting in the early 1980s, the Department of Orthopaedic Surgery initiated a weekly, didactic topic-related fracture case conference. This conference consisted of a short lecture presented by a senior resident on pertinent anatomy, fracture mechanism, radiographic and clinical evaluation, classification, and treatment options and was followed by a series of cases that were used to clarify further the options for fracture care. The senior resident was also responsible for preparing a handout on the fracture topic that was distributed prior to the lecture.

Over time, those of us who worked there realized that these topic-related fracture handouts were useful as a reference for later study and that incoming residents used them as an aid in the Emergency Department. This realization resulted in the compilation of *Fractures and Dislocations: A Manual of Orthopaedic Trauma*, which was derived from these handouts. We originally organized and prepared it as an "in house" publication with the help of two senior residents, Scott Alpert and Ari Ben-Yishay, and an editorial associate, William Green. Initially, we also distributed the book. With its increasing popularity, it then became part of the Lippincott Williams & Wilkins publishing program.

This new volume is a modification of *Fractures and Dislocations: A Manual of Orthopaedic Trauma*, which was updated with the able assistance of Andrew Chen, M.D. It has been made possible by the hard work and effort of the many residents who trained at the Hospital for Joint Diseases. It is intended as a companion handbook for *Rockwood, Green, and Wilkins' Fractures in Adults* and *Fractures in Children,* and has been revised with this usage in mind. We have made efforts to include Orthopaedic Trauma Association classifications wherever possible to present a more standardized approach to the fractures discussed. We have also used some of the excellent illustrations from *Fractures in Adults* and *Fractures in Children*. Our hope is that this book will serve as a quick reference for clinicians, who can then refer to the texbook for more complete discussions.

Kenneth J. Koval, M.D.
Joseph D. Zuckerman, M.D.

ACKNOWLEDGMENTS

We thank the many people who made the writing of this book possible. In particular, we acknowledge the work of Andrew Chen, M.D., who updated the material from the previous edition of *Fractures and Dislocations: A Manual of Orthopaedic Trauma*; William Green, for his editorial insight; and the people of Lippincott Williams & Wilkins, who gave us the opportunity to produce this manuscript.

I. GENERAL CONSIDERATIONS

1. MULTIPLE TRAUMA

High velocity trauma is the number one cause of death worldwide in the 18- to 44-year age group. In the 1990s, in the United States alone, income loss due to death and disability secondary to high velocity trauma totaled 75 billion dollars annually; despite this, trauma research received less than 2% of the total national research budget.

FIELD TRIAGE

Management priorities are as follows:

- Assessment and establishment of airway and ventilation;
- Assessment of circulation and perfusion;
- Control of hemorrhaging;
- Extrication of the patient;
- Management of shock;
- Stabilization of the fracture;
- Transport of the patient.

Trauma Deaths

Trauma deaths tend to occur in three phases:

1. Immediate: usually due to severe brain injury or disruption of the heart, aorta, or large vessels; amenable to public health measures and education, such as the use of safety helmets and passenger restraints.
2. Early: minutes to a few hours after injury; usually due to intracranial bleed, hemopneumothorax, splenic rupture, liver laceration, or multiple injuries with significant blood loss. These represent correctable injuries for which immediate, coordinated, definitive care at a level 1 trauma center is most beneficial.
3. Late: days to weeks after injury; related to sepsis or multiple organ failure.

Golden Hour

- Rapid transport of the severely injured patient to a trauma center for appropriate assessment and treatment.
- Patient's chance of survival rapidly diminished after 1 hour. There is a threefold increase in mortality for every 30 minutes of elapsed time without care in the patient with severe multiple injuries.

RESUSCITATION

Airway Control

- Inspect the upper airway to ensure patency.
- Remove foreign objects and suction secretions.
- Establish a nasal, endotracheal, or nasotracheal airway as necessary. A tracheostomy may be necessary.
- Manage the patient as if a cervical spine injury is present; however, no patient should expire from lack of an airway because of a concern over a possible cervical spine injury. Gentle maneuvers, such as axial traction, usually allow for safe intubation without neurologic compromise.

Breathing

- Evaluate ventilation (breathing) and oxygenation.
- Recognize the most common reasons for ineffective ventilation after establishment of an airway, including malposition of the endotracheal tube, pneumothorax, and hemothorax.
  1. Tension pneumothorax
     Diagnosis. Tracheal deviation, unilateral absent breath sounds, tympany, and distended neck veins.
     Treatment. Insert large-bore needle into the second intercostal space at the midclavicular line, followed by a chest tube.

2. Open pneumothorax
   Diagnosis. Sucking chest wound.
   Treatment. Occlusive dressing should not be taped on one side to allow air to escape; follow with surgical wound closure and a chest tube.
3. Flail chest with pulmonary contusion
   Diagnosis. Paradoxical movement of the chest wall with ventilation.
   Treatment. Fluid resuscitation (beware of overhydration); intubation; positive end-expiratory pressure may be necessary.
4. Endotracheal tube malposition
   Diagnosis. Malposition evident on chest radiograph; unilateral breath sounds; asymmetric chest excursion.
   Treatment. Adjustment of the endotracheal tube and/or reintubation.
5. Hemothorax
   Diagnosis. Opacity on chest radiograph, diminished/absent breath sounds.
   Treatment. Chest tube placement.

CIRCULATION

- *Hemodynamic stability* is defined as normal vital signs that are sustained with only maintenance fluid volumes.
- In trauma patients, shock is hemorrhagic until proven otherwise.
- At a minimum, two large-bore intravenous lines should be placed in the antecubital fossae or groin with avoidance of injured extremities. Alternatively, saphenous vein cutdowns for adults and intraosseous (tibia) infusions for children younger than age 6 years may be used.
- Serial monitoring of blood pressure and urine output is necessary, with possible central access required for central venous monitoring or Swan-Ganz catheter placement for hemodynamic instability. Serial hematocrit monitoring should be undertaken until hemodynamic stability is documented.

INITIAL MANAGEMENT OF A PATIENT IN SHOCK

- Direct control of obvious bleeding: direct pressure control is preferable to tourniquets or blind clamping.
- Large-bore venous access, Ringer lactate resuscitation, monitoring of urine output, central venous pressure, and pH.
- Blood replacement as indicated by serial hematocrit monitoring.
- Traction with Thomas splints or distal extremity splints to limit hemorrhage from unstable fractures.
- Consideration of angiography (and/or embolization) or immediate operative intervention for hemorrhage control.

DIFFERENTIAL DIAGNOSIS OF HYPOTENSION IN A TRAUMA PATIENT

Cardiogenic Shock

Cardiac arrhythmias, myocardial damage, pericardial tamponade
Diagnosis. Distended neck veins, hypotension, muffled heart sounds (Beck triad).
Treatment. Pericardiocentesis through subxiphoid approach.

Neurogenic Shock

Thoracic level spinal cord injury in which sympathetic disruption results in an inability to maintain vascular tone.
Diagnosis. Hypotension without tachycardia or vasoconstriction; consider in head-injured or spinal cord-injured patient who does not respond to fluid resuscitation.
Treatment. Volume restoration followed by vasoactive drugs (beware of fluid overload).

Septic Shock

A consideration in patients with gas gangrene, missed open injuries, and contaminated wounds closed primarily.
Diagnosis. Hypotension accompanied by fever, tachycardia, cool skin, multiorgan failure. Occurs in the early to late phases but not in the acute presentation.
Treatment. Fluid balance, vasoactive drugs, antibiotics.

Hemorrhagic Shock

A finding in patients with large open wounds, active bleeding, pelvic and/or femoral fractures, blunt abdominal trauma, or thoracic trauma.

Diagnosis. Hypotension, tachycardia. In the absence of open hemorrhage, bleeding into voluminous spaces (chest, abdomen, pelvis, thigh) must be ruled out. May require diagnostic peritoneal lavage, angiography, computed tomography (CT), magnetic resonance imaging, and so forth as dictated by the patient presentation.

Treatment. Aggressive fluid resuscitation, blood replacement, angiographic embolization, operative intervention, fracture stabilization, and so on as dictated by the source of hemorrhage.

CLASSIFICATION OF HEMORRHAGE

Class I: Less than 15% loss of circulating blood volume.
Diagnosis: no change in blood pressure, pulse, or capillary refill.
Treatment: crystalloid.

Class II: 15% to 30% loss of circulating blood volume.
Diagnosis: tachycardia with normal blood pressure.
Treatment: crystalloid.

Class III: 30% to 40% loss of circulating blood volume.
Diagnosis: tachycardia, tachypnea, and hypotension.
Treatment: rapid crystalloid replacement, then blood.

Class IV: More than 40% loss of circulating blood volume.
Diagnosis: marked tachycardia and hypotension.
Treatment: immediate blood replacement.

BLOOD REPLACEMENT

- Fully cross-matched blood is preferable; approximately 1 hour is required for laboratory cross-match and unit preparation.
- Saline cross-matched blood may be ready in 10 minutes; it may have minor antibodies.
- Type O negative blood is used for life-threatening exsanguination.
- Warming the blood helps prevent hypothermia.
- Coagulation factors, platelets, and calcium levels must be monitored.

PNEUMATIC ANTISHOCK GARMENT

- Use: control hemorrhage associated with pelvic fractures.
- Systolic blood pressure: may support by increasing peripheral vascular resistance.
- Central venous pressure: may support by diminishing lower extremity pooling.
- Advantages: simple, rapid, and reversible; immediate fracture stabilization.
- Disadvantages: limited access to the abdomen, pelvis, and lower extremities; exacerbation of congestive heart failure; decreased vital capacity; potential for compartment syndrome.

INDICATIONS FOR IMMEDIATE SURGERY

Hemorrhage secondary to the following:

1. Liver, splenic, and/or renal parenchymal injury; laparotomy.
2. Aortic, caval, or pulmonary vessel tears; thoracotomy.
3. Depressed skull fracture or acute subdural hemorrhage; craniotomy.
4. Pelvic fracture; stabilization.

DISABILITY (NEUROLOGIC ASSESSMENT)

- The initial survey consists of an assessment of the patient's level of consciousness, pupillary response, sensation and motor response in all extremities, and rectal tone and sensation.
- The Glasgow coma scale (Table 1.1) assesses level of consciousness, severity of brain function, brain damage, and potential patient recovery by measuring three behavioral responses: eye opening, best verbal response, and best motor response.

Table 1.1. Glasgow coma scale (GCS)

Parameter	Score
A. Eye opening (E)	
1. Spontaneous	4
2. To speech	3
3. To pain	2
4. None	1
B. Best motor response (M)	
1. Obeys commands	6
2. Localizes to stimulus	5
3. Withdraws to stimulus	4
4. Flexor posturing	3
5. Extensor posturing	2
6. None	1
C. Verbal response (V)	
1. Oriented	5
2. Confused conversation	4
3. Inappropriate words	3
4. Incomprehensible phonation	2
5. None	1

GCS = E + M + V (range, 3–15).
Note: Patients with a Glasgow coma scale of <13, a systolic blood pressure of <90, or a respiratory rate of >29 or <10/min should be sent to a trauma center. These injuries cannot be adequately evaluated by physical exam.

- A revised trauma score results from the sum of respiratory rate, systolic blood pressure, and Glasgow coma scale and can be used to decide which patients should be sent to a trauma center (Table 1.2).

RADIOGRAPHIC EVALUATION

A radiographic trauma series consists of the following:

- Lateral cervical spine (C-spine)
  Must see all seven vertebrae and top of T-1.
  Can perform swimmer's view or CT, as needed. In the absence of adequate C-spine views of all vertebrae, the C-spine cannot be "cleared" from possible injury, and a rigid cervical collar must be maintained until adequate views or a CT can be obtained. Clinical clearance cannot occur if the patient has a depressed level of consciousness for any reason (e.g., ethanol intoxication).
- Anteroposterior chest
- Anteroposterior pelvis
- Possibly lateral thoracolumbar spine
- Possibly, CTs of the head, C-spine (if not cleared by plain radiographs), thorax, abdomen, and pelvis with or without contrast as dictated by the injury pattern

STABILIZATION

- The stabilization phase occurs immediately after the initial resuscitation and may encompass hours to days, during which medical optimization is sought. It consists of the following:
  1. Restoration of stable hemodynamics;
  2. Restoration of adequate oxygenation and organ perfusion;
  3. Restoration of adequate kidney function;
  4. Treatment of bleeding disorders.
- Risk of deep venous thrombosis is highest in this period; it may be as high as 58% in patients with multiple injuries. Highest risk injuries include spinal cord injuries,

Table 1.2. Revised trauma score (RTS)

Parameter	Rate	Score
A. Respiratory rate (breaths/min)	10–29	4
	>29	3
	6–9	2
	1–5	1
	0	0
B. Systolic blood pressure (mm Hg)	>89	4
	76–89	3
	50–75	2
	1–49	1
	0	0
C. Glasgow coma scale conversion	13–15	4
	9–12	3
	6–8	2
	4–5	1
	3	0

RTS = A + B + C.

femur fractures, tibia fractures, and pelvic fractures. A high index of suspicion must be followed by duplex ultrasonography.

- Subcutaneous heparin, low molecular weight heparin, and low dose warfarin have been shown to be more effective than sequential compression devices in preventing thromboses but are contraindicated in patients at risk for hemorrhage, especially after head trauma. Prophylaxis should be continued until adequate mobilization of the patient out of bed is achieved.
- Venacaval filters may be placed at the time of angiography; they are effective in patients with proximal venous thrombosis.
- Pulmonary injuries (e.g., contusion), sepsis, multiorgan failure (e.g., due to prolonged shock), massive blood replacement, and pelvic or long bone fractures may result in the adult respiratory distress syndrome.

DECISION TO OPERATE

- Most patients are safely stabilized from a cardiopulmonary perspective within 4 to 6 hours of presentation.
- Early intervention is indicated for the following:
  1. Femoral or pelvic fractures that carry a high risk of pulmonary complications (e.g., fat embolus syndrome, adult respiratory distress syndrome);
  2. Active or impending compartment syndrome, most commonly associated with tibia or forearm fractures;
  3. Open fractures;
  4. Vascular disruption;
  5. Unstable cervical or thoracolumbar spine injuries;
  6. Possibly with fractures of the femoral neck, talar neck, or other bones in which a fracture has a high risk of osteonecrosis.
- Patients that are hemodynamically stable without immediate indication for surgery should receive medical optimization (i.e., cardiac risk stratification and clearance) before operative intervention.
- Soft tissue status must be considered, because blistering, massive swelling, and tissue necrosis may result in wound compromise and dehiscence (see Chapter 2).

TSCHERNE CLASSIFICATION OF SOFT TISSUE INJURY (CLOSED FRACTURES)

Grade 0: minimal soft tissue damage; indirect violence; simple fracture pattern.

Grade 1: superficial abrasion or contusion caused by pressure from within; mild to moderately severe fracture configuration.

Grade 2: deep, contaminated abrasion associated with localized skin or muscle contusion; impending compartment syndrome; severe fracture configuration.
Grade 3: extensive skin contusion or crush; underlying muscle damage possibly severe; subcutaneous avulsion; decompensated compartment syndrome; associated major vascular injury; severe or comminuted fracture configuration.

CONCOMITANT INJURIES

Head Injuries

- The diagnosis and initial management of head injuries takes priority in the earliest phase of treatment.
- Mortality rates in trauma patients are associated with severe head injury more than with any other organ system.
- Neurologic assessment is accomplished by use of the Glasgow coma scale (Table 1.1).
- Intracranial pressure monitoring may be necessary.

Evaluation
Emergent CT either with or without intravenous contrast is indicated to radiographically characterize the injury after the initial neurologic assessment.

Cerebral Contusion
Diagnosis. History of prolonged unconsciousness with focal neurologic signs.
Treatment. Close observation.

Epidural Hemorrhage (Tear of Middle Meningeal Artery)
Diagnosis. Loss of consciousness with intervening lucid interval, followed by severe loss of consciousness.
Treatment. Surgical decompression.

Subdural Hemorrhage (Tear of Subdural Veins)
Diagnosis. Neurologic signs are slow to appear; lucid intervals may be accompanied by progressive depressed level of consciousness.
Treatment. Surgical decompression.

Subarachnoid Hemorrhage (Continuous with Cerebrospinal Fluid)
Diagnosis. Signs of meningeal irritation.
Treatment. Close observation.

Thoracic Injuries

- These may result from blunt (e.g., crush), penetrating (e.g., gunshot), or deceleration (e.g., motor vehicle accident) mechanisms.
- Injuries may include disruption of the great vessels, aortic dissection, sternal fracture, or cardiac or pulmonary contusions.
- A high index of suspicion for thoracic injuries must accompany scapular fractures.
- Emergent thoracotomy may be indicated for severe hemodynamic instability.
- Chest tube placement may be indicated for hemothorax or pneumothorax.

Evaluation
An anteroposterior chest radiograph may reveal mediastinal widening, hemothorax, pneumothorax, or musculoskeletal injuries.
Obtaining a CT with intravenous contrast is indicated with suspected thoracic injuries and may demonstrate thoracic vertebral injuries.

Abdominal Injuries

May accompany blunt or penetrating trauma.

Evaluation
A CT with oral and intravenous contrast may be used to diagnose intraabdominal or intrapelvic injury. Pelvic fractures, lumbosacral fractures, or hip pathology may be observed.

Diagnostic peritoneal lavage remains the gold standard for diagnosing operable intraabdominal injury.
Peritoneal lavage is needed in any patient with blunt trauma who cannot be adequately evaluated by physical examination.
CT of the abdomen is not as sensitive, as specific, or as accurate as diagnostic peritoneal lavage.
Ultrasound has been used to evaluate fluid present in the abdominal cavity.

Positive Peritoneal Lavage
Gross blood, bile, or fecal material;
More than 100,000 red blood cells per mL;
More than 500 white blood cells per mL.

Genitourinary Injuries

Fifteen percent of abdominal trauma results in genitourinary injury.

Evaluation
If genitourinary injury is suspected (e.g., blood seen at the urethral meatus), a retrograde urethrogram should be performed before insertion of an indwelling bladder catheter. Urethral injury may necessitate the placement of a suprapubic catheter.
If hematuria is present, a voiding urethrogram, cystogram, and intravenous pyelogram are indicated.

2. OPEN FRACTURES

- An *open fracture* refers to osseous disruption in which a break in the skin and underlying soft tissue communicates directly with the fracture and its hematoma. A *compound fracture* refers to the same injury, but its use is archaic.
- One-third of patients with open fractures are multiply injured.
- Any wound occurring on the same limb segment as a fracture must be suspected to be a consequence of an open fracture until proven otherwise.
- Soft tissue injuries in an open fracture may have the following three important consequences:
  1. Contamination of the wound and fracture by exposure to the external environment.
  2. Crushing, stripping, and devascularization resulting in soft tissue compromise and increased susceptibility to infection.
  3. Destruction or loss of the soft tissue envelope affecting the method of fracture immobilization, compromising the contribution of the overlying soft tissues to fracture healing (e.g., contribution of osteoprogenitor cells), and resulting in the loss of function due to muscle, tendon, nerve, vascular, ligament, or skin damage.

MECHANISM OF INJURY

- Open fractures result from the application of a violent force. The applied kinetic energy ($\frac{1}{2}mv^2$; m, mass; v, velocity) is dissipated by the soft tissue and osseous structures.
- The amount of osseous displacement and comminution is suggestive of the degree of soft issue injury and is proportional to the applied force.

CLINICAL EVALUATION

1. Patient assessment: airway, breathing, circulation, and disability (mnemonic—ABCD).
2. Initiate resuscitation: address life-threatening injuries.
3. Evaluate injuries to the head, chest, abdomen, pelvis, and spine.
4. Identify all injuries to extremities.
5. Assess neurovascular status of injured limb(s).
6. Assess skin and soft tissue damage: exploration of the wound in the emergency setting is not indicated if operative intervention is planned because it risks further contamination with limited capacity to provide useful information; it may also precipitate further hemorrhage.
   - Obvious foreign bodies that are easily accessible may be removed under sterile conditions.
   - The open wound should be covered with a sterile, saline-soaked gauze pad.
   - Sterile injection of joints with saline or methylene blue may be undertaken to determine egress from wound sites to evaluate possible continuity.
7. Identify skeletal injury and obtain necessary radiographs.

Compartment Syndrome

- Open fractures are not immune from the potentially disastrous consequences of a compartment syndrome, particularly with severe blunt trauma or crush injuries.
- Severe pain, decreased sensation, pain from a passive stretch of fingers or toes, and a tense extremity are all clues to the diagnosis. A strong suspicion or an unconscious patient in the appropriate clinical setting warrants monitoring of compartment pressures.
- Compartment pressures greater than 30 mm Hg or within 30 mm Hg of the diastolic blood pressure indicate compartment syndrome; immediate fasciotomies should be performed.
- Distal pulses may remain present long after muscle and nerve ischemia and damage are irreversible. The apparatus for measuring compartment syndrome is illustrated in Fig. 2.1.

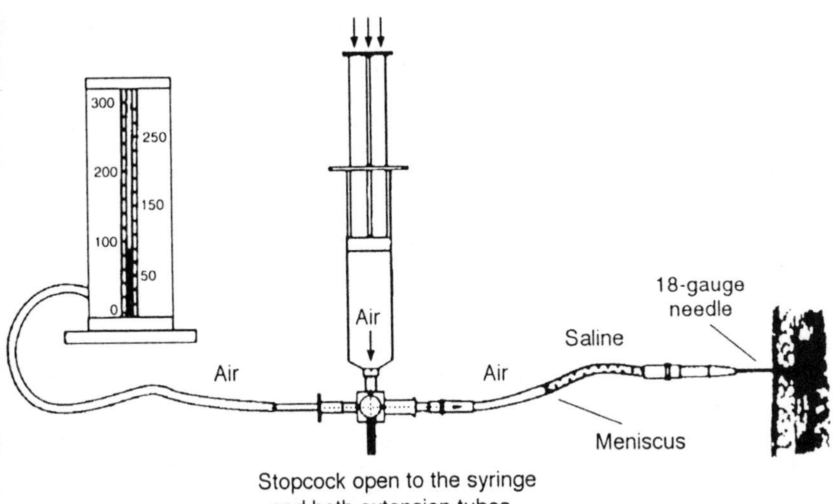

FIG. 2.1. Apparatus for measuring compartment pressures. (From Whitesides TE Jr, Haney TC, Morimoto K, Harada H. Tissue pressure measurements as a determinant for the need of fasciotomy. *Clin Orthop Rel Res* 1975;113:43, with permission.)

Vascular Injury

- An angiogram should be obtained if vascular injuries are suspected.
- Indications for angiogram include the following:
  - Knee dislocation;
  - Cool pale foot with poor distal capillary refill;
  - High energy injury in an area of compromise (e.g., trifurcation of the popliteal artery);
  - Documented ankle-brachial index less than 0.9 associated with a lower extremity injury.
  - (Note: Preexisting peripheral vascular disease may result in abnormal ankle-brachial indices; comparison with the contralateral extremity may reveal underlying vascular disease.)

RADIOGRAPHIC EVALUATION

- Trauma survey: lateral cervical spine film; anteroposterior views of the chest, abdomen, and pelvis.
- Extremity radiographs as indicated by clinical setting, injury pattern, and patient complaints.
- Including the joint above and below an apparent limb injury is important.
- Additional studies: computed tomography either with or without intravenous or oral contrast, cystogram, urethrogram, intravenous pyelogram, and angiography, as indicated clinically.

GUSTILO AND ANDERSON CLASSIFICATION (OPEN FRACTURES)

- Originally designed to classify soft tissue injuries associated with open tibial shaft fractures; later extended to all open fractures.
- Useful for communicative purposes despite variability in interobserver reproducibility.

Grade I: Clean skin opening of less than 1 cm, usually from inside to outside; minimal muscle contusion; simple transverse or short oblique fractures.

Grade II: Laceration more than 1 cm long, with extensive soft tissue damage; minimal to moderate crushing component; simple transverse or short oblique fractures with minimal comminution.

Grade III: Extensive soft tissue damage, including muscles, skin, and neurovascular structures; often a high energy injury with a severe crushing component.

IIIA: Extensive soft tissue laceration, adequate bone coverage; segmental fractures, gunshot injuries; minimal periosteal stripping.

IIIB: Extensive soft tissue injury with periosteal stripping and bone exposure requiring soft tissue flap closure; usually associated with massive contamination.

IIIC: Vascular injury requiring repair.

TSCHERNE CLASSIFICATION OF OPEN FRACTURES

Takes into account size of wound, level of contamination, and mechanism of fracture.

Grade I: Small puncture wound without associated contusion, negligible bacterial contamination, low energy mechanism of fracture.

Grade II: Small laceration, skin and soft tissue contusions, moderate bacterial contamination, variable mechanisms of injury.

Grade III: Large laceration with heavy bacterial contamination, extensive soft tissue damage, frequent associated arterial or neural injury.

Grade IV: Incomplete or complete amputation with variable prognosis based on location of and nature of injury (e.g., cleanly amputated middle phalanx versus crushed leg at proximal femoral level).

TSCHERNE CLASSIFICATION OF CLOSED FRACTURES

Classifies soft tissue injury in closed fractures, taking into account indirect versus direct injury mechanisms.

Grade 0: Injury from indirect forces with negligible soft tissue damage.

Grade I: Closed fracture caused by low to moderate energy mechanisms, with superficial abrasions or contusions of soft tissues overlying the fracture.

Grade II: Closed fracture with significant muscle contusion, with possible deep contaminated skin abrasions associated with moderate to severe energy mechanisms and skeletal injury. High risk for compartment syndrome.

Grade III: Extensive crushing of soft tissues, subcutaneous degloving or avulsion, arterial disruption or established compartment syndrome.

TREATMENT

Emergency Room Management

After initial trauma survey and resuscitation for life-threatening injuries (see Chapter 1), the following should occur:

1. Perform a careful clinical and radiographic evaluation as outlined above.
2. Address wound hemorrhage with direct pressure rather than with limb tourniquets or blind clamping.
3. Initiate parenteral antibiosis (see below).
4. Assess skin and soft tissue damage; place a saline-soaked sterile dressing on the wound.
5. Perform provisional reduction of the fracture and place splint.
6. Operate: open fractures constitute orthopedic emergencies, because intervention less than 8 hours after injury may result in a lower incidence of wound infection and osteomyelitis. The patient should undergo formal wound exploration, irrigation,

and debridement before fracture stabilization, with the understanding that the wound may require multiple debridements.

IMPORTANT:

- Do not irrigate, debride, or probe the wound in the emergency room if immediate operative intervention is planned. Doing so may further contaminate the tissues and may force debris further into the wound. Only obvious foreign bodies that are easily accessible may be removed, especially if they are causing further contamination or injury.
- Bone fragments should not be removed, no matter how seemingly nonviable they may be.
- Wound closure should not be performed in the emergency setting. A saline-soaked sterile dressing should be placed on the wound instead.

Antibiotic Coverage

Grades I and II: use a first-generation cephalosporin.
Grade III: add an aminoglycoside.
Farm injuries: add penicillin and an aminoglycoside.

Tetanus Prophylaxis

This should also be given in the emergency room (Table 2.1). The current dose of toxoid is 0.5 mL regardless of age; for immune globulin the dose is 75 U for patients less than the age of 5 years, 125 U for ages from 5 to 10 years, and 250 U for an age of more than 10 years. Both shots are administered intramuscularly, each from a different syringe and into a different site.

Irrigation and Debridement

Adequate irrigation and debridement is the most important step in open fracture treatment. The following steps should be taken:

- The wound should be extended proximally and distally to examine the zone of injury.
- The clinical utility of intraoperative cultures has been highly debated and remains controversial.
- A meticulous debridement should be performed, starting with the skin and subcutaneous fat.
  1. Large skin flaps should not be developed as this further devitalizes tissues that receive vascular contributions from vessels arising vertically from fascial attachments.
  2. A traumatic skin flap with a base to length ratio of 1:2 will frequently have a devitalized tip, particularly if it is distally based.
  3. Tendons, unless severely damaged or contaminated, should be preserved.

Table 2.1. Requirements for tetanus prophylaxis

	Clean minor wounds (<6 hr old)		All other wounds	
Immunization history	dT	TIG	dT	TIG
Incomplete (<3 doses) or not known	+	–	+	+
Complete: >10 years since last dose	+	–	+	–
Complete: <10 years since last dose	–	–	–[a]	–

+, Prophylaxis required; –, prophylaxis not required; dT, diphtheria and tetanus toxoids; TIG, tetanus immune globulin.
[a] Required if >5 years since last dose.

4. Osseous fragments devoid of soft tissue may be discarded.
5. Extension into adjacent joints mandates joint exploration, irrigation, and debridement.

- The fracture surfaces should be exposed, with recreation of the injury.
- Pulsatile low pressure lavage irrigation, with or without antibiotic solution, should be performed. Some authors have demonstrated decreased infection rates with more than 10 L of irrigation under pulsatile lavage.
- Meticulous hemostasis must be maintained, as blood loss may already be significant and the generation of clots may contribute to dead space and nonviable tissue.
- Fasciotomy should be considered, especially in the forearm or leg.
- Traumatic wounds should not be closed. Close the surgically extended part of the wound only.
- The wound should be dressed with a saline-soaked gauze or synthetic dressing.
- Serial debridement(s) may be performed every 24 to 48 hours, as necessary, until no evidence of necrotic soft tissue or bone is found.
- The role of dressing changes on the patient floor is controversial, but many clinicians advocate twice daily wet-to-dry sterile gauze dressing changes.

Foreign Bodies

Foreign bodies, especially organic ones, must be sought and removed because they are sources of contamination and additional morbidity. (Note: gunshot injuries are discussed separately; see Chapter 3.)

- Wood may become blood soaked and may therefore be difficult to differentiate from muscle.
- Cloth and leather are usually found between tissue planes and may be found in areas remote from the site of injury.
- The foreign material itself usually incites an inflammatory response, while intrinsic crevices may harbor pathogenic organisms or spores.

Fracture Stabilization

In open fractures with extensive soft tissue injury, fracture stabilization (internal or external fixation) provides protection from additional soft tissue injury, as well as maximum access for wound management and maximum limb and patient mobilization (see individual chapters for specific fracture management).

Soft Tissue Coverage and Bone Grafting

- Wound coverage is performed once no further evidence of necrosis is found (preferably by the third debridement).
- The type of coverage—delayed primary closure, split-thickness skin graft, rotational or free muscle flaps—depends on the severity and location of the soft tissue injury.
- Bone grafting can be performed when the wound is clean, closed, and dry. The timing of bone grafting after free flap coverage is controversial. Some advocate bone grafting at the time of coverage; others wait until the flap has healed (normally 6 weeks).

Limb Salvage

Choice of limb salvage versus amputation in Gustilo grade III injuries is controversial. Immediate or early amputation may be considered if any of the following are seen:

1. The limb is nonviable as evidenced by irreparable vascular injury, warm ischemia time greater than 8 hours, or severe crush with minimal remaining viable tissue.
2. Even after revascularization the limb remains so severely damaged that function will be less satisfactory than that afforded by a prosthesis.
3. The severely damaged limb may constitute a threat to the patient's life, especially in patients with severe, debilitating, chronic disease.
4. The severity of the injury would demand multiple operative procedures and prolonged reconstruction time that is incompatible with the personal, sociologic, and economic consequences the patient is willing to withstand.

Table 2.2. Mangled Extremity Severity Score (MESS) for prediction of amputation

	Points
A. Skeletal/soft-tissue injury	
1. Low energy (stab, simple fracture, low velocity gunshot wound)	1
2. Medium energy (open/multiple fractures or dislocations)	2
3. High energy (close-range shotgun, high velocity gunshot, crush)	3
4. Very high energy (above plus gross contamination, soft tissue avulsion)	4
B. Limb ischemia	
1. Pulse reduced or absent, but perfusion normal	1[a]
2. Pulseless, paresthesias, diminished capillary refill	2[a]
3. Cool, paralyzed, insensate, numb	3[a]
C. Shock	
1. Systolic blood pressure always >90 mm Hg	0
2. Hypotensive transiently	1
3. Persistent hypotension	2
D. Age (yr)	
1. <30	0
2. 30–50	1
3. >50	2

MESS was designed to predict the likelihood of amputation based on four criteria. A score of >7 accurately predicted amputation in 100% of limbs in both retrospective and prospective studies. MESS = total points.

[a] Score doubles for ischemia >6 hours.

5. The patient presents with a severe multiple organ system trauma in whom salvage of a marginal extremity may result in a high metabolic cost or large necrotic/inflammatory load that could precipitate pulmonary or multiple organ failure.
6. The expected postsalvage function does not justify salvage.

The Mangled Extremity Severity Score in Table 2.2 can be used to predict the need for amputation.

COMPLICATIONS

- *Infection.* Open fractures may result in cellulitis or osteomyelitis despite aggressive serial debridements, copious lavage, appropriate antibiosis, and meticulous wound care. Gross contamination at the time of injury is causative, although retained foreign bodies, soft tissue compromise, and multisystem injury are risk factors for infection.
- *Compartment syndrome.* A devastating complication resulting in severe loss of function, especially in tight fascial compartments, including the forearm and leg. This may be avoided by a high index of suspicion with serial neurovascular examinations accompanied by compartmental pressure monitoring, prompt recognition of impending compartment syndrome, and fascial release at the time of surgery.

3. GUNSHOT FRACTURES

BALLISTICS

- Low velocity (<2,000 ft/s): includes all handguns.
- High velocity (>2,000 ft/s): includes all military rifles and most hunting rifles.
- Shotgun wounding potential depends on the following:
  1. Chote (shot pattern);
  2. Load (size of the individual pellet);
  3. Distance from target.

ENERGY

- The kinetic energy (KE) of any moving object is directly proportional to its mass (m) and the square of its velocity (v^2) and is defined by the equation $KE = \frac{1}{2}(mv^2)$.
- The energy delivered by a missile to a target depends on the following factors:
  1. The energy of the missile on impact (striking energy);
  2. The energy of the missile upon exiting the tissue (exit energy);
  3. The behavior of the missile while traversing the target: tumbling, deformation, or fragmentation.

TISSUE PARAMETERS

- The wounding potential of a bullet depends on the missile parameters, including caliber, mass, velocity, range, composition, and design, and the target tissue parameters.
- The degree of injury created by the missile generally depends on the specific gravity of the traversed tissue: higher specific gravity = greater damage.
- A missile projectile achieves a high kinetic energy due to its relatively high velocity. The impact area is relatively small, resulting in a small area of entry with a momentary vacuum created by the soft tissue shock wave. This can draw adjacent material, such as clothing and skin, into the wound.
- The direct passage of the missile through the target tissue becomes the permanent cavity. The permanent cavity is small, and its tissues are subjected to crush.
- The temporary cavity (cone of cavitation) is the result of a stretch-type injury from the dissipation of imparted kinetic energy (i.e., shock wave). It is large, and its size distinguishes high energy from low energy wounds.
- Gases are compressible, whereas liquids are not. Therefore, penetrating missile injuries to the chest may produce destructive patterns only along the direct path of impact due to air-filled structures, whereas similar injuries to fluid-filled structures (e.g., liver, muscle) produce considerable displacement of the incompressible liquid with shock-wave dissipation, resulting in significant momentary cavities. This may lead to regions of destruction that are apparently distant to the immediate path of the missile with resultant soft tissue compromise.

CLINICAL EVALUATION

- After initial trauma survey and management (see Chapter 1), specific evaluation of the gunshot injury will vary based on the location of injury and patient presentation. Careful neurovascular examinations must be undertaken to rule out the possibility of disruption of vascular or neural elements.
- Attention must also be paid to possible injuries sustained after the missile impact, such as those that may occur after a fall from a height.

RADIOGRAPHIC EVALUATION

- Standard anteroposterior and lateral radiographs of the injured sites should be obtained.
- Specific attention must be paid to retained missile fragments, degree of fracture comminution, and the presence of other foreign bodies (e.g., gravel).
- Missile fragments can often be found distant to the site of missile entry or exit.

TREATMENT OF ORTHOPEDIC GUNSHOT INJURIES

Low Velocity Wounds

Victims may be able to be treated as outpatients.

Steps in Treatment

1. Administer antibiotics (first-generation cephalosporin), tetanus toxoid, and antitoxin.
2. Irrigate and debride the entrance and exit skin edges.
3. Indications for operative debridement include the following:
   - Retention in the subarachnoid space;
   - Articular involvement (intraarticular bone or missile fragments);
   - Vascular disruption;
   - Gross contamination;
   - Missile superficial on palm or sole;
   - Massive hematoma;
   - Foreign body or material;
   - Severe tissue damage;
   - Compartment syndrome;
   - Gastrointestinal contamination.
4. Treat fractures as closed fractures in general.

High Velocity and Shotgun Wounds

These should be treated as high energy injuries with significant soft tissue damage.

Steps in Treatment

1. Administer antibiotics (first-, second-, or third-generation cephalosporin versus vancomycin and aminoglycoside), tetanus toxoid, and antitoxin.
2. Perform extensive and multiple operative debridements.
3. Stabilize fractures.
4. Delay wound closure with possible skin grafts or flaps for extensive soft tissue loss.

IMPORTANT:

Gunshot wounds that pass through the abdomen and then exit through the soft tissues with bowel contamination deserve special attention. These require debridement of the intraabdominal and extraabdominal missile paths, along with the administration of broad-spectrum antibiotics covering gram-negative and anaerobic pathogens.

COMPLICATIONS

- *Retained missile fragments.* These are generally tolerated well by the patient and do not warrant a specific indication for surgery or a hunt for fragments at the time of surgery unless they are causing symptoms (pain, loss of function); are superficial in location, especially on the palms or soles; are involved in an infected wound; or are intraarticular in location. Occasionally, the patient will develop a draining sinus through which fragments will be expressed.
- *Infection.* Studies have demonstrated that gunshot injuries are not necessarily "sterile injuries" as was once thought. This is secondary to skin flora, clothing, and other foreign bodies that are drawn into the wound at the time of injury. Furthermore, missiles that pass through the mouth or abdomen are seeded with pathogens that are then dispersed along the missile path. Meticulous debridement and copious irrigation will minimize the possibility of wound infection, abscess formation, and osteomyelitis.
- *Neurovascular disruption.* The incidence of damage to neurovascular structures is much higher in high velocity injuries (military weapons, hunting rifles) due to the energy dissipation through tissues created by the shock wave. Temporary cavitation may produce traction or avulsion injuries to structures remote from the immediate path of the missile. These may result in injuries ranging from neuropraxia and thrombosis to frank disruption of neural and vascular structures.
- *Lead poisoning.* Synovial or cerebrospinal fluid is caustic to the lead components of bullet-missiles, resulting in lead breakdown products that may produce severe synovitis and low-grade lead poisoning. Intraarticular or subarachnoid retention of missiles or missile fragments are thus indications for exploration and removal.

4. PATHOLOGIC FRACTURES

EPIDEMIOLOGY

- The incidence of pathologic fracture is unknown due to underreporting and inaccuracies of diagnosis.
- A total of 75,000 cases of hypercalcemia are diagnosed in the United States each year; approximately 40% are secondary to malignancy, causing the elevated calcium level.

DEFINITION

- A pathologic fracture is one that occurs when the normal integrity and strength of bone have been compromised by invasive disease or destructive processes.
- Etiologies include neoplasm, necrosis, metabolic disease, disuse, infection, metastatic disease, iatrogenic causes (e.g., surgical defect), or primary bone tumor.

MECHANISM OF INJURY

- Pathologic fractures may occur as a result of minimal trauma or during normal activities.
- Alternatively, pathologic fractures may occur during high energy trauma involving a region that is predisposed to fracture.

CLINICAL EVALUATION

- *History.* Suspicion of pathologic fracture should be raised in patients presenting with fracture involving the following:
  Normal activity or minimal trauma;
  Excessive pain at the site of fracture before injury;
  Patients with a known primary malignancy or metabolic disease;
  A history of multiple fractures;
  Risk factors, such as smoking and environmental exposure to carcinogens.
- *Physical examination.* In addition to the standard physical examination performed for the specific fracture encountered, attention should be directed to evaluation of a possible soft-tissue mass at the fracture site, evidence of primary disease (e.g., lymphadenopathy, thyroid nodules, breast masses, prostate nodules, rectal lesions), and an examination of other painful regions to rule out impending fractures.

LABORATORY EVALUATION

- Complete blood cell count with differential, red blood cell indices, and peripheral smear.
- Erythrocyte sedimentation rate.
- Chemistry panel: electrolytes, plus calcium, phosphate, albumin, globulin, alkaline phosphatase.
- Acid phosphatase: males with unknown primary tumor.
- Urinalysis.
- Stool guaiac.
- Serum and urine protein electrophoresis (rules out possible myeloma).
- 24-hour urine hydroxyproline: Paget disease.
- Specific tests: thyroid function tests, carcinoembryonic antigen, parathyroid hormone, prostate-specific antigen.

RADIOGRAPHIC EVALUATION

- *Plain radiographs.* As with all fractures, include the joint above and below the fracture. Measuring size accurately is difficult, particularly with permeative lesions. More than 30% of bone must be lost before it is detectable by plain radiography.
- *Chest radiograph.* Rule out primary lung tumor or metastases in all cases.
- *Bone scan.* This is the most sensitive indicator of skeletal disease because it gives information on the presence of multiple lesions. "Hot" areas can be correlated with plain x-rays but may be "cold" with myeloma.

- Other useful tests in evaluating a patient with suspected pathologic fracture of unknown etiology include the following:
  - Upper/lower gastrointestinal series;
  - Endoscopy;
  - Mammography;
  - Computed tomography of the chest, head, and abdomen;
  - Liver, spleen, and thyroid scans;
  - Intravenous pyelogram and renal ultrasound.

Despite an elaborate workup, including all the tests outlined above, the primary disease process will not be identified in 15% of patients with suspected metastatic disease.

THE SPRINGFIELD CLASSIFICATION

The Springfield classification is based on the pattern of bone invasion.

Systemic

- Osteoporosis: most common cause of pathologic fractures in the elderly population.
- Metabolic bone disease: osteomalacia, hyperparathyroidism.
- Paget disease: present in 5% to 15% of the elderly population. Pathologic fracture is the most common orthopedic complication, seen in 10% to 30% of Paget disease patients—often the first manifestation of unrecognized Paget disease.

Localized

Accounts for most pathologic fractures and includes the following:

Primary malignancy of bone;
Hematopoietic disorders, such as myeloma, lymphoma, leukemia;
Metastatic disease:

- Most pathologic fractures (80%) from metastatic disease arise from lesions of the breast, lung, thyroid, kidney, or prostate.
- The most common locations include the spine, ribs, pelvis, femur, and humerus.

CLASSIFICATION BY PATHOLOGIC PROCESS

Systemic Skeletal Disease

Bones are weak and predisposed to fracture. Healing and callus formation are normal.

- Correctable disorders: osteomalacia, disuse osteoporosis, hyperparathyroidism, renal osteodystrophy, and steroid-induced osteoporosis.
- Noncorrectable disorders: osteogenesis imperfecta, polyostotic fibrous dysplasia, osteopetrosis, postmenopausal osteoporosis, Paget disease, rheumatoid arthritis, and Gaucher disease.

Benign Local Disease

- Nonossifying fibroma, unicameral bone cyst, aneurysmal bone cyst, enchondroma, chondromyxoid fibroma;
- Giant cell tumor, osteoblastoma, and chondroblastoma.

Malignant Primary Bone Tumors

Ewing sarcoma, multiple myeloma, non-Hodgkin lymphoma, osteosarcoma, chondrosarcoma, fibrosarcoma, and malignant fibrous histiocytoma.

Carcinoma Metastasized to Bone

Breast, lung, thyroid, kidney, prostate, and gastrointestinal malignancy.

Miscellaneous

Irradiated bone, congenital pseudarthrosis, and localized structural defects.

TREATMENT

Initial Treatment

- Standard fracture care—reduction and immobilization.
- Evaluation of underlying pathologic process.
- Optimization of medical condition.

Nonoperative Treatment

- In general, fractures through primary benign lesions of bone will heal without surgical management.
- Healing time is slower than in normal bone, particularly after radiation therapy or chemotherapy.
- Contrary to popular belief, the fracture will not stimulate involution of the lesion.

Operative Treatment

- Goals of surgical intervention are the following:
  - Prevention of disuse osteopenia;
  - Mechanical support for weakened or fractured bone to permit the patient to perform daily activities;
  - Alleviation of pain;
  - Decreased length and cost of hospitalization.
- Internal fixation, with or without cement augmentation, is the standard of care for most pathologic fractures, particularly of long bones. Internal fixation will eventually fail if the bone does not heal.
- Loss of fixation, due to poor bone quality, is the most common complication in the treatment of pathologic fractures.
- Contraindications to surgical management of pathologic fractures are the following:
  - General condition inadequate for tolerating anesthesia and the surgical procedure;
  - Mental obtundation or decreased level of consciousness that precludes the need for local measures to relieve pain;
  - Life expectancy of less than 1 month (controversial).
- Adequate management requires multidisciplinary care by oncologists, internal medicine physicians, and radiation therapists.
  - Radiation and chemotherapy are useful adjunctive therapies in the treatment of pathologic fractures and are potential mainstays of therapy in cases of metastatic disease.
  - Radiation and chemotherapy are used to decrease the size of the lesion, stop lesion progression, and alleviate symptoms.
  - Radiation and chemotherapy delay soft tissue healing and should not be administered until 10 to 21 days postoperatively.

Management of Specific Pathologic Fractures

Femur Fractures

- The proximal femur is involved in over 50% of long bone pathologic fractures due to its high weight-bearing stresses.
- Pathologic fractures of the femoral neck generally do not unite regardless of the degree of displacement; these require proximal femoral replacement. If the acetabulum is intact, a hemiarthroplasty may be indicated; however, with acetabular involvement, total hip replacement is required.
- Pathologic femoral shaft fractures may be managed with intramedullary nailing.
- Indications for prophylactic fixation are as follows:
  - Cortical bone destruction ≥50%;
  - Proximal femoral lesion ≥2.5 cm;
  - Pathologic avulsion of the lesser trochanter;
  - Persistent pain after irradiation.
- Advantages of prophylactic fixation include the following:
  - Decreased morbidity;

Shorter hospital stay;
Easier rehabilitation;
Pain relief;
Faster and less complicated surgery;
Decreased surgical blood loss.

Humerus Fractures

- The humeral shaft is frequently involved with metastatic disease, increasing the possibility of a humeral shaft fracture.
- Prophylactic fixation of impending pathologic fractures is not recommended on a routine basis.
- Operative stabilization of pathologic fractures of the humerus may be performed to alleviate pain, to reduce the need for nursing care, and to optimize patient independence.

Adjuvant Therapy: Radiation Therapy and Chemotherapy

The role in treatment of pathologic fractures is as follows:

- To palliate symptoms;
- To diminish lesion size;
- To prevent advancement of the lesion.

5. PERIPROSTHETIC FRACTURES

TOTAL HIP ARTHROPLASTY

Femoral Shaft Fractures

Epidemiology

- The overall incidence of intraoperative fractures is 0.8% to 2.3%, including cemented and uncemented components.
- Postoperative fracture has an incidence of 0.1%.
- Fractures occur more frequently with noncemented components, with an incidence from 2.6% to 4% to as high as 17.6% for noncemented revisions.

Risk Factors

- Osteopenia: may be osteoporosis or bone loss secondary to osteolysis.
- Stress risers of bone-cortical defects.
- Revision surgery.
- Inadequate implant site preparation: large implant with inadequate reaming or broaching.
- Pericapsular pathology: scarred capsule with inadequate release that may result in intraoperative fracture.
- Loose components: loose femoral components may be responsible for up to 33% of periprosthetic femur fractures.

Surgical Considerations

To avoid periprosthetic fractures during revision surgery, one should incorporate the following:

- Use a longer stem prosthesis, spanning two times the bone diameter beyond the defect.
- Consider bone grafting the defect.
- Place cortical windows in an anterolateral location on the femur in line with the neutral bending axis.
- Leave windows less than 30% of the bone diameter.
- Choose the correct starting point for reaming and broaching.

JOHANSSON CLASSIFICATION

Type I: Fracture proximal to prosthetic tip with the stem remaining in the medullary canal.

Type II: Fracture extending beyond distal stem with dislodgement of the stem from the distal canal.

Type III: Fracture entirely distal to the tip of the prosthesis.

COOKE AND NEWMAN CLASSIFICATION (FIG. 5.1) (MODIFICATION OF BETHEA ET AL.)

Type I: Explosion type with comminution around the stem; the prosthesis is always loose, and the fracture is inherently unstable.

Type II: Oblique fracture around the stem; fracture pattern is stable, but prosthetic loosening usually is present.

Type III: Transverse fracture at the distal tip of the stem; the fracture is unstable, but prosthetic fixation is usually unaffected.

Type IV: Fracture entirely distal to prosthesis; fracture is unstable, but prosthetic fixation usually is unaffected.

Treatment

Recommendations are as follows:

- Cooke and Newman type I periprosthetic fractures should be treated operatively (see below).

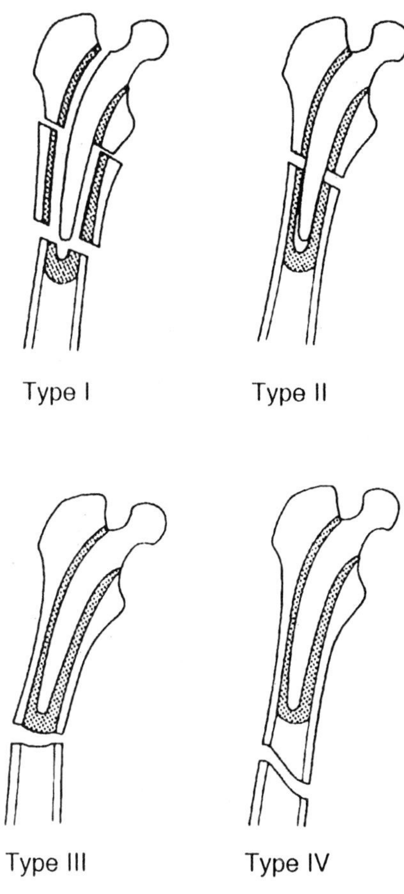

FIG. 5.1. Cooke and Newman classification of periprosthetic fractures about total hip implants. (From Cooke PH, Newman JH. Fractures of the femur in relation to cemented hip prostheses. *J Bone Joint Surg Br* 1988;70B:386, with permission.)

- Type II periprosthetic fractures may be treated nonoperatively but are associated with a high incidence of subsequent loosening.
- Type III periprosthetic fractures are unstable; nonoperative treatment is often unsatisfactory with an increased incidence of nonunion and malunion.
- Type IV periprosthetic fractures may be treated operatively or nonoperatively with a good union rate.

Nonoperative treatment follows these general principles:

- Alignment is important for possible future revision.
- Options include skeletal traction versus a spica cast for 4 to 7 weeks.

Operative treatment follows these general guidelines:

- Bone is frequently osteoporotic and may compromise adequate fixation.
- Operative treatment often leads to greater periosteal stripping. This may increase the likelihood of nonunion in cases where the endosteal blood supply is already compromised by prior canal preparation and stem insertion.
- Options include the following:
  Longer stem prosthetic revision;

Open reduction and internal fixation with plate, screws, Parham bands, and bone grafting;
Cerclage wiring with allograft struts;
Condylocephalic nails (noncemented stems).

Treatment for acetabular fractures is as follows:

- Nondisplaced fractures should be observed and should be treated with crutches and limited weight bearing. A very high incidence of late loosening of the acetabular component is found and requires revision.
- Displaced fractures should be treated by open reduction and internal fixation, and the component should be revised.

TOTAL KNEE ARTHROPLASTY

Supracondylar Femur Fractures

Epidemiology

- The postoperative incidence is 0.6% to 2.5%.
- These generally occur within 10 years after surgery, usually with relatively minor trauma.
- Fracture of the patella after total knee arthroplasty may occur, with a prevalence of 0.1% to 8.5%.
- Fragments are generally angulated anteriorly (which is opposite to normal supracondylar femur fractures). This is most likely caused by a posteriorly directed force and relative hamstring weakness.

Risk Factors

Supracondylar fractures after total knee replacement are multifactorial in origin:

- Osteoporosis;
- Preexisting neurologic disease;
- Notching of the anterior cortex:
  - Biomechanical analysis: 3 mm of anterior notching reduces torsional strength by 29%.
  - A high correlation exists between notching and supracondylar fractures in patients with rheumatoid arthritis and significant osteopenia.
  - No correlation between notching and supracondylar fractures is found in the absence of significant osteopenia.

NEER CLASSIFICATION, WITH MODIFICATION BY MERKEL (FIG. 5.2)

Type I: Minimally displaced supracondylar fracture.
Type II: Displaced supracondylar fracture.
Type III: Comminuted supracondylar fracture.
Type IV: Fracture at the tip of the prosthetic femoral stem of the diaphysis above the prosthesis.
Type V: Any fracture of the tibia.

Treatment

Recommendations are as follows:

- Anatomic and mechanical alignment are critical.
- Nondisplaced fractures may be treated nonoperatively.
- Open reduction and internal fixation are indicated if the alignment is unacceptable by closed means and if bone stock is adequate for fixational devices.
- The fracture should be treated nonoperatively, despite poor alignment, with clinical and radiographic reevaluation after healing if bone quality is poor.
- Immediate prosthetic revision is indicated in selected cases.

Nonoperative treatment includes the following:

- Skeletal traction, long-leg casting, or cast bracing for 4 to 8 weeks may be used to treat type I fractures.

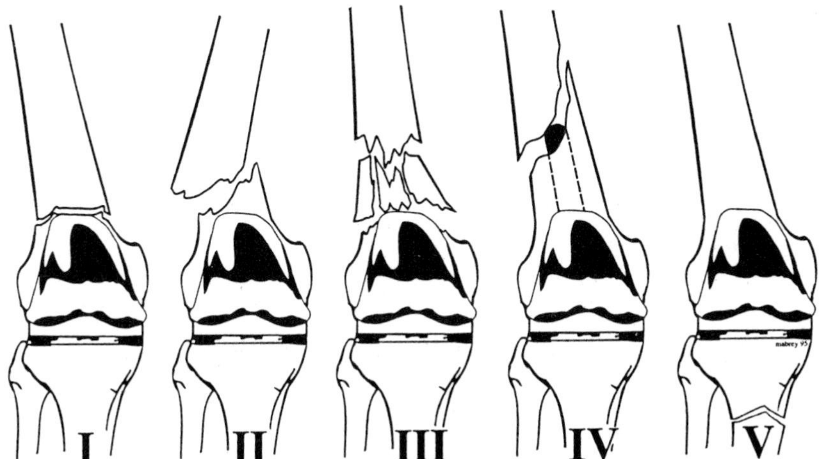

FIG. 5.2. Classification scheme for periprosthetic fracture of the knee. (Types I, II, and III from Neer C, Grantham S, Shelton M. Supracondylar fracture of the adult femur. A study of 110 cases. *J Bone Joint Surg Am* 1967;49A:591, with permission; and from Merkel KD, Johnson EW. Supracondylar fracture of the femur after total knee arthroplasty. *J Bone Joint Surg Am* 1986; 68A:29–43, with permission.)

Operative treatment includes the following:

- Type II fractures are almost always managed with open reduction and internal fixation because of the difficulties in maintaining acceptable alignment after displacement.
  - A fixed angle plate, dynamic compression plate, condylar buttress plate, or retrograde intramedullary nailing may be used for operative stabilization.
  - Primary revision with a stemmed component may be considered if involvement of the bone-implant interface exists.
  - Bone loss may be addressed with autologous grafting.
  - Cases of severe bone loss, especially in the metaphyseal region, may be addressed with distal femoral replacement with a specialized prosthesis designed for oncology management.
- Type III fractures are particularly suited for retrograde intramedullary nailing, as dissection of the individual fragments may devascularize them. Consideration may be given to a distal femoral replacement prosthesis designed for tumor management in cases with extensive comminution or bone loss.
- Type IV fractures around the diaphysis or the tip of a femoral component may be treated with cortical strut grafts and cerclage wiring, a dynamic compression plate, or a combination of techniques.
- Alignment guidelines are as follows:
  - Angulation <5 to 10 degrees in either plane.
  - Translation <5 mm.
  - Rotation <10 degrees.
  - Shortening <1 cm.

Tibial Fractures (Neer and Merkel Type V)

Epidemiology

- Tibial plateau fractures are most common (medial are more common than lateral).
- Shaft fractures are uncommon and are related to press-fit stems.

Risk Factors

- Significant trauma (shaft fractures).
- Tibial component malalignment associated with increased medial plateau stress fractures.
- Revision surgery with press-fit stems.

Treatment

Nonoperative treatment is as follows:

- Closed reduction and cast immobilization may be performed for most shaft fractures after alignment is restored.
- Early conversion to a cast brace to preserve knee range of motion is advised.

Operative treatment is as follows:

- Periprosthetic tibial fractures not involving the plateau may require open cerclage wiring and bone grafting if closed reduction and cast immobilization are unsuccessful.
- Type V fractures of the tibia typically involve the bone-implant interface, necessitating revision of the tibial component. Plateau fractures are usually associated with loosening; early component revision is recommended to maintain an acceptable functional result.

Patella Fractures

Epidemiology

The postoperative incidence is 0.3% to 5.4% (reported as high as 21%).

Risk Factors

- Large central peg component;
- Excessive resection of the patella during prosthetic implantation;
- Lateral release, with devascularization of the patella;
- Malalignment;
- Thermal necrosis (secondary to the use of methylmethacrylate).

GOLDBERG CLASSIFICATION

Type I: Fractures not involving cement/implant composite or quadriceps mechanism.
Type II: Fractures involving cement/implant composite and/or quadriceps mechanism.
Type IIIA: Inferior pole fractures with patellar ligament disruption.
Type IIIB: Inferior pole fractures without patellar ligament disruption.
Type IV: Fracture-dislocations.

Treatment

Nonoperative treatment is as follows:

- Fractures without component loosening, extensor mechanism rupture, or malalignment of the implant (type I or IIIB) may be treated nonoperatively.
- The patient may be placed in a knee immobilizer for 4 to 6 weeks; partial weight bearing with crutches is acceptable.

Operative treatment is as follows:

- Surgery is indicated for patients with disruption of the extensor mechanism, patellar dislocation, or prosthetic loosening.
- Treatment options include the following:
  - Open reduction and internal fixation with revision of the prosthetic patella, which are indicated for type II, IIIA, and IV fractures.
  - Fragment excision, which may be undertaken for small fragments that do not compromise implant stability or patellar tracking.

Patellectomy, which may be necessary in cases of extensive comminution or devascularization with osteonecrosis.

- A cadaveric study, by intraarterial contrast injection, demonstrated impaired patellar blood flow after medial arthrotomies within 1 cm of the patellar margin and lateral releases within 1.5 cm.
- Surgical considerations include adequate medial arthrotomy margin, adequate lateral release margin, preservation of the superior lateral geniculate artery, and preservation of the patellar fat pad.

Total Shoulder Arthroplasty

Epidemiology

- Periprosthetic fractures of the shoulder complicate approximately 2% of cases.

Risk Factors

- Excessive reaming of the proximal humerus.
- Overimpaction of the humeral component.
- Excessive torque placed on the humerus during implant insertion.

UNIVERSITY OF TEXAS AT SAN ANTONIO CLASSIFICATION OF PERIPROSTHETIC SHOULDER FRACTURES (FIG. 5.3)

Type I: Fractures occurring proximal to the tip of the humeral prosthesis.
Type II: Fractures occurring in the proximal portion of the humerus with distal extension beyond the tip of the humeral prosthesis.
Type III: Fractures occurring entirely distal to the tip of the humeral prosthesis.
Type IV: Fractures occurring adjacent to the glenoid prosthesis.

Treatment

Choice of treatment is controversial. Some advocate nonoperative treatment with surgical intervention indicated for compromise of prosthetic fixation and intraopera-

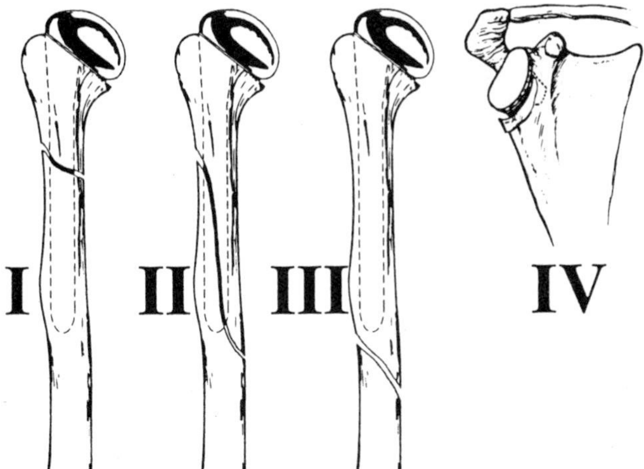

FIG. 5.3. Classification of periprosthetic shoulder fractures. Type I: Fractures occurring in the proximal portion of the prosthesis. Type II: Fractures occurring in the proximal portion of the humerus with distal extension beyond the tip of the prothesis. Type III: Fractures occurring entirely distal to the tip of the prosthesis. Type IV: Fractures occurring adjacent to the glenoid prosthesis. (From Rockwood CA, Green DP, Bucholz RW, Heckman JD. *Rockwood and Green's fractures in adults*, 4th ed. Philadelphia: Lippincott-Raven, 1996:543, with permission.)

tive fractures. Others advocate aggressive operative stabilization of all periprosthetic fractures of the shoulder.

Nonoperative treatment is as follows:

- Closed treatment involves fracture brace, isometric exercises, and early range of motion exercises until radiographic evidence of healing.

Operative treatment is as follows:

- Primary goals include fracture union, prosthesis stability, and maintenance of motion.
- Open reduction and internal fixation may be performed with cerclage wiring with possible bone grafting.
- Revision to a long-stem prosthesis may be required for cases with gross implant loosening.
- Options for postoperative immobilization range from sling immobilization for comfort until range-of-motion exercises can be instituted to shoulder spica casting for 6 weeks in cases of tenuous fixation.

Total Elbow Arthroplasty

Epidemiology

- Overall prevalence of periprosthetic fractures of the elbow is approximately 8%.
- Most fractures are preceded by prosthetic loosening and thinning of the cortices. These occur more commonly in the humerus than in the ulna.

Risk Factors

- Osteoporosis.
- Paucity of bone between the medial and lateral columns of the distal humerus.
- Abnormal humeral bowing in the sagittal plane.
- The size and angulation of the humeral and ulnar medullary canals.
- Excessive reaming to accommodate the prostheses.
- Revision elbow surgery.

CLASSIFICATION (FIG. 5.4)

Type I: Fracture of the humerus proximal to the humeral component.
Type II: Fracture of the humerus or ulna in any location along the length of the prosthesis.
Type III: Fracture of the ulna distal to the ulnar component.
Type IV: Fracture of the implant.

Treatment

Nonoperative treatment is as follows:

- All nondisplaced periprosthetic fractures that do not compromise implant stability may be initially addressed with splinting at 90 degrees and early isometric exercises.
- The patient may then be changed to a fracture brace for 3 to 6 weeks.

Operative treatment is as follows:

- Displaced type I or type II fractures may be managed with open reduction and internal fixation with cerclage wire fixation, Parham bands, or plates and screws. Alternatively, revision to a long-stem humeral component may be performed, with the component extending at least two diameters proximal to the tip of the implant. Supplemental bone grafting may be used as necessary.
- Type III fractures are usually amenable to cerclage wiring.

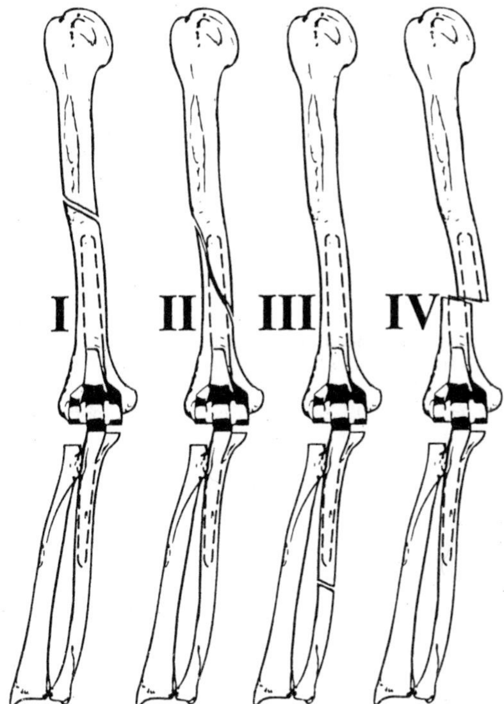

FIG. 5.4. Classification of periprosthetic elbow fractures. Type I: Fracture of the humerus proximal to the humeral component. Type II: Fracture of the humerus or ulna in any location along the length of the prosthesis (including those fractures that extend proximal and distal to the humeral and ulnar components, respectively). Type III: Fracture of the ulna distal to the ulnar component. Type IV: Fracture of the implant. (From Heckman JD, Bucholz RW, eds. *Rockwood, Green, and Wilkins' Fractures in Adults*. Philadelphia: Lippincott Williams & Wilkins, 2001.)

- Consideration should be given to more constrained prostheses if rigid fixation of implant components cannot be obtained.
- All Type IV fractures require component revision.
- Displaced olecranon fractures should be fixed with a tension band and cement.

Fractures About Large-Segment Allografts

Epidemiology

- These occur in 16% to 40% of cases, mostly in the distal femur, proximal tibia, and distal tibia.
- Risk increases four- to fivefold with plate fixation and adjuvant chemotherapy.

Mechanism of Injury

- Most are spontaneous, occur 2 to 3 years after implantation, and are not related to trauma.
- A possible cause is nonunion at the graft-host junction.
- These fractures generally occur through defects in the graft (i.e., screw holes) and in areas where revascularization and host-tissue ingrowth are absent.

BERREY ET AL. CLASSIFICATION

Type I: Rapid dissolution of the graft (rare).
Type II: Fracture of the shaft (most common).
Type III: Intraarticular fracture of an osteochondral allograft.

Treatment

Immobilization is generally ineffective.

Autogenous bone graft should be placed at the graft-host junction (if a nonunion is present) and at the fracture site. The creation of stress risers should be avoided.

Type I. Revise with either a new allograft, a vascularized fibular graft (if feasible), or a prosthesis.

Type II. Revise with new allograft; intramedullary fixation is recommended if the fracture is >0 cm from the joint line; fixation can be augmented with methylmethacrylate; prosthetic replacement may be considered.

Type III. Revise with osteochondral allograft and intramedullary fixation; consider prosthetic replacement.

Good results are expected in 50% to 80% of cases; the prognosis is better than for infection or tumor recurrence.

II. AXIAL SKELETON FRACTURES

6. GENERAL SPINE

EPIDEMIOLOGY

- Approximately 11,000 new spinal cord injuries requiring treatment occur each year.
- Delayed diagnosis of vertebral injury is frequently associated with loss of consciousness secondary to multiple trauma or intoxication with alcohol or drugs.
- The ratio of males to females sustaining vertebral fractures is 4 : 1.
- In older patients (>75 years of age), 60% of vertebral fractures are caused by falls.

ANATOMY

- The spinal cord occupies approximately 35% of the canal at the level of the atlas (C-1) and 50% of the canal in the lower cervical spine and thoracolumbar segments. The remainder of the canal is filled with epidural fat, cerebrospinal fluid, and dura mater.
- A *myelomere* is a segment of cord from which a nerve root arises. Each myelomere lies one level above the same numbered vertebral body until T-10. The lumbar myelomeres are concentrated between the T-11 and L-1.
- The *conus medullaris* represents the caudal termination of the spinal cord. It contains the sacral and coccygeal myelomeres and lies dorsal to the L-1 body and L1-2 intervertebral disk.
- The *cauda equina* (literally translated as horse's tail) represents the motor and sensory roots of the lumbosacral myelomeres. These roots are less likely to be injured because they have more room in the canal and are not tethered to the same degree as the spinal cord. Furthermore, the motor nerve roots are composed of lower motor neurons that are more resilient to injury than are the upper motor neurons of the brain and spinal cord.
- A *reflex arc* is a simple sensorimotor pathway that can function without using either ascending or descending white matter long-tract axons. A spinal cord level that is anatomically and physiologically intact may demonstrate a functional reflex arc at that level despite dysfunction of the spinal cord cephalad to that level.

MECHANISM OF INJURY

Primary

- Contusion: a sudden brief compression by a displaced structure. This accounts for most primary injuries and is thus responsible for most neurologic deficits. Contusion injuries are potentially reversible, although irreversible neuronal death occurs along with vascular injury and intramedullary hemorrhage.
- Compression: injury resulting from decreased size of the spinal canal. This may occur with translation or angulation of the spinal column, as with burst injuries, or with epidural hematomas. Injury occurs by mechanical deformation interrupting axonal flow or interruption of spinal vascularity, resulting in ischemia of neurologic structures.
- Stretch: injury resulting in longitudinal traction, as in the case of a flexion-distraction injury. Injury occurs as a result of capillary and axonal collapse secondary to tensile distortion.
- Laceration: caused by penetrating foreign bodies, missile fragments, or displaced bone.

Secondary

This refers to injuries to the spinal cord that result from the ischemia and edema that accompany all spinal cord injuries due to vascular disruption at the time of injury and the release of vasoactive substances in response to injury. This results in further compromise of the spinal microvasculature, with resultant cell membrane disruption, edema, and progressive neurologic deficit.

CLINICAL EVALUATION

1. Assess the patient: **A**irway, **B**reathing, **C**irculation, **D**isability.
2. Initiate resuscitation: address life-threatening injuries.
3. Evaluate level of consciousness.
4. Evaluate injuries to head, chest, abdomen, pelvis, and spine. Log roll patient to assess spinal column, examine skin for bruising and abrasions, and palpate spinous processes for tenderness and diastasis. Evaluate for noncontiguous spinal injuries; many authors have emphasized the need to evaluate the spinal column for injuries to more than one level.
   - Calenoff found a 5% incidence of multiple noncontiguous vertebral injuries. Half of the secondary lesions were initially missed, with a mean delay of 53 days in their diagnosis; 40% of second-degree lesions occurred above the first-degree lesion and 60%, below. The region T2-7 accounted for 47% of primary lesions in this population but for only 16% of reported spinal injuries in general.
   - Three common patterns of noncontiguous spinal injuries are as follows:

     Pattern A: first-degree injury at C5-7, second-degree injuries at T-12 or in the lumbar spine.

     Pattern B: first-degree injury at T2-4 with second-degree injuries in the cervical spine.

     Pattern C: first-degree injury at Tl2-L2 with second-degree injury at L4-5.
5. Assess injuries to extremities.
6. Complete neurologic examination to evaluate reflexes, sensation (touch, pain), and motor function. Figure 6.1 illustrates the pain-temperature dermatone chart.
7. Perform a rectal exam to test for perianal sensation, resting tone, and the bulbocavernosus reflex.

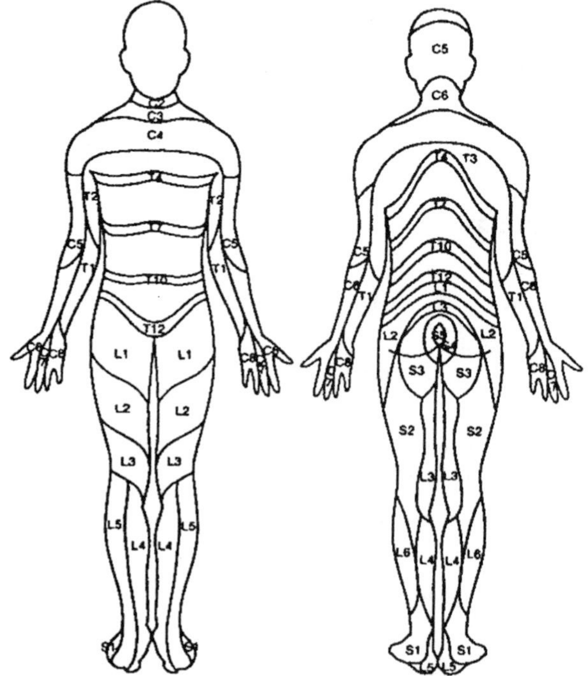

FIG. 6.1. Pain-temperature dermatone chart. Note that C-4 includes the upper chest just superior to T-2. The rest of the cervical and T-1 roots are located in the upper extremities. (From Benson DR, Keenan TL. Evaluation and treatment of trauma to the vertebral column. *Instr Court Lect* 1990;39:584, with permission.)

Spinal Shock

Spinal shock is defined as a spinal cord nervous tissue dysfunction based on physiologic rather than structural disruption. Resolution of spinal shock may be recognized when reflex arcs caudal to the level of injury begin to function again, usually within 24 hours of injury.

Bulbocavernosus Reflex

- The bulbocavernosus reflex refers to contraction of the anal sphincter in response to stimulation of the trigone of the bladder with either a squeeze on the glans penis, a tap on the mons pubis, or a pull on a urethral catheter.
- Absence of this reflex indicates spinal shock.
- The return of the bulbocavernosus reflex, generally within 24 hours of the initial injury, hallmarks the end of spinal shock.
- The presence of a complete lesion after spinal shock has resolved portends a virtually nonexistent chance of neurologic recovery.
- The bulbocavernosus reflex is not prognostic for lesions involving the conus medullaris or the cauda equina.

Neurogenic Shock

- Refers to flaccid paralysis, areflexia, and lack of sensation secondary to physiologic spinal cord "shut-down" in response to injury.
- Most common in cervical and upper thoracic injuries.
- Almost always resolves within 24 to 48 hours.
- Bulbocavernosus reflex (S2-3) first to return.
- Occurs secondary to sympathetic outflow disruption (T1-L2) with resultant unopposed vagal (parasympathetic) tone.
- Initial tachycardia and hypertension immediately after injury, followed by hypotension accompanied by bradycardia and venous pooling.
- Hypotension from neurogenic shock differentiated from cardiogenic, septic, and hypovolemic shock by the presence of associated bradycardia (as opposed to tachycardia).
- Treatment based on administration of isotonic fluids, with careful assessment of fluid status (beware of overhydration).

RADIOGRAPHIC EVALUATION

- Lateral cervical spine radiograph is routine in the standard evaluation of trauma patients. Patients complaining of neck pain should undergo complete radiographic evaluation of the cervical spine, including anteroposterior and odontoid views.
- Lateral radiographic examination of the entire spine is recommended in patients with spine fractures where complete clinical assessment is impaired due to neurologic injury or other associated injuries.
- Computed tomography or tomogram may be necessary for cervical spine clearance in patients with questionable or inadequate plain radiographs or to assess the occipitocervical and cervicothoracic junction.
- Magnetic resonance imaging may aid in assessing spinal cord/root injury and the degree of canal compromise.

NEUROLOGIC INJURY CLASSIFICATION

Complete Spinal Cord Injury

- No sensation or voluntary motor function caudal to the level of injury in the presence of an intact bulbocavernosus reflex (indicating intact S2-3 and resolution of spinal shock).
- Reflex return below level of cord injury.
- Named by last spinal level of partial neurologic function.
- Can expect up to one to two levels of additional root return, although prognosis for recovery is extremely poor.

Incomplete Spinal Cord Injury (Fig. 6.2)

- Some neurologic function persists caudal to the level of injury after the return of the bulbocavernosus reflex.

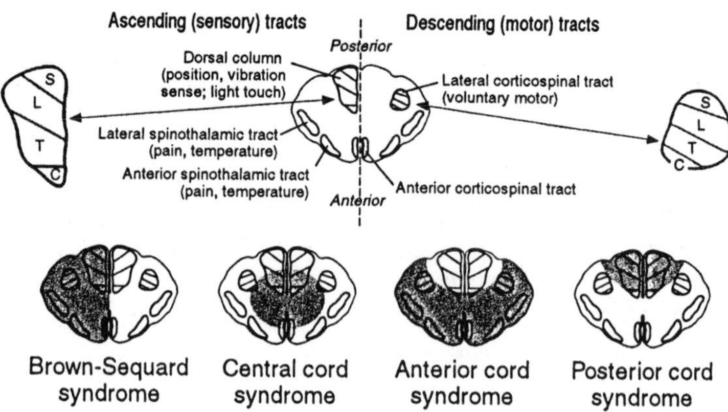

FIG. 6.2. Patterns of incomplete spinal cord injury. Abbreviations: *S*, sacral; *L*, lumbar; *T*, thoracic; *C*, cervical.

- As a rule, the greater the function distal to the lesion and the faster the recovery, the better the prognosis.
- Sacral sparing is represented by perianal sensation, voluntary rectal motor function, and great toe flexor activity; it indicates at least partial continuity of white matter long tracts (corticospinal and spinothalamic) with implied continuity between the cerebral cortex and lower sacral motor neurons. Indicates incomplete cord injury, with the potential for a greater return of cord function after resolution of spinal shock.

TYPES OF INJURIES

Specific Syndromes

1. Brown-Sequard syndrome
   - Presents as hemicord injury with ipsilateral muscle paralysis, loss of proprioception and light touch sensation, and contralateral hypesthesia to pain and temperature.
   - Prognosis good, with >90% of patients regaining bowel and bladder function and ambulatory capacity.
2. Central cord syndrome
   - Most common type of syndrome; frequently associated with an extension injury to an osteoarthritic spine in a middle-aged person.
   - Presents with flaccid paralysis of upper extremities (more involved) and spastic paralysis of lower extremities (less involved), with the presence of sacral sparing.
   - Radiographs frequently demonstrate no fracture or dislocation, as the lesion is created by a pincer effect between anterior osteophytes and posterior infolding of the ligamentum flavum.
   - Prognosis is fair, with 50% to 60% of patients regaining motor and sensory function to the lower extremities, although permanent central gray matter destruction results in poor hand function.
3. Anterior cord syndrome
   - This syndrome is common: motor and pain/temperature loss (corticospinal and spinothalamic tracts) with preserved light touch and proprioception (dorsal columns).
   - Prognosis is good if recovery is evident and progressive within 24 hours of injury. After 24 hours, the absence of sacral sensation to temperature or pinprick portends a poor outcome, with functional recovery in 10% of patients.
4. Posterior cord syndrome
   - This syndrome is rare: loss of deep pressure, deep pain, and proprioception with full voluntary power, pain, and temperature sensation.

5. Conus medullaris syndrome
   - Seen in T12-L1 injuries: loss of voluntary bowel and bladder control (S2-4 parasympathetic control) with preserved lumbar root function.
   - May be complete or incomplete; the bulbocavernosus reflex may be permanently lost.
   - Uncommon as a pure lesion; more common with an associated lumbar root lesion (mixed conus-cauda lesion).

Nerve Root Lesions
- Isolated root lesions may occur at any level; may accompany spinal cord injury.
- May be partial or complete and may result in radicular pain, sensory dysfunction, weakness, hyporeflexia, or areflexia.

Cauda Equina Syndrome
- Caused by multilevel lumbosacral root compression within the lumbar spinal canal.
- Clinical manifestations: saddle anesthesia, bilateral radicular pain, numbness, weakness, hyporeflexia or areflexia, and loss of voluntary bowel/bladder function.

CLASSIFICATION: GRADING SYSTEMS FOR SPINAL CORD INJURY

Frankel Classification
Grade A: Absent motor and sensory function.
Grade B: Absent motor function; sensation present.
Grade C: Motor function present but not useful (2/5 or 3/5); sensation present.
Grade D: Motor function present and useful (4/5); sensation present.
Grade E: Normal motor (5/5) and sensory function.

American Spinal Injury Association Impairment Scale
Grade A: Complete—no motor or sensory function preserved in sacral segments S4-5.
Grade B: Incomplete—sensory but not motor function preserved below the neurologic level and extending through the sacral segments S4-5.
Grade C: Incomplete—motor function preserved below the neurologic level; most key muscles below the neurologic level have a muscle grade <3.
Grade D: Incomplete—motor function preserved below the neurologic level; most key muscles below the neurologic level have a muscle grade >3.
Grade E: Normal—motor and sensory function normal.

American Spinal Injury Association Motor Index Score
Ten key muscle segments corresponding to innervation by C5-8, T-1, L2-3, L4-5, and S-1 are each given a functional score of 0–5. Both right and left sides are graded for a total of 100 points.

TREATMENT
Note: Specific fractures of the cervical and thoracolumbar spines are covered in Chapters 7 and 8, respectively.

Immobilization
1. A rigid cervical collar is used until the patient is cleared radiographically and clinically. A patient with a depressed level of consciousness (e.g., due to ethanol intoxication) cannot be cleared clinically.
2. A special backboard with a head cutout must be used for children to accommodate a proportionally larger head size and prominent occiput.
3. The patient should be removed from the backboard (by log rolling) as soon as possible to minimize pressure sore formation.

Medical Management of Acute Spinal Cord Injury
- Methlyprednisolone
  May improve recovery of neurologic injury.

Is currently considered "standard of care" for spinal cord injury if administered within 8 hours of injury as it improves motor recovery among complete and partial cord injuries.

Is given in a loading dose of 30 mg/kg within 8 hours of spinal cord injury and then 5.4 mg/kg/h over the next 24 hours.

Is not indicated for pure root lesions.

- Experimental pharmacologic agents include the following:

  Naloxone (opiate receptor antagonist);

  Thyrotropin-releasing hormone;

  G_{M1} gangliosides, which are membrane glycolipids that, when administered within 72 hours of injury, result in a significant increase in motor scores. Administer 100 mg/day for up to 32 days postinjury. Not recommended for simultaneous use with methylprednisolone.

COMPLICATIONS

- *Gastrointestinal.* Ileus, regurgitation and aspiration, and hemorrhagic gastritis are common early complications, occurring as early as the second day postinjury. Gastritis is thought to be the result of sympathetic outflow disruption with subsequent unopposed vagal tone resulting in increased gastric activity. Passage of a nasogastric tube and administration of H_2 receptor antagonists should be used as prophylaxis against these potential complications.
- *Urologic.* Urinary tract infections are recurrent problems in the long-term management of paralyzed patients. An indwelling urinary catheter should remain in the patient during the acute initial management only to monitor urinary output, which is generally low with neurogenic shock due to venous pooling and a low-flow state. After this, sterile intermittent catheterization should be undertaken to minimize potential infectious sequelae.
- *Pulmonary.* Acute quadriplegic patients are able to inspire only using the diaphragm, because abdominal and intercostal muscles are paralyzed. Vital capacity ranges from 20% to 25% of normal, and the patient is unable to forcibly expire, cough, or clear pulmonary secretions. Management of fluid balance is essential in the neurogenic shock patient, as volume overload rapidly results in pulmonary edema with resolution of shock. Positive pressure or mechanical ventilation may be necessary for adequate pulmonary function. Without an aggressive pulmonary toilet, pooling of secretions, atelectasis, and pneumonia are common and are associated with high morbidity and mortality.
- *Skin.* Problems associated with pressure ulceration are common in spinal cord injured patients due to anesthesia of the skin. Turning the patient every 2 hours, careful inspection and padding of bony prominences, and aggressive treatment of developing decubiti are essential to prevent long-term sequelae of pressure ulceration.

7. CERVICAL SPINE

EPIDEMIOLOGY

- Cervical spine injuries occur most frequently in association with high energy mechanisms, including motor vehicle accidents (45%) and falls from a height (20%).
- Less commonly, cervical spine injuries occur during athletic participation (15%), most notably during American football and diving events, and as a result of acts of violence (15%).
- Neurologic injury occurs in 40% of patients with cervical fractures.

ANATOMY

- The *atlas* refers to the first cervical vertebra, which has no body. The two large lateral masses provide the only two weight-bearing articulations between the skull and the vertebral column.
  - The tectorial membrane is the main stabilizer of the atlanto-occipital joint.
  - The anterior tubercle is held adjacent to the odontoid process of C-2 by the transverse atlantal ligament.
  - Fifty percent of total neck flexion and extension occurs at occiput–C-1.
  - The vertebral artery emerges from the foramen transversarium and passes between C-1 and the occiput, traversing a depression on the superior aspect of the C-1 ring. Fractures are common in this location.
- The *axis* refers to the second cervical vertebra, whose body is the largest of the cervical vertebrae.
  - The transverse atlantal ligament (cruciform ligament) provides primary support for the atlantoaxial joint.
  - The alar ligaments are secondary stabilizers of the atlantoaxial joint.
  - The facet joint capsules at occiput–C-1 and C1-2 provide very little support.
  - Fifty percent of total neck rotation occurs at C1-2.
- C3-7 can be conceptualized as a three-column system (Denis) (Fig. 7.1):
  - *Anterior column.* The anterior vertebral body and intervertebral disk resist compressive loads, whereas the anterior longitudinal ligament and annulus fibrosis are the most important checkreins to distractive forces (extension).
  - *Middle column.* The posterior vertebral body and uncovertebral joints resist compression, whereas the posterior longitudinal ligament and annulus fibrosis limit distraction.
  - *Posterior column.* The facet joints and lateral masses resist compressive forces, whereas the facet joint capsules, interspinous ligaments, and supraspinous ligaments counteract distractive forces.
- The vertebral artery bypasses the empty foramen transversarium of C-7 to enter the vertebral foramina of C6-C1. Injuries to the vertebral arteries are uncommon due to redundancy of the vessel.

MECHANISM OF INJURY

Motor vehicle accidents (primarily in young patients), falls (primarily in older patients), diving accidents, and blunt trauma account for most cervical spine injuries. Forced flexion or extension due to unrestrained deceleration forces, with or without distraction or axial compression, also cause injuries.

CLINICAL EVALUATION

1. Assess the patient: **A**irway, **B**reathing, **C**irculation, **D**isability.
2. Initiate resuscitation: address life-threatening injuries. Maintain rigid cervical immobilization.
3. Evaluate level of consciousness and neurologic impairment (Glasgow coma scale).
4. Assess head, neck, chest, abdominal, pelvic, and extremity injuries.
5. Ascertain history: mechanism of injury, witnessed head trauma, movement of extremities/level of consciousness immediately after trauma, and so on.

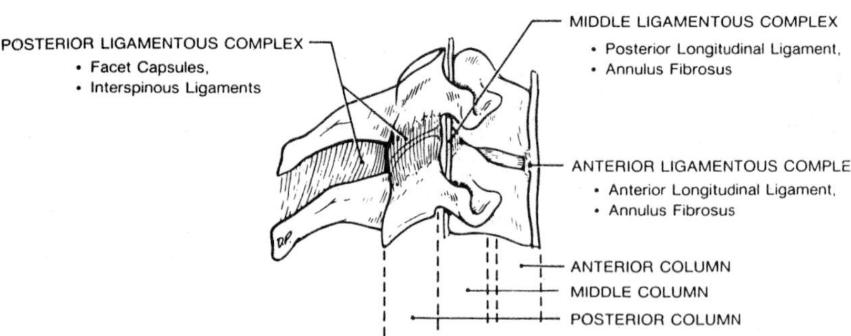

FIG. 7.1. The components of the cervical three-column spine. The ligamentous complexes resist distractive forces. The bony structures counteract compression. (From Rockwood CA Jr, Green DP, Bucholz RW, Heckman JD, eds. *Rockwood and Green's fractures in adults,* 4th ed. Vol. 2. Philadelphia: Lippincot-Raven; 1996:1489, with permission.)

6. Perform a physical examination:
   - Neck pain.
   - Lacerations and contusions on scalp, face, and neck.
7. Perform a neurologic examination as follows:
   - Cranial nerves.
   - Complete sensory and motor exam.
   - Upper and lower extremity reflexes.
   - Rectal exam: perianal sensation and rectal tone.
   - Bulbocavernosus reflex (see Chapter 6).

RADIOGRAPHIC EVALUATION

- A lateral cervical spine radiograph is taken; one must visualize the atlanto-occipital junction, all seven cervical vertebrae, and the cervicothoracic junction (as inferior as the superior aspect of T-1). This may necessitate downward traction on bilateral upper extremities or a swimmer's view (upper extremity proximal to the x-ray beam abducted 180 degrees, axial traction on the contralateral upper extremity, and the beam directed 60 degrees caudad). Patients complaining of neck pain should undergo complete radiographic evaluation of the cervical spine, including anteroposterior and odontoid views. On the lateral cervical spine radiograph, one may appreciate the following:
  1. Acute kyphosis or loss of lordosis;
  2. Continuity of radiographic "lines": anterior vertebral line, posterior vertebral line, facet joint line, and spinous process line;
  3. Widening or narrowing of disk spaces;
  4. Increased distance between spinous processes or facet joints;
  5. Rotation;
  6. Abnormal retropharyngeal swelling, which depends on the level in question:
     At C-1: >10 mm.
     At C3-4: >4 mm.
     At C5-7: >15 mm.
  7. Radiographic markers of cervical spine instability (Fig. 7.2), which include the following:
     Compression fractures with >25% loss of height.
     Angular displacements >11 degrees between adjacent vertebrae.
     Translation >3.5 mm.
     Intervertebral disk space separation greater than 1.7 mm.
- Computed tomography (CT), tomograms, and/or magnetic resonance imaging (MRI) may be valuable for assessing the upper cervical spine or the cervicothoracic junction, especially if either is inadequately visualized by plain radiography.

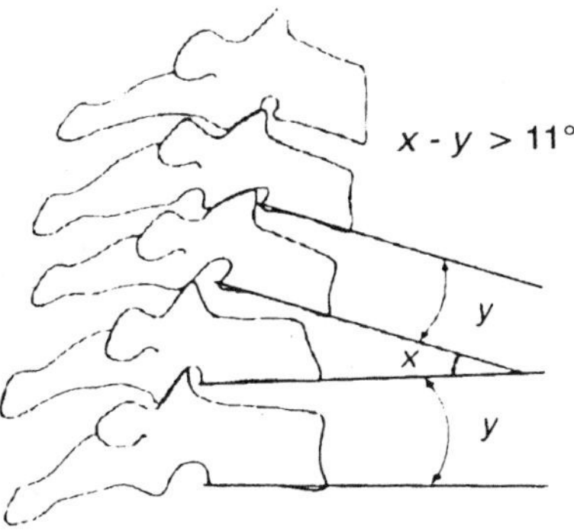

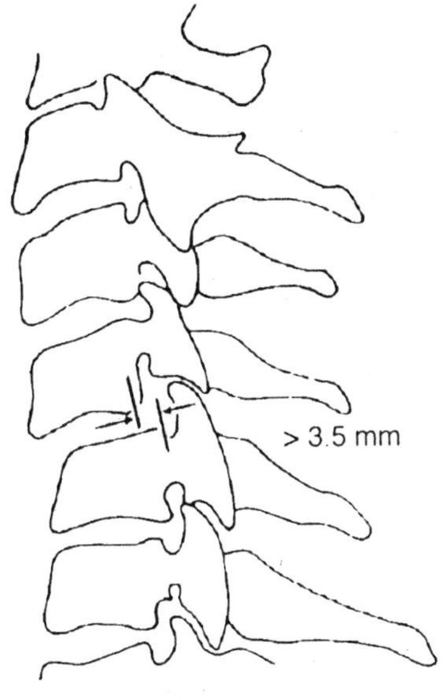

FIG. 7.2. Instability in cervical spine trauma. **Top:** Angular displacement. **Bottom:** Vertebral body translation. (From White AA 3rd, Johnson RM, Panjabi MM, Southwick WO. Biomechanical analysis of clinical stability in the cervical spine. *Clin Orthop Rel Res* 1975;109:85, with permission.)

- Stress flexion/extension radiographs may be performed if instability is suspected but should be performed in the awake and alert patient only. The atlantodens interval (ADI) should be <3 mm in adults and <5 mm in children.
- Traction x-rays should be used during reductions only.
- Atlantoaxial offset may be measured on an odontoid view: $x + y > 6.9$ mm (Fig. 7.3); indicates C1-2 instability and rupture of the transverse ligament.

ORTHOPAEDIC TRAUMA ASSOCIATION (OTA) CLASSIFICATION OF CERVICAL SPINE INJURIES

Type A: Compression injuries of the body (compressive forces)
- Type A1: Impaction fractures
- Type A2: Split fractures
- Type A3: Burst fractures

Type B: Distraction injuries of the anterior and posterior elements (tensile forces)
- Type B1: Posterior disruption predominantly ligamentous (flexion-distraction injury)

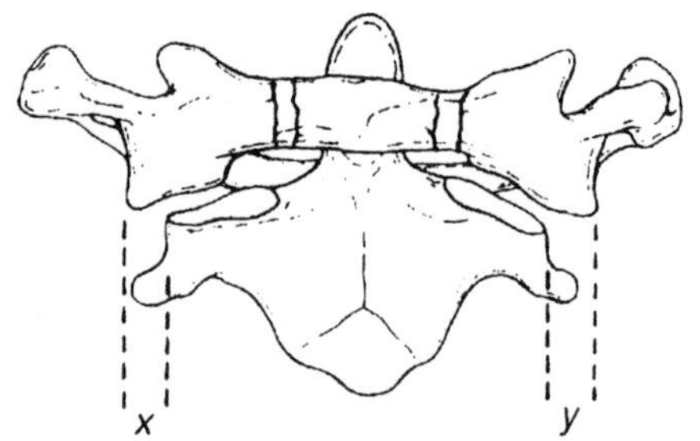

FIG. 7.3. Atlantoaxial offset. (From Browner BD, Jupiter JB, Levine AM, eds. *Skeletal trauma*. Philadelphia: W.B. Saunders, 1992:672, with permission.)

Type B2: Posterior disruption predominantly osseous (flexion-distraction injury)
Type B3: Anterior disruption though the disk (hyperextension-shear injury)

Type C: Multidirectional injuries with translation affecting the anterior and posterior elements (axial torque causing rotation injuries)
Type C1: Rotational wedge, split, and burst fractures
Type C2: Flexion subluxation with rotation
Type C3: Rotational shear injuries (Holdsworth slice rotation fracture)

INJURIES TO THE OCCIPUT–C1-2 COMPLEX

Occipital Condyle Fractures

- Frequently associated with C-1 fractures and cranial nerve palsies.
- Mechanism of injury—compression and lateral bending involved; this causes either compression fracture of the condyle as it presses against the superior facet of C-1 or avulsion of the alar ligament with extremes of atlanto-occipital rotation.
- CT frequently necessary for diagnosis.
- Type I, impaction of condyle; type II, associated with basilar or skull fractures; type III, condylar avulsion.
- Treatment—rigid cervical collar immobilization for 8 weeks for stable injuries and halo immobilization or occipital-cervical fusions for unstable injuries.

Occipitoatlantal Dislocation (Craniovertebral Dissociation)

- Almost always fatal; rare survivors have severe neurologic deficits ranging from complete C-1 flaccid quadriplegia to mixed incomplete syndromes, such as Brown-Sequard syndrome.
- Twice as common in children due to inclination of the condyles.
- Associated with submental lacerations, mandibular fractures, and posterior pharyngeal wall lacerations.
- Associated with injury to the cranial nerves, the first three cervical nerves, and the vertebral arteries.
- Mechanism—high-energy injury resulting from a combination of hyperextension, distraction, and rotation at the craniocervical junction.
- Diagnosis on the basis of the lateral cervical spine radiograph as follows:
  The tip of the odontoid should be in line with basion.
  The odontoid-basion distance is 4 to 5 mm in adults and up to 10 mm in children.
  Translation of the odontoid on the basion is never greater than 1 mm in flexion/extension views.
  The powers' ratio (BC/OA) should be <1 (Fig. 7.4).
- Classified based on position of the occiput in relation to C-1:
  Type I: Occipital condyles anterior to the atlas; most common.
  Type II: Condyles longitudinally dissociated from atlas without translation; result of pure distraction.
  Type III: Occipital condyles posterior to the atlas.
- Immediate treatment—halo vest application with strict avoidance of traction. Reduction maneuvers are controversial and should ideally be undertaken with fluoroscopic visualization. Long-term stabilization involves fusion between the occiput and the upper cervical spine.

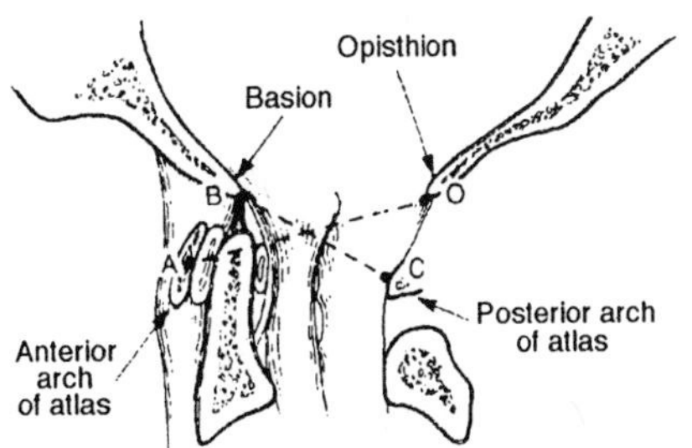

FIG. 7.4. Powers' ratio. (From Browner BD, Jupiter JB, Levine AM, eds. *Skeletal trauma*. Philadelphia: W.B. Saunders, 1992:668, with permission.)

Atlas Fractures

- Rarely associated with neurologic injury.
- Fifty percent are associated with other C-spine fractures, especially odontoid fractures and spondylolisthesis of the axis.
- Cranial nerve lesions of VI–XII and neurapraxia of the suboccipital and greater occipital nerves may be associated.
- Vertebral artery injuries may cause symptoms of basilar insufficiency, such as vertigo, blurred vision, and nystagmus.
- Patients may present with neck pain and a subjective feeling of "instability."
- Mechanism of injury is axial compression with elements of hyperextension and asymmetric loading of condyles causing variable fracture patterns.
- Treatment is as follows:
  - Initial treatment includes halo traction/immobilization.
  - Stable fractures (posterior arch or nondisplaced fractures involving the anterior and posterior portions of the ring) may be treated with a rigid cervical orthosis.
  - Less stable configurations (asymmetric lateral mass fracture with "floating" lateral mass, burst fractures) may require prolonged rigid halo immobilization.
  - C1-2 fusion may be necessary to alleviate chronic instability and/or pain.

CLASSIFICATION (FIG. 7.5)

- *Burst fractures* (Jefferson fracture) (33%). Axial load injury resulting in multiple fractures of the ring; low incidence of neurologic injury.

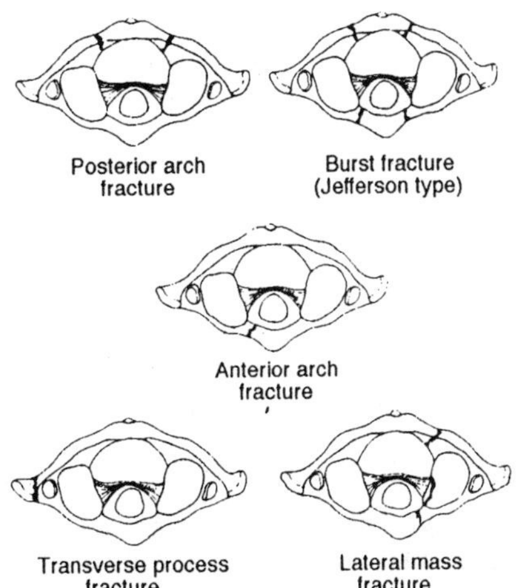

FIG. 7.5. Atlas fractures. (From Browner BD, Jupiter JB, Levine AM, eds. *Skeletal trauma*. Philadelphia: W.B. Saunders, 1992:669, with permission.)

- *Posterior arch fractures* (28%). Hyperextension injury; associated with odontoid and axis fractures.
- *Anterior arch fractures.* Hyperextension injury.
- *Lateral mass fractures.* Axial load and lateral bending injury.
- *Comminuted fractures* (28%). Axial load and lateral bending injury; associated with high nonunion rate and poor clinical result.
- *Transverse process fracture.* Avulsion injury.
- *Inferior tubercle fracture.* Avulsion of the longus colli muscle.

Transverse Ligament Rupture (Traumatic C1-2 Instability)

- This is a rare, usually fatal, injury seen mostly in an older age group (aged 50 to 60).
- Mechanism of injury is forced flexion.
- Clinical picture ranges from severe neck pain to complete neurologic compromise.
- Rupture of the transverse ligament may be determined by the following:
  1. Visualizing the avulsed lateral mass fragment on CT.
  2. Atlantoaxial offset >6.9 mm on the odontoid radiograph.
  3. ADI >3 mm in adults. An ADI >5 mm in adults also implies rupture of the alar ligaments (Fig. 7.6).
  4. Direct visualization of the rupture on MRI.
- Treatment is as follows:
  Initial treatment includes halo traction/immobilization.
  In the case of avulsion, halo immobilization is continued until osseous healing is documented.
  C1-2 fusion is indicated for tears of the transverse ligament without bony avulsion, for chronic instability, or for pain.

Atlantoaxial Rotary Subluxation and Dislocation

- This is a rare injury, with patients presenting with confusing complaints of neck pain, occipital neuralgia, and occasionally symptoms of vertebrobasilar insufficiency. In chronic cases, the patient may present with torticollis.
- This injury is infrequently associated with neurologic injury.
- The mechanism of injury is flexion/extension with a rotational component, although in some cases, it can occur spontaneously with no reported history of trauma.
- Odontoid radiographs may show asymmetry of C-1 lateral masses with unilateral facet joint narrowing or overlap (wink sign). The C-2 spinous process may be rotated from the midline on an anteroposterior view.
- The subluxation may be documented on dynamic CT; failure of C-1 to reposition on a dynamic CT indicates fixed deformity.

FIELDING CLASSIFICATION (FIG. 7.7)

Type I: Odontoid as a pivot point; no neurologic injury; ADI <3 mm. Transverse ligament intact (47%).

Type II: Opposite facet as a pivot; ADI <5 mm. Transverse ligament insufficient (30%).

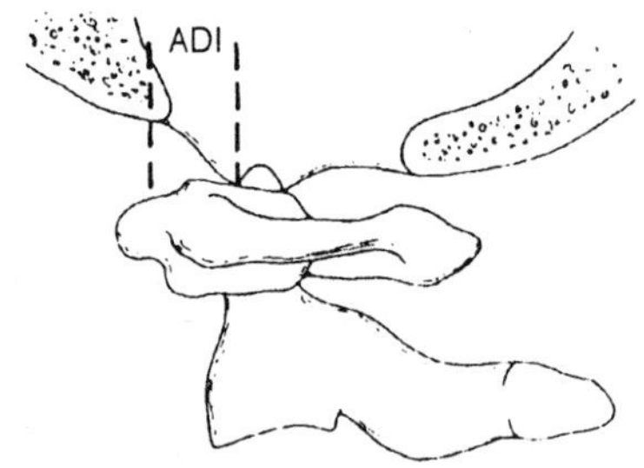

FIG. 7.6. Atlantodens interval (ADI). (From Browner BD, Jupiter JB, Levine AM, et al. *Skeletal trauma*. Philadelphia: W.B. Saunders, 1992:672, with permission.)

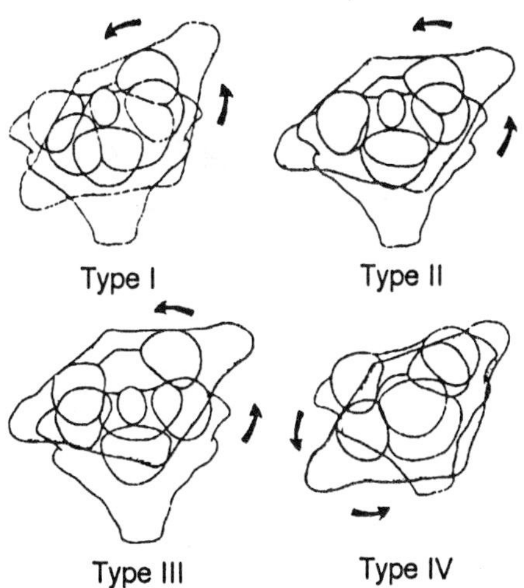

FIG. 7.7. Atlantoaxial rotatory subluxation. (From Browner BD, Jupiter JB, Levine AM, eds. *Skeletal trauma*. Philadelphia: W.B. Saunders, 1992:676, with permission.)

Type III: Both joints anteriorly subluxed; ADI >5 mm. Transverse and alar ligaments incompetent.
Type IV: Rare; both joints posteriorly subluxed.
Type V: Levine and Edwards—frank dislocation; extremely rare.

- Treatment is as follows:
  - Cervical halter traction in the supine position should be supplemented by active range-of-motion exercises for 24 to 48 hours initially, followed by ambulatory orthotic immobilization with active range-of-motion exercises until free motion returns.
  - Rarely, fixed rotation with continued symptoms and lack of motion indicates a C1-2 posterior fusion.

Fractures of the Odontoid Process (Dens)

- This injury has a high association with other C-spine fractures.
- Five percent to 10% incidence of neurologic involvement is found, with presentation ranging from Brown-Sequard syndrome to hemiparesis, cruciate paralysis, and quadriparesis.
- Vascular supply arrives through the apex of the odontoid and through the base with a watershed area in the neck of the odontoid.
- Mechanism of injury comprises high energy mechanisms involving motor vehicles or falls with avulsion of the apex of the dens by the alar ligament or lateral/oblique forces that cause fracture through the body and base of the dens.

ANDERSON AND D'ALONZO CLASSIFICATION (FIG. 7.8)

Type I: Oblique avulsion fracture of the apex (5%).
Type II: Fracture at the junction of the body and the neck; high nonunion rate (60%).
Type III: Fracture extends into the body of C-2 and may involve the lateral facets (30%).

- Treatment is as follows:
  - Type I: If injury is isolated, stability of the fracture pattern allows for immobilization in a cervical orthosis.
  - Type II: Treatment is controversial because lack of periosteum and cancellous bone and presence in watershed area results in high incidence of nonunion

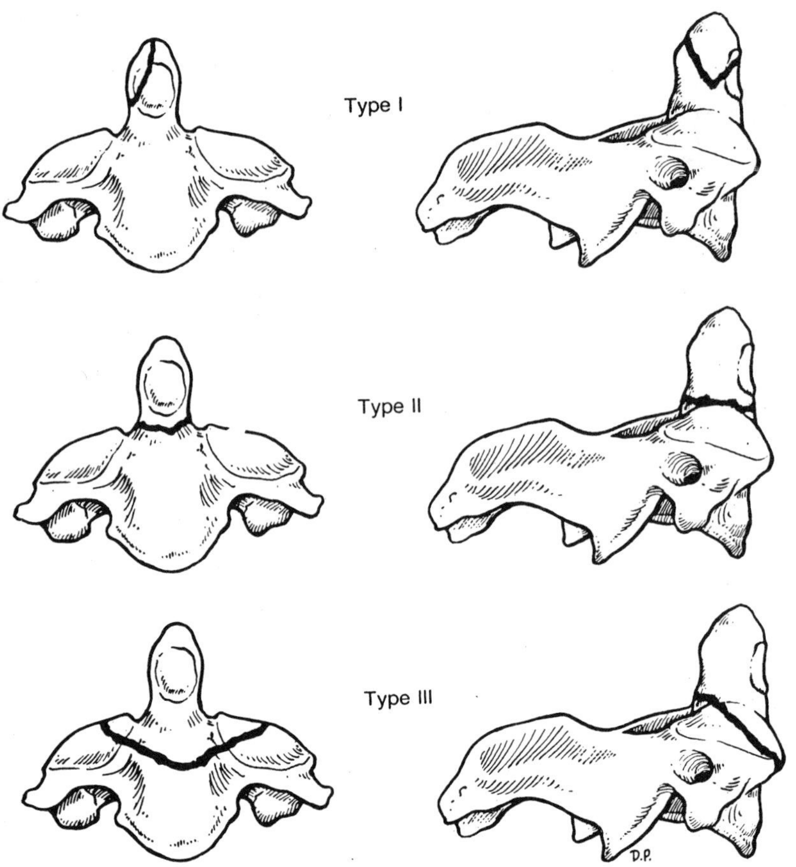

FIG. 7.8. Anderson and D'Alonzo classification of odontoid fractures. (Adapted from Anderson LD, Alonzo RT. Fractures of the odontoid process of the axis. *J Bone Joint Surg Am* 1974;56A:1663–1674, with permission.)

(36%) despite recumbent traction. Risk factors include age >50 years, >5 mm displacement, and posterior displacement. May require screw fixation of the odontoid or C1-2 posterior fusion for adequate treatment. Reduce fracture and hold in a halo.

Type III: High likelihood of union is found with halo immobilization due to cancellous bed of fracture site.

C-2 Lateral Mass Fractures

- Patients often present with neck pain, limited range of motion, and no neurologic injury.
- Mechanism of injury is axial compression and lateral bending.
- CT is helpful in diagnosis. A depression fracture of the C-2 articular surface is common.
- Treatment ranges from collar immobilization to late fusion for chronic pain.

Traumatic Spondylolisthesis of C-2 (Hangman Fracture)

- Thirty percent incidence of concomitant C-spine fractures. May be associated with cranial nerve, vertebral artery, and craniofacial injuries.

- Low incidence of spinal cord injury with types I and II; high with type III injuries.
- Mechanism of injury—motor vehicle accidents and falls with flexion, extension, and axial loads. May be associated with varying degrees of intervertebral disk disruption. Hanging mechanisms involve hyperextension and distraction injury, in which the patient may experience bilateral pedicle fractures and complete disruption of disk and ligaments between C-2 and C-3.

LEVINE AND EDWARDS; EFFENDI CLASSIFICATION (FIG. 7.9)

Type I: Nondisplaced, no angulation; translation < 3 mm; stable; C2-3 disk intact (29%).

Type II: Significant angulation at C2-3; translation >3 mm; most common injury pattern; unstable; C2-3 disk disrupted (56%). Subclassified into flexion, extension, and listhetic types.

Type IIA: Avulsion of entire C2-3 intervertebral disk in flexion, leaving the anterior longitudinal ligament intact. Results in severe angulation. No translation; unstable; probably due to flexion-distraction injury (6%).

Type III: Rare; results from initial anterior facet dislocation of C-2 on C-3 followed by extension injury fracturing the neural arch. Results in severe angulation and translation with unilateral or bilateral facet dislocation of C2-3; unstable (9%).

- Treatment is as follows:
  - Type I: Usually requires rigid cervical orthosis for up to 6 weeks.
  - Type II: Determined by stability; usually requires halo traction/immobilization with serial radiographic confirmation of reduction for at least 6 weeks.
  - Type IIA: Traction may exacerbate condition; therefore, only immobilization may be indicated.

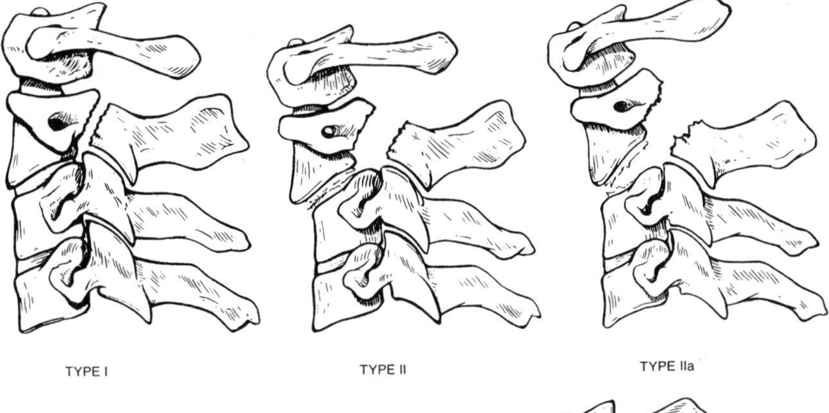

FIG. 7.9. Types of traumatic spondylolistheses of the axis. (Adapted from Levine AM, Edwards CC. The management of traumatic spondylolisthesis of the axis. *J Bone Joint Surg Am* 1985;67A:217–226, with permission.)

Type III: Initial halo traction is followed by open reduction and posterior fusion of C2-3, with possible anterior fusion.

INJURIES TO C3-7

- Vertebral bodies have a superior cortical surface that is concave laterally and convex anteroposteriorly, allowing for flexion, extension, and lateral tilt by the gliding motion of the facets.
- The uncinate process projects superiorly from the lateral aspect of the vertebral body. With degenerative changes, these may articulate with the superior vertebra, resulting in an uncovertebral joint (of Luschka).
- Mechanism of injury includes motor vehicle accidents, falls, diving accidents, and blunt trauma.
- Radiographic evaluation consists of anteroposterior, lateral, and odontoid views of the cervical spine (see "Radiographic Evaluation" above).
  - If cervical spine instability is suspected, flexion/extension views may be obtained in a willing, conscious, and cooperative patient without neurologic compromise. A "stretch" test (Panjabi and White) may be performed with longitudinal cervical traction. An abnormal test is indicated by greater than 1.7 mm interspace separation or >7.5-degree change between vertebrae.
  - CT with reconstructions may be obtained to characterize the fracture pattern and degree of canal compromise better.
  - MRI may be undertaken to further delineate spinal cord, disk, and canal abnormalities.

ALLEN CLASSIFICATION

1. Compressive flexion (shear mechanism resulting in "teardrop" fractures)
   - Stage I: Blunting of anterior body; posterior elements intact.
   - Stage II: "Beaking" of the anterior body; loss of anterior vertebral height.
   - Stage III: Fracture line passing from anterior body through the inferior subchondral plate.
   - Stage IV: Inferoposterior margin displaced <3 mm into the neural canal.
   - Stage V: Teardrop fracture; inferoposterior margin >3 mm into the neural canal; posterior ligaments and the posterior longitudinal ligament have failed.
2. Vertical compression (burst fractures)
   - Stage I: Fracture through superior or inferior endplate with no displacement.
   - Stage II: Fracture through both endplates with minimal displacement.
   - Stage III: Burst fracture; displacement of fragments peripherally and into the neural canal.
3. Distractive flexion (dislocations)
   - Stage I: Failure of the posterior ligaments, divergence of spinous processes, and facet subluxation.
   - Stage II: Unilateral facet dislocation; translation is always <50%.
   - Stage III: Bilateral facet dislocation; translation of 50% and "perched" facets.
   - Stage IV: Bilateral facet dislocation with 100% translation.
4. Compressive extension
   - Stage I: Unilateral vertebral arch fracture.
   - Stage II: Bilateral laminar fracture without other tissue failure.
   - Stages III and IV: Theoretical continuum between stages II and V.
   - Stage V: Bilateral vertebral arch fracture with full vertebral body displacement anteriorly; ligamentous failure at the posterosuperior and anteroinferior margins.
5. Distractive extension
   - Stage I: Failure of anterior ligamentous complex or transverse fracture of the body; widening of the disk space and no posterior displacement.
   - Stage II: Failure of posterior ligament complex and superior displacement of the body into the canal.
6. Lateral flexion
   - Stage I: Asymmetric unilateral compression fracture of the vertebral body plus a vertebral arch fracture on the ipsilateral side without displacement.

Stage II: Displacement of the arch on the anteroposterior view or failure of the ligaments on the contralateral side with articular process separation.

7. Miscellaneous C-spine fractures
   - *"Clay shoveler's" fracture:* Avulsion of spinous processes of the lower cervical and upper thoracic vertebrae. It historically occurred as a result of muscular avulsion due to using a shovel in unyielding clay with force transmission through a contracted shoulder girdle. Treatment includes restricted motion and symptomatic treatment until clinical improvement or radiographic healing of the spinous process occurs.
   - *Sentinel fracture:* Fracture through lamina on either side of spinous process. A loose posterior element may impinge on the cord. Symptomatic treatment only unless spinal cord compromise exists.
   - *Ankylosing spondylitis:* May result in calcification and ossification of the ligamentous structures of the spine, resulting in "chalk stick" fractures that occur as a result of trivial injuries. These fractures are notoriously unstable because they tend to occur through brittle ligamentous structures. Treatment includes traction with minimal weight in flexion, with aggressive immobilization with either halo vest or open stabilization.
   - *Gunshot injuries:* Missile impact against bony elements may cause high velocity fragmentation frequently associated with gross instability and complete spinal cord injury. Surgical extraction of missile fragments is rarely indicated in the absence of canal compromise. Missiles that traverse the esophagus or pharynx should be removed, with aggressive exposure and debridement of the missile tract. These injuries carry high incidences of abscess formation, osteomyelitis, and mediastinitis.

TREATMENT: GENERAL CERVICAL SPINE

Initial Treatment

- Immobilization with a cervical orthosis (for stable fractures) or Gardner-Wells tong traction (for unstable injuries) should be maintained in the emergency setting before CT for evaluation of spinal and other system injuries.

  Orthoses for immobilization.
  - Soft cervical orthosis: no significant immobilization; supportive treatment for minor injuries.
  - Rigid cervical orthosis (Philadelphia collar): effective in controlling flexion and extension but provides little rotational or lateral bending stability.
  - Poster braces: effective in controlling midcervical flexion; fair control in other planes of motion.
  - Cervicothoracic orthoses: effective in flexion and extension and rotational control; limited control of lateral bending.
  - Halo device: provides most rigid immobilization (of external devices) in all planes.

  Gardner-Wells tongs: applied one finger's width above the pinna of the ear in line with the external auditory canal. Slight anterior displacement will apply an extension force, whereas posterior displacement will apply a flexion force. Useful when reducing facet dislocations.
- Patients with neural deficits due to burst-type injuries should have traction to stabilize and indirectly decompress the canal.
- Patients with unilateral or bilateral facet dislocations and complete neural deficits should have Gardner-Wells tong traction and reduction by sequentially increasing the amount of traction.
- Patients with incomplete neural deficits or who are neurologically intact with unilateral and bilateral facet dislocations require an MRI before reduction to evaluate for a herniated disk.
- A halo ring should be applied 1 cm above the ears. Anterior pin sites should be placed below the equator of the skull above the supraorbital ridge, anterior to the temporalis muscle, and over the lateral two-thirds of the orbit. Posterior sites are variable and are placed to maintain horizontal orientation of the halo. Pin pressure should be

6 to 8 pounds in the adult and should be tightened at 48 hours and monthly thereafter. Pin care is essential.

Operative Treatment

Fusion of the Upper Cervical Spine (C1-2)

- Fusion of the occiput–C-1 limits 50% of flexion and extension.
- Fusion of C1-2 limits 50% of rotation.
- Posterior approach is as follows:
  - Modified Brooks or Gallie arthrodesis using sublaminar wires and a bone graft between the arches of C-1 and C-2 is most effective.
  - Flexion control is obtained via the wires, extension via the bone blocks, and rotation via friction between the bone blocks and the posterior arches.
  - Transarticular screws are effective, especially if the posterior elements of C-1 and C-2 are fractured.

Anterior Stabilization of the Dens

- Useful in type II and type III odontoid fractures and nonunions.
- Preserves range of motion.
- Must maintain reduction of the fracture.
- Anteromedial approach to the upper cervical spine used.
- Insertion of two small fragment cancellous lag screws under fluoroscopic imaging.
- Postoperative immobilization with a rigid cervical orthosis.
- Stabilization not indicated for fixation of anteriorly displaced fractures.

Stabilization of the Lower Cervical Spine (C3-7)

- Fifty percent of flexion and extension and 50% of rotation are evenly divided between each of the facet articulations.
- Fusion of each level reduces motion by a proportionate amount.
- Rogers technique of posterior interspinous wiring is as follows:
  - Effective for isolated posterior ligamentous disruption complicated by associated facet or anterior column disruptions.
  - Neutralizes flexion but provides no rotational or extension control.
  - Involves decortication and wiring between adjacent spinous processes with bone grafting.
- The triple-wire technique is as follows:
  - Useful in bilateral facet dislocations.
  - Provides significant stability over posterior midline wiring alone.
  - Does not apply to fractures of the spinous processes, laminae, or lateral masses.
  - Uses two wires passed through drill holes at the base of the adjacent spinous processes in addition to an interspinous wire to secure bilateral corticocancellous grafts to the spinous processes and laminae.
- Bilateral-lateral mass plating is as follows:
  - Can be used for a variety of fractures, including facet fractures, facet dislocations, and teardrop (compressive flexion stage V) fractures.
  - Single-level fusions sufficient for dislocations; multilevel fusions possibly required for more unstable patterns.
  - Can stop fusion at levels with fractured spinous processes or laminae, thus avoiding the fusion of extra levels with consequent loss of motion.
- Anterior decompression and fusion is as follows:
  - This is used for vertebral body burst fractures with spinal cord injury and persistent anterior cord compression.
  - MRI, myelography, and CT are valuable in the preoperative assessment of bony and soft-tissue impingement on the spinal cord.
  - Disk and osseous fragments are removed from the canal and a tricortical iliac or fibular graft is placed between the vertebral bodies by a variety of techniques.
  - Anterior plating or halo vest immobilization adds stability during healing.

COMPLICATIONS

Complications of spinal cord injury are covered in Chapter 6.

8. THORACOLUMBAR SPINE

EPIDEMIOLOGY

- Neurologic injury complicates 15% to 20% of fractures at the thoracolumbar level.
- Sixty-five percent of thoracolumbar fractures occur as a result of motor vehicle trauma and falls from a height, with the remainder caused by athletic participation and acts of violence.

ANATOMY (SEE CHAPTER 6 FOR A GENERAL DEFINITION OF TERMS)

- The thoracolumbar spine consists of 12 thoracic vertebrae and 5 lumbar vertebrae.
- The thoracic level is kyphotic, whereas the lumbar region is lordotic. The thoracolumbar region, as a transition zone, is especially prone to injury.
- The thoracic spine is much stiffer than the lumbar spine in flexion-extension and lateral bending, reflecting the restraining effect of the rib cage and the thinner intervertebral disks of the thoracic spine.
- Rotation about the craniocaudal axis is greater in the thoracic spine, achieving a maximum at T8-9.
- This is due to the orientation of the lumbar facets, which limit the rotation arc to approximately 10 degrees for the lumbar spine versus 75 degrees for the thoracic spine.
- The conus medullaris is found at the L1-2 level. Caudal to this is the cauda equina, which are the motor and sensory roots of the lumbosacral myelomeres.
- The corticospinal tracts demonstrate polarity, with cervical fibers distributed centrally and sacral fibers peripherally.
- Neurologic deficits secondary to skeletal injury from the first through tenth thoracic levels are frequently complete, primarily related to spinal cord injury with varying levels of root injury. The proportion of root injury increases with more caudal injuries, with skeletal injuries caudal to L-1 causing injury entirely to the root.

SPINAL STABILITY

A spinal injury is unstable if normal physiologic loads cause further neurologic damage, chronic pain, and unacceptable deformity.

White and Panjabi

Tables 8.1 and 8.2 define the scoring criteria for the assessment of clinical instability of spinal fractures.

Denis

Figure 8.1 shows the three-column model of spinal stability:

1. Anterior column: anterior longitudinal ligament, anterior half of the vertebral body, and anterior annulus.
2. Middle column: posterior half of vertebral body, posterior annulus, and posterior longitudinal ligament.
3. Posterior column: posterior neural arches (pedicles, facets, and laminae) and posterior ligamentous complex (supraspinous ligament, interspinous ligament, ligamentum flavum, and facet capsules).
    - Instability exists with disruption of any two of the three columns.
    - Thoracolumbar stability usually follows the middle column; if it is intact, then the injury is usually stable.

Degrees of Instability

1. First degree (mechanical instability): potential for late kyphosis
    - Severe compression fractures
    - Seat belt-type injuries
2. Second degree (neurologic instability): potential for late neurologic injury
    - Burst fractures without neurologic deficit

Table 8.1. Thoracic and thoracolumbar spine stability scale

Element	Point value
Anterior elements unable to function	2
Posterior elements unable to function	2
Disruptions of costovertebral articulations	1
Radiographic criteria	4
Sagittal displacement >2.5 mm (2 pts)	
Relative sagittal plane angulation >5 degrees (2 pts)	
Spinal cord or cauda equina damage	2
Dangerous loading anticipated	1

Instability: total of ≥5 points.
From White A, Panjabi M. *Clinical biomechanics of the spine*. Philadelphia: Lippincott, 1990:335, with permission.

3. Third degree (mechanical and neurologic instability)
   - Fracture-dislocations
   - Severe burst fractures with neurologic deficit

McAfee

1. Researchers have noted that burst fractures can be unstable with early progression of neurologic deficits and spinal deformity and late onset of neurologic deficits and mechanical back pain.
2. Factors indicative of instability in burst fractures are as follows:
   >50% canal compromise.
   >15 to 25 degrees of kyphosis.
   >40% loss of anterior body height.

MECHANISM OF INJURY (TABLE 8.3)

- Generally represent high-energy injuries, typically from motor vehicle accidents or falls from heights.

Table 8.2. Lumbar spine stability scale

Element	Point value
Anterior elements unable to function	2
Posterior elements unable to function	2
Radiographic criteria	4
Flexion/extension x-rays	
Sagittal plane translation >4.5 mm or 15% (2 pts)	
Sagittal plane rotation (2 pts)	
>15 degrees at L1-2, L2-3, and L3-4	
>20 degrees at L4-5	
>25 degrees at L5-S1	
—or—	
Resting x-rays	
Sagittal plane displacement >4.5 mm or 15% (2 pts)	
Relative sagittal plane angulation >22 degrees (2 pts)	
Spinal cord or cauda equina damage	2
Cauda equina damage	3
Dangerous loading anticipated	1

Instability: total of ≥5 points.
From White A, Panjabi M. *Clinical biomechanics of the spine*. Philadelphia: Lippincott, 1990:352, with permission.

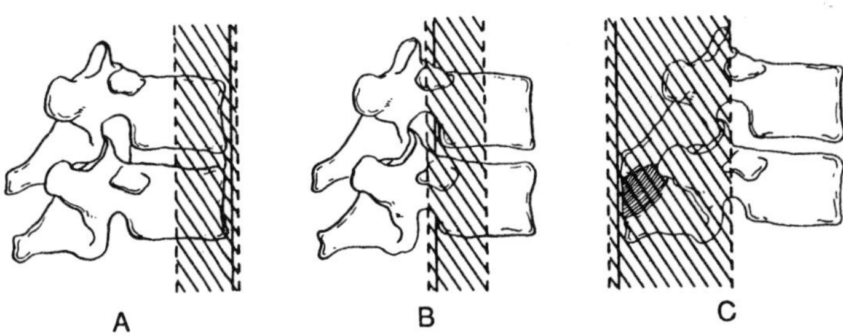

FIG. 8.1. The three columns of the spine, as proposed in Denis' three-column theory, are illustrated. **A:** The anterior column consists of the anterior longitudinal ligament, anterior part of the vertebral body, and the anterior portion of the annulus fibrosis. **B:** The middle column consists of the posterior longitudinal ligament, posterior part of the vertebral body, and posterior portion of the annulus. **C:** The posterior column consists of the bony and ligamentous posterior elements. (From Denis F. The three-column spine and its significance in the classification of acute thoracolumbar spinal injuries. *Spine* 1983;8:817-831, with permission.)

- May represent a combination of flexion, extension, compression, distraction, torsion, and shear.

CLINICAL EVALUATION

The patient should arrive via emergency transport with rigid cervical orthosis and backboard in place.

1. Assess the patient: **A**irway, **B**reathing, **C**irculation, **D**isability.
2. Initiate resuscitation: address life-threatening injuries.
3. Evaluate level of consciousness.
4. Evaluate injuries to the head, chest, abdomen, pelvis, and spine. Log roll patient to assess spinal column; assess presence of gross deformity; examine skin for bruising and abrasions; and palpate spinous processes for tenderness, step-off, or diastasis.
5. Evaluate for noncontiguous spinal injuries.

Table 8.3. Basic types of spinal fractures and columns involved in each

	Column involvement		
Type of fracture	Anterior	Middle	Posterior
Compression	Compression	None	None or distraction (in severe fractures)
Burst	Compression	Compression	None or distraction
Seat-belt	None or compression	Distraction	Distraction
Fracture-dislocation	Compression and/or rotation, shear	Distraction and/or rotation, shear	Distraction and/or rotation, shear

From Denis F. The three-column spine and its significance in the classification of acute thoracolumbar spinal injuries. *Spine* 1983;8:817-831, with permission.

6. Perform a complete neurologic examination:
   - Cranial nerves.
   - Complete sensory and motor examination.
   - Upper and lower extremity reflexes.
   - Rectal examination: perianal sensation and rectal tone.
   - Bulbocavernosus reflex: not prognostic in injuries to the conus medullaris or cauda equina (see Chapter 6).
7. Administer pharmacologic treatment (e.g., corticosteroids), if indicated (see Chapter 6).

RADIOGRAPHIC EVALUATION

- Anteroposterior and lateral views of the thoracic and lumbar spine should be obtained.
- Chest and abdominal radiographs obtained during the initial trauma survey are not adequate for assessing vertebral column injury.
- Computed tomography and/or magnetic resonance imaging of the injured area may be obtained to characterize the fracture further, assess for canal compromise, and evaluate the degree of neural compression.
- Myelography is seldom used in the acute trauma setting, although it may be helpful in cases in which a neurologic deficit is present that is unexplained by the osseous lesion. The major problem encountered is manipulation of the patient for instillation of the dye. Magnetic resonance imaging has largely obviated the need for myelographic evaluation in the acute trauma setting.

ORTHOPAEDIC TRAUMA ASSOCIATION (OTA) CLASSIFICATION OF THORACIC AND LUMBAR SPINE INJURIES

Type A: Compression injuries of the vertebral body (compressive forces)
- A1: Impaction fractures
- A2: Split fractures
- A3: Burst fractures

Type B: Distraction injuries of the anterior and posterior elements (tensile forces)
- B1: Posterior disruption predominantly ligamentous (flexion-distraction injury)
- B2: Posterior disruption predominantly osseous (flexion-distraction injury)
- B3: Anterior disruption thorough the disk (hyperextension-shear injury)

Type C: Multidirectional injuries with translation affecting the anterior and posterior elements (axial torque causing rotation injuries)
- C1: Rotational wedge, split, and burst fractures
- C2: Flexion subluxation with rotation
- C3: Rotational shear injuries (Holdsworth slice rotation fracture)

MCAFEE ET AL. CLASSIFICATION

Classification is based on the failure mode of the middle osteoligamentous complex (posterior longitudinal ligament, posterior half of the vertebral body, and posterior annulus fibrosus):

- Axial compression
- Axial distraction
- Translation within the transverse plane

The six injury patterns are the following:

1. Wedge-compression fracture;
2. Stable burst fracture;
3. Unstable burst fracture;
4. Chance fracture;
5. Flexion-distraction injury;
6. Translational injuries.

Denis

Minor Spinal Injuries
Articular process fractures (1%)
Transverse process fractures (14%)
Spinous process fractures (2%)
Pars interarticularis fractures (1%)
Major spinal injuries (Table 8.3)
Compression fractures (48%)
Burst fractures (14%)
Fracture-dislocations (16%)
Seat belt-type injuries (5%)

Compression Fractures
- Fractures can be anterior (89%) or lateral (11%).
- Fractures are rarely associated with neurologic compromise.
- These are generally stable injuries, although they can be considered unstable if loss of >50% vertebral body height or angulation >20 degrees occurs or if they are associated with multiple adjacent compression fractures.
- The middle column remains intact; it may act as a hinge with a posterior column distraction injury (seen with compression in 40% to 50%).
- Four subtypes described on the basis of endplate involvement (Fig. 8.2) are as follows:

Type A:	fracture of both endplates (16%)
Type B:	fracture of the superior endplate (62%)
Type C:	fracture of the inferior endplate (6%)
Type D:	both endplates intact (15%)

- Treatment includes a hyperextension orthosis with early ambulation for stable fractures.
- Unstable fractures may require hyperextension casting or open reduction and internal fixation.
- Upper thoracic fractures are not amenable to casting or bracing and require surgical management to prevent significant kyphosis.

Burst Fractures
- No direct relationship is seen between the percent of canal compromise and degree of neurologic injury.

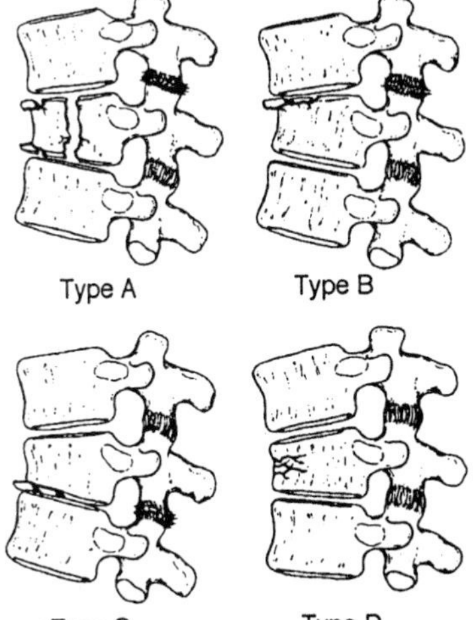

FIG. 8.2. Compression fractures. (From Browner BD, Jupiter JD, Levine AM, eds. *Skeletal trauma*. Philadelphia: W.B. Saunders, 1992:746, with permission.)

- Mechanism is compression failure of anterior and middle columns under axial load.
- An association between lumbar burst fractures associated with longitudinal laminar fractures and neurologic injury exists.
- These fractures result in loss of posterior vertebral body height and the splaying of pedicles on radiographic evaluation.
- The five types (Fig. 8.3) are as follows:

Type A:	fracture of both endplates (24%)
Type B:	fracture of the superior endplate (49%)
Type C:	fracture of the inferior endplate (7%)
Type D:	burst rotation (15%)
Type E:	burst lateral flexion (5%)

- Treatment may consist of hyperextension casting if no neurologic compromise exists and if the fracture pattern is stable. However, early posterior stabilization is advocated to restore sagittal and coronal plane alignment in cases with the following characteristics:
  Neurologic deficits;
  Loss of vertebral body height >50%;
  Angulation >20 degrees;
  Canal compromise >50%;
  Scoliosis >10 degrees.
- Instrumentation should provide distraction and extension moments. Harrington rods tend to produce kyphosis and are thus contraindicated for use in the lower lumbar spine.

Flexion-Distraction Injuries (Chance Fractures, Seat Belt-Type Injuries)
- These injuries are usually neurologically intact.

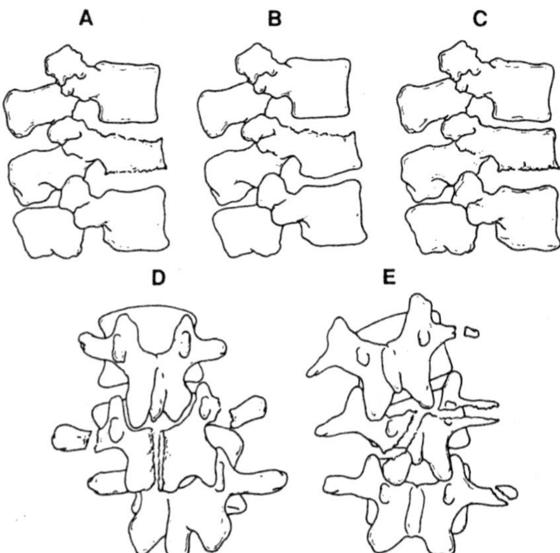

FIG. 8.3. Five types of burst fractures, according to Denis. **(A)** Type A burst fractures involves both endplates, whereas **(B)** type B involves only the superior endplate. **(C)** Type C is a fracture of only the inferior endplate, whereas **(D)** type D shows rotation. **(E)** Type E fracture is characterized by lateral wedging of the vertebral body. (From Rockwood CA Jr, Green DP, Bucholz RW, Heckman JD, eds. *Rockwood and Green's fractures in adults.* Vol. 2. Philadelphia: Lippincott-Raven, 1996:1536, with permission.)

- Flexion injury appears with axis of rotation at the anterior column, with compression failure of the anterior column, and with tension failure of posterior and middle columns.
- Increased interspinous distance on the anteroposterior view may be seen.
- Four types (Fig. 8.4) are as follows:

Type A:	one-level bony injury (47%)
Type B:	one-level ligamentous injury (11%)
Type C:	two-level injury through bony middle column (26%)
Type D:	two-level injury through ligamentous middle column (16%)

- Treatment consists of hyperextension casting for type A injuries. For injuries with compromise of the middle and posterior columns with ligamentous disruption, posterior spinal fusion with compression should be performed. Particular attention should be paid to the ability of the middle column to bear load because retropulsion of bone or disk fragments into the neural canal could occur.

Fracture Dislocations

- Failure of all three columns under compression, tension, rotation, or shear.
- Three types, with different mechanisms (Denis) (Fig. 8.5), as follows:
  - Type A—flexion-rotation. Posterior and middle column fail in tension and rotation; anterior column fails in compression and rotation; 75% have neurologic deficits, 52% of these are complete lesions.
  - Type B—shear. Shear failure of all three columns, most commonly in the posteroanterior direction; all cases with complete neurologic deficits.
  - Type C—flexion-distraction. Tension failure of posterior and middle columns, with anterior tear of annulus fibrosus and stripping of the anterior longitudinal ligament; 75% with neurologic deficits (all incomplete).

FERGUSON AND ALLEN (MECHANISTIC) CLASSIFICATION

The seven types are as follows:

1. Compressive flexion. Type I lesions do not progress; type II lesions may progress; type III lesions are likely to progress.
   I: anterior wedge fracture (middle and posterior elements intact)

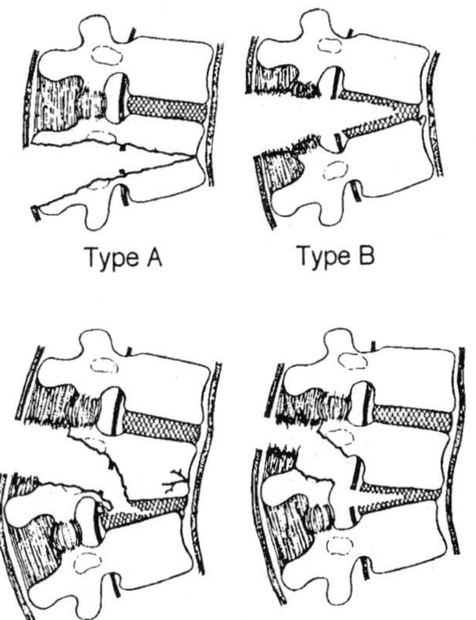

FIG. 8.4. Seat belt-type fractures. (From Browner BD, Jupiter JB, Levine AM, eds. *Skeletal trauma.* Philadelphia: W.B. Saunders, 1992:754, with permission.)

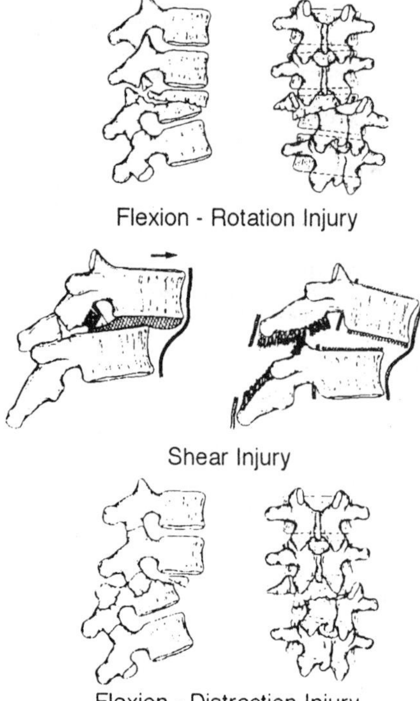

FIG. 8.5. Fracture-dislocations. (From Browner BD, Jupiter JB, Levine AM, eds. *Skeletal trauma*. Philadelphia: Saunders, 1992:758, with permission.)

II: posterior tension failure with anterior compression wedge fracture
III: middle element failure plus above = "blowout"

2. Distractive flexion: chance fracture and variants
3. Lateral flexion
   I: unilateral anterior and middle element compression failure
   II: above with posterior element injury, ipsilateral compression, and contralateral distraction. Only type II lesions are likely to have progressive deformity.
4. Translation: displacement anteriorly, posteriorly, or laterally; usually associated with other injury mechanisms.
5. Torsional flexion: torsion and compression failure of the anterior and middle elements and torsion and tension failure of the posterior elements.
6. Vertical compression: compression failure of anterior and middle elements ± posterior element compression; no progression of deformity or neurologic injury.
7. Distractive extension: tension failure of anterior elements and compression failure of posterior elements; rare in thoracolumbar spine and common in cervical spine.

TREATMENT

Nonoperative Treatment

- This is the standard of care for vertebral compression fractures and some burst fractures.
- Not equating instability with operative management is important; some unstable compression fractures (see above) may respond well to hyperextension casting if sagittal alignment is restored.
- Treatment includes the use of thoracolumbar spinal orthoses, lumbosacral corsets, hyperextension braces, Jewett braces, and hyperextension casting.
- A brace should not be considered a substitute for a well-molded hyperextension cast. Severe kyphosis may adversely affect the results of hyperextension casting.

- A Jewett brace provides minimal stabilization below the thoracolumbar junction.
- A well-molded jacket from the lower rib cage to the pubis can immobilize the upper lumbar vertebrae; adding a thigh cuff immobilizes the lower lumbar vertebrae.

Operative Treatment

- The presence of a neurologic deficit indicates that the spine has been deformed beyond the normal range and that compromise of a neurologic structure has occurred; these injuries may require operative stabilization, especially if the deficit is progressive or if the injury is inherently unstable (e.g., posterior ligamentous injuries).
- Operative indications for a lumbar burst are as follows:
    - >15 to 25 degrees of kyphosis;
    - >40% loss of vertebral height;
    - >50% canal compromised;
    - Presence of neurologic injury.
- For thoracic burst, the operative indications are the same as above. The index of suspicion for an unstable injury requiring surgery would be even higher if the ribs at the level of the thoracic spinal injury were also injured.
- A low lumbar burst is best treated with pedicle screw fixation to preserve levels and to maintain lumbar lordosis.
- Posterior spinal fusions may be performed to stabilize the injury and to prevent further compromise with indirect canal decompression. A high failure rate exists if short-segment pedicle screw constructs are used.
- Direct decompression can also be performed through a posterolateral approach (transpedicular) or through a laminectomy (dangerous above L-3).
- Anterior spinal decompression and fusion may be performed as a primary or secondary procedure in patients where posterior reduction fails to decompress the spinal canal adequately and a partial neurologic deficit remains. Anterior plating is safe above L-4.

PROGNOSIS AND NEUROLOGIC RECOVERY

Bradford and McBride

- These authors modified the Frankel grading system of neurologic injury for thoracolumbar injuries, dividing Frankel D types (impaired but functional motor function) based on the degree of motor function and bowel and bladder function as follows:
    - Type A: complete motor and sensory loss.
    - Type B: preserved sensation, no voluntary motor.
    - Type C: preserved motor, nonfunctional.
    - Type D1: low functional motor (3+/5+) and/or bowel or bladder paralysis.
    - Type D2: mid-functional motor (3+ to 4+/5+) and/or neurogenic bowel or bladder dysfunction.
    - Type D3: high functional motor (4+/5+) and normal voluntary bowel or bladder function.
    - Type E: complete motor and sensory function normal.
- In patients with thoracolumbar spine fractures and incomplete neurologic injuries, greater neurologic improvement (including return of sphincter control) was found in patients treated by anterior spinal decompression versus posterior or lateral spinal decompression.

Dall and Stauffer

- These researchers prospectively examined neurologic injury and recovery patterns for T12-L1 burst fractures with partial paralysis and >30% initial canal compromise.
- Their conclusions were as follows:
    1. Severity of neurologic injury did not correlate with fracture pattern or amount of computed tomographically measured canal compromise.
    2. Neurologic recovery did not correlate with the treatment method or amount of canal decompression.

3. Neurologic recovery did correlate with the initial fracture pattern (four types):
   Type I: <15 degrees of kyphosis; maximal canal compromise at level of ligamentum flavum.
   Type II: <15 degrees of kyphosis; maximal compromise at the bony posterior arch.
   Type III: >15 degrees of kyphosis; maximal compromise at the bony arch.
   Type IV: >15 degrees of kyphosis; maximal compromise at the level of the ligamentum flavum.

- Type I or type II: Significant neurologic recovery occurred in >90% of cases, regardless of the severity of the initial paralysis or treatment method.
- Type III: Significant neurologic recovery occurred in <50% of patients.
- Type IV: Variable response.

Camissa et al.
- Associated dural tears in 37% of burst fractures with associated laminar fractures; all had neurologic deficits.
- Concluded that the presence of a preoperative neurologic deficit in a patient who had a burst fracture and an associated laminar fracture was a sensitive (100%) and specific (74%) predictor of dural laceration, as well as a predictor of risk for associated entrapment of neural elements.

Keenen et al.
- Demonstrated an 8% incidence of dural tears in all surgically treated spine fractures and 25% in lumbar burst fractures.
- Of patients with burst fractures and dural tears, 86% had neurologic deficits versus 42% in those without dural tears.

COMPLICATIONS
Complications of spinal cord injury are covered in Chapter 6.

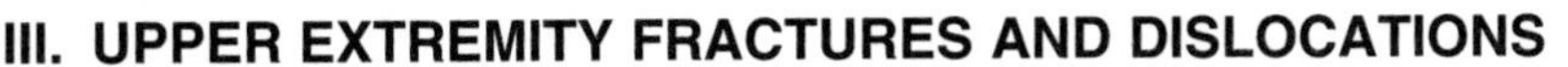

III. UPPER EXTREMITY FRACTURES AND DISLOCATIONS

9. CLAVICLE

EPIDEMIOLOGY

The trimodal distribution described by Allman is as follows:

Group I: median age of 13 years, accounting for 76% of clavicular fractures.
Group II: median age of 47 years, accounting for 21%.
Group III: median age of 59 years, accounting for 3%.

ANATOMY

- The clavicle is the first bone to ossify (fifth week of gestation) and the last ossification center (sternal end) to fuse at 22 to 25 years of age.
- It is the only long bone to ossify by intramembranous ossification without a cartilaginous stage.
- The clavicle is the only osseous strut connecting the trunk to the shoulder and arm.
- The flat outer third is the attachment site for the trapezius and deltoid muscles and the acromioclavicular and coracoclavicular ligaments.
- The tubular medial one-third protects the brachial plexus, the subclavian and axillary vessels, and the superior lung. It is strongest in axial load.
- The junction between the two cross-sectional configurations occurs in the middle third and constitutes a vulnerable area to fracture, especially with axial loading. Moreover, the middle third lacks reinforcement by muscles or ligaments distal to the subclavius insertion, resulting in additional vulnerability.

MECHANISM OF INJURY

- No correlation exists between the fracture location and the mechanism of injury.
- Falls onto the affected shoulder account for most (87%) clavicular fractures, with direct impact accounting for only 7% and falls onto an outstretched hand accounting for 6%.
- Uncommonly, clavicular fractures occur with aberrant muscle contractions during seizures or atraumatically from pathologic mechanisms or stress fractures.

CLINICAL EVALUATION

- The patient usually presents with splinting of the affected extremity, with the arm adducted across the chest and supported by the contralateral hand to unload the injured clavicle.
- A careful neurovascular examination is necessary to ensure the integrity of neural and vascular elements lying posterior to the clavicle.
- The proximal fracture end is usually prominent and may tent the skin. Crepitus may be present. Assessment of skin integrity is essential to rule out an open fracture.
- The chest should be auscultated for symmetric breath sounds. Tachypnea may be present due to pain with inspiratory effort; this should not be confused with diminished breath sounds, which may be present from an ipsilateral pneumothorax due to apical lung injury.
- Associated skeletal injuries, including head, neck, coracoid, acromioclavicular, sternoclavicular, scapulothoracic, and rib injuries, should be ruled out.

RADIOGRAPHIC EVALUATION

- Proximal third fractures are uncommon and may represent epiphyseal injury if the sternal ossification center is not fused. An anteroposterior view and a 45-degree caudal tilt view may demonstrate injury.
- With middle third fractures, an anteroposterior view and a 45-degree caudal tilt view are usually sufficient to demonstrate the injury.
- With distal third fractures, standard radiographs typically overexpose the distal clavicle. In addition, evaluation of ligamentous integrity is essential. Neer recommends three views:
  - Anteroposterior view of both shoulders with 10-lb weights strapped to the wrists: compare the distance between coracoid and medial fragments.

Anterior 45-degree oblique: taken with the patient erect and the affected shoulder placed flat on the radiographic plate; provides lateral view of scapula and demonstrates the proximal fragment posteriorly and the distal fragment anteriorly.
Posterior 45-degree oblique.

- Computed tomography may be useful in the evaluation of a fracture, especially in cases of proximal third fractures, to differentiate sternoclavicular dislocation from epiphyseal injury or in distal third fractures to identify articular involvement.

DESCRIPTIVE CLASSIFICATION

Clavicle fractures may be classified according to anatomic description, including location, displacement, angulation, pattern (i.e., greenstick, oblique, transverse), and comminution.

ALLMAN CLASSIFICATION

- Group I: fracture of the middle third (80%). Most common fracture in both children and adults; proximal and distal segments are secured by ligamentous and muscular attachments.
- Group II: fracture of the distal third (15%) (Figs. 9.1 through 9.4). Subclassified according to the location of coracoclavicular ligaments relative to the fracture as follows:
  - Type I: minimal displacement—interligamentous fracture between conoid and trapezoid or between the coracoclavicular and acromioclavicular ligaments (Fig. 9.1).
  - Type II: displaced secondary to a fracture medial to the coracoclavicular ligaments—higher incidence of nonunion.
    - IIA: conoid and trapezoid attached to the distal segment (Fig. 9.2)

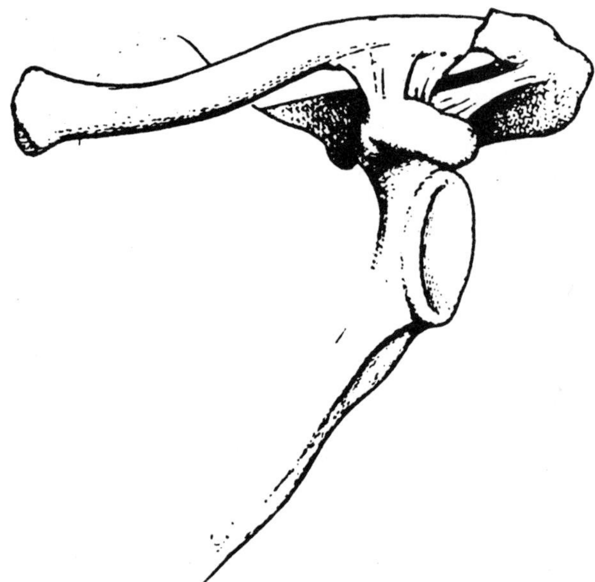

FIG. 9.1. A type I fracture of the distal clavicle (group II). The intact ligaments hold the fragments in place. (From Rockwood CA Jr, Green DP, Bucholz RW, Heckman JD, eds. *Rockwood and Green's fractures in adults*, 4th ed. Vol. 1. Philadelphia: Lippincott-Raven, 1996:1117, with permission.)

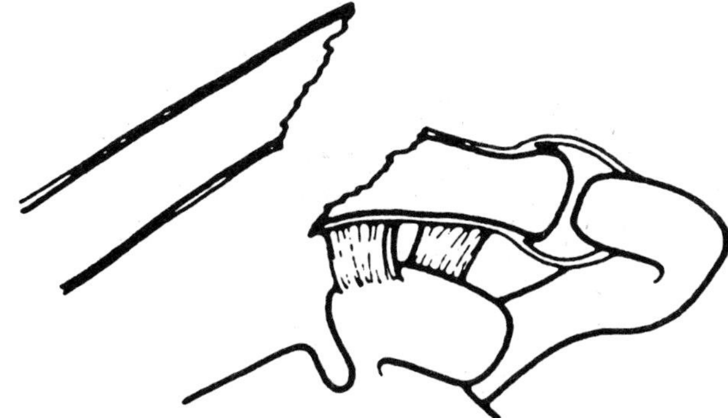

FIG. 9.2. A type IIA distal clavicle fracture. In type IIA, both conoid and trapezoid ligaments are on the distal segment, whereas the proximal segment, without ligamentous attachments, is displaced. (From Rockwood CA Jr, Green DP, Bucholz RW, Heckman JD, eds. *Rockwood and Green's fractures in adults*, 4th ed. Vol. 1. Philadelphia: Lippincott-Raven, 1996:1118, with permission.)

IIB: conoid torn, trapezoid attached to the distal segment (Fig. 9.3)

Type III: fracture of the articular surface of the acromioclavicular joint with no ligamentous injury—may be confused with first-degree acromioclavicular joint separation (Fig. 9.4).

- Group III: fracture of the proximal third (5%). Minimal displacement results if the costoclavicular ligaments remain intact. May represent epiphyseal injury in children and teenagers. Subgroups include the following:
  - Type I: minimal displacement.
  - Type II: displaced.
  - Type III: intraarticular.
  - Type IV: epiphyseal separation.
  - Type V: comminuted.

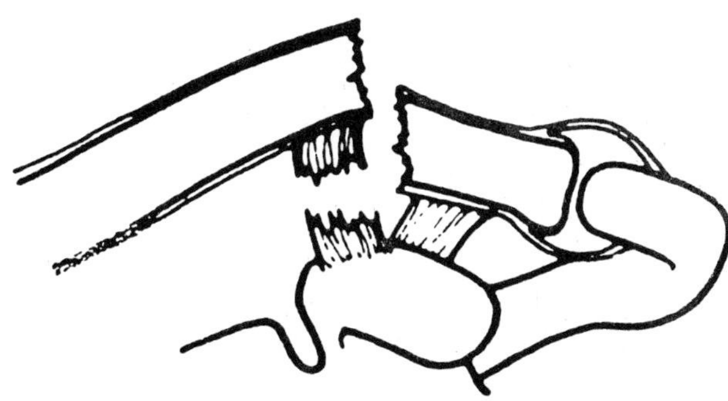

FIG. 9.3. A type IIB fracture of the distal clavicle. The conoid ligament is ruptured, whereas the trapezoid ligament remains attached to the distal segment. The proximal fragment is displaced. (From Rockwood CA Jr, Green DP, Bucholz RW, Heckman JD, eds. *Rockwood and Green's fractures in adults*, 4th ed. Vol. 1. Philadelphia: Lippincott-Raven, 1996:1118, with permission.)

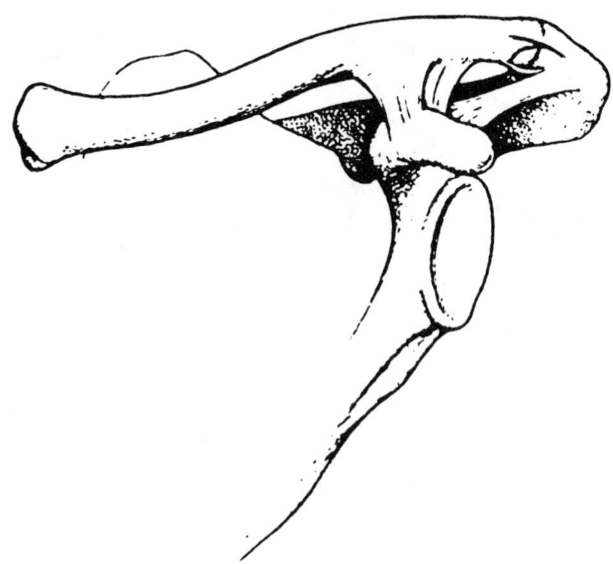

FIG. 9.4. A type III distal clavicle fracture, involving only the articular surface of the acromioclavicular joint. No ligamentous disruption or displacement occurs. These fractures present as late degenerative changes of the joint. (From Rockwood CA Jr, Green DP, Bucholz RW, Heckman JD, eds. *Rockwood and Green's fractures in adults*, 4th ed. Vol. 1. Philadelphia: Lippincott-Raven, 1996:1119, with permission.)

ORTHOPAEDIC TRAUMA ASSOCIATION (OTA) CLASSIFICATION OF CLAVICLE FRACTURES

- Clavicle fracture, medial end
  - Type A: metaphyseal
    - A1: extraarticular, impacted
    - A2: extraarticular, displaced
    - A3: extraarticular, multifragmentary
- Clavicle fracture, diaphyseal
  - Type A: simple
    - A1: spiral
    - A2: oblique
    - A3: transverse
  - Type B: wedge
    - B1: spiral wedge
    - B2: bending wedge
    - B3: fragmented wedge
  - Type C: complex
    - C1: spiral
    - C2: segmental
    - C3: irregular
- Clavicle fracture, lateral end
  - Type A: extraarticular metaphysis
    - A1: impacted
    - A2: displaced (coracoclavicular ligaments intact)
    - A3: multifragmentary (coracoclavicular ligaments intact)
  - Type B: intraarticular
    - B1: slight displacement (no dislocation)

B2: wedge fracture with dislocation
B3: multifragmentary fracture with dislocation

TREATMENT

Nonoperative Treatment

- The management goal is to brace the shoulder girdle with sling immobilization for 4 to 6 weeks to ensure adequate reduction while allowing for ipsilateral use of the elbow, wrist, and hand.
- Closed treatment is successful in most cases, with no need for reduction. Comfort and pain relief are the main goals. A sling has been shown to give the same results as figure-of-eight bandages, while providing more comfort and fewer skin problems.

Operative Treatment

- Operative intervention with stable fixation should be considered for the following:
  - Open fractures;
  - Fractures with associated neurovascular injury;
  - Fractures with severe associated injuries, such as a flail chest with multiple rib fractures or a scapulothoracic dissociation;
  - Group II, type II fractures—controversial because these have a high nonunion rate if treated closed;
  - Cosmetic reasons, such as uncontrolled deformity due to malunion, although the resultant operative scar may result in greater cosmetic disturbance than the deformity itself.
- Stable fixation may be accomplished via the use of the following:
  - Plate fixation: subcutaneous location may result in prominence of hardware.
  - Intramedullary devices (Hagie pins, Steinmann pins): may be prone to migration of hardware.
  - Cerclage suturing or wiring.
  - External fixation (Hoffman device).

COMPLICATIONS

- Neurovascular: laceration of subclavian vessels and brachial plexus; exuberant callus may form in middle third, causing neurovascular compression.
- Malunion: may cause unsightly prominence, but operative management may result in unacceptable scar or painful nonunion.
- Nonunion: rare; predisposing factors include the following:
  - Inadequate immobilization (multiple injuries);
  - Operative treatment;
  - Group II, type II fractures;
  - Soft tissue interposition.
- Posttraumatic arthritis: may occur after intraarticular injuries to the sternoclavicular or acromioclavicular joints.

10. ACROMIOCLAVICULAR AND STERNOCLAVICULAR JOINTS

ACROMIOCLAVICULAR JOINT

Epidemiology

- Most common in the second decade of life, associated with contact athletic activities.
- More common in males by a ratio between 5 to 1 and 10 to 1.

Anatomy (Fig. 10.1)

- The acromioclavicular (AC) joint is a diarthrodial joint, with fibrocartilage-covered articular surfaces, located between the lateral end of the clavicle and the medial acromion.
- Inclination of the plane of the joint may be vertical or may be inclined medially 50 degrees.
- The AC ligaments (anterior, posterior, superior, inferior) strengthen the thin capsule. Fibers of the deltoid and trapezius muscles blend with the superior AC ligament to strengthen the joint.
- The AC joint has minimal mobility through a meniscoid intraarticular disk that demonstrates an age-dependent degeneration until it is essentially nonfunctional beyond the fourth decade.
- The horizontal stability of the AC joint is conferred by the AC ligaments, whereas the vertical stability is maintained by the coracoclavicular ligaments. The average coracoclavicular distance is 1.1 to 1.3 cm.

Mechanism of Injury

- Direct force: most common cause, resulting from a fall onto the shoulder with the arm adducted, driving the acromion medially and inferiorly (Fig. 10.2).
- Indirect force: fall onto an outstretched hand with force transmission up the arm, through the humeral head, and into the AC articulation.

Clinical Evaluation

- The patient should be examined in the standing or sitting position with the upper extremity in a dependent position, thus stressing the AC joint and emphasizing any deformity.
- A standard shoulder examination should be performed, including assessment of neurovascular status and possible associated upper extremity injuries. Inspection may reveal an apparent step-off deformity of the injured AC joint, with possible tenting of the skin overlying the distal clavicle.
- Range of motion may be limited by pain. Tenderness may be elicited over the AC or coracoclavicular spaces.

Radiographic Evaluation

- A standard trauma series of the shoulder (anteroposterior, scapular-Y, and axillary views) is usually sufficient for the recognition of an AC injury, although closer evaluation requires targeted views of the AC joint, which necessitates one-third to one-half the radiation to avoid overpenetration.
- Ligamentous injury to the coracoclavicular joints may be assessed via stress radiographs, in which weights (10 to 15 lb) are strapped to the wrists and an anteroposterior radiograph is taken of both shoulders to compare coracoclavicular distances.

CLASSIFICATION (FIG. 10.3)

- Type I: sprain of the AC ligament.
  AC joint tenderness, minimal pain with arm motion, no pain in coracoclavicular interspace.
  No abnormality on radiographs.
- Type II: AC ligament tear with joint disruption, coracoclavicular ligaments sprained.
  Distal clavicle is slightly superior to acromion and mobile to palpation; tenderness is found in the coracoclavicular space.

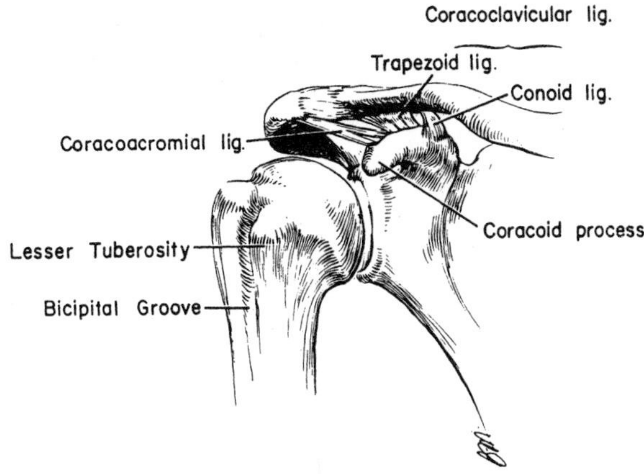

FIG. 10.1. Normal anatomy of the acromioclavicular joint. (From Rockwood CA Jr, Green DP, Bucholz RW, Heckman JD, eds. *Rockwood and Green's fractures in adults,* 4th ed. Vol. 2. Philadelphia: Lippincott-Raven, 1996:1343, with permission.)

Radiographs demonstrate slight elevation of the distal end of the clavicle and AC joint widening. Stress films show the coracoclavicular space unchanged from the normal shoulder as the coracoclavicular ligaments are sprained but integrity is maintained.

- Type III: AC and coracoclavicular ligaments torn with AC joint dislocation; deltoid and trapezius muscles usually detached from the distal clavicle.

The upper extremity and distal fragment are depressed, and the distal end of the proximal fragment may tent the skin. The AC joint is tender, and coracoclavicular widening is evident.

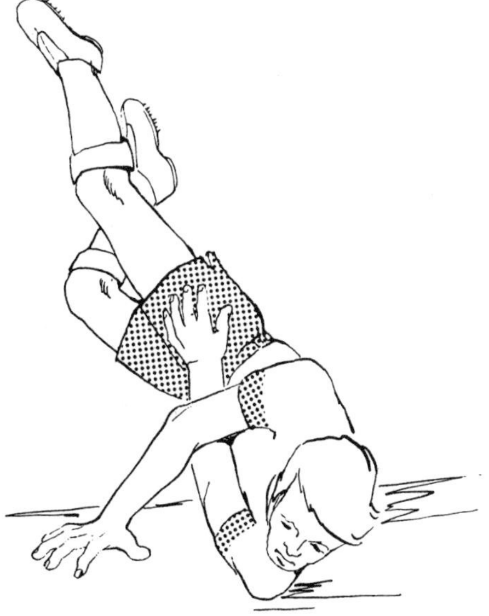

FIG. 10.2. The most common mechanism is a direct force that occurs from a fall on the point of the shoulder. (From Rockwood CA Jr, Green DP, Bucholz RW, Heckman JD, eds. *Rockwood and Green's fractures in adults,* 4th ed. Vol. 2. Philadelphia: Lippincott-Raven, 1996: 1351, with permission.)

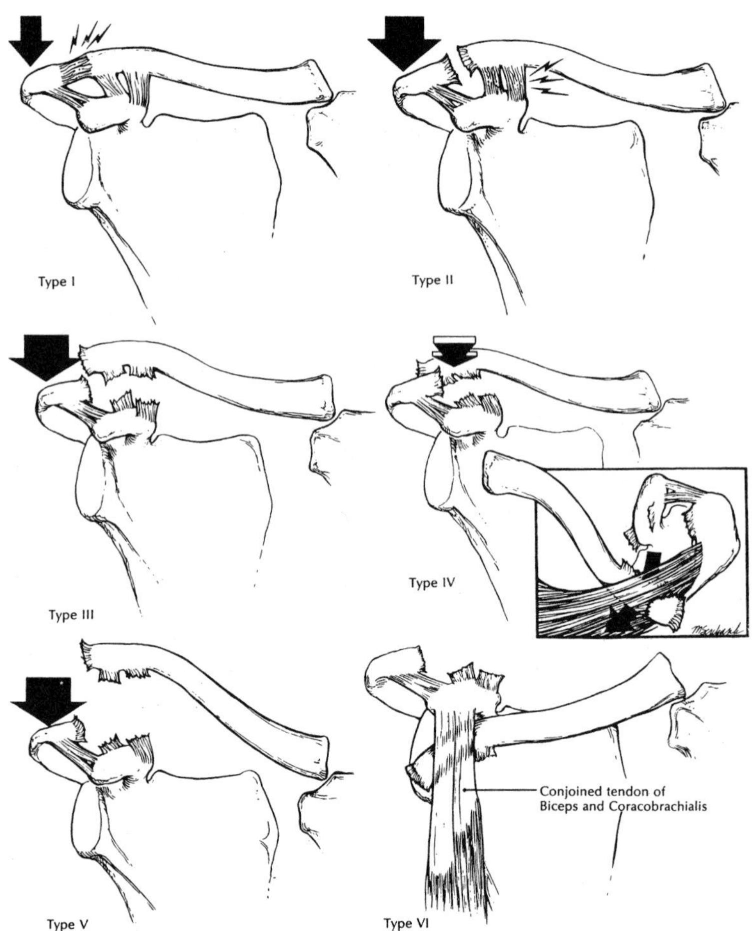

FIG. 10.3. Schematic drawings of the classification of ligamentous injuries to the acromioclavicular joint. **Top left:** In a type I injury, a mild force applied to the point of the shoulder does not disrupt either the acromioclavicular or coracoclavicular ligaments. **Top right:** A moderate to heavy force applied to the point of the shoulder will disrupt the acromioclavicular ligaments, but the coracoclavicular ligaments remain intact. **Center left:** When a severe force is applied to the point of the shoulder, both the acromioclavicular and coracoclavicular ligaments are disrupted. **Center right:** In a type IV injury, not only are the ligaments disrupted, but the distal end of the clavicle is also displaced posteriorly into or through the trapezium muscle. **Bottom left:** A violent force applied to the point of the shoulder not only ruptures the acromioclavicular and coracoclavicular ligaments but also disrupts the muscle attachments and creates a major separation between the clavicle and the acromion. **Bottom right:** This represents an inferior dislocation of the distal clavicle in which the clavicle is inferior to the coracoid process and posterior to the biceps and coracobrachialis tendons. The acromioclavicular and coracoclavicular ligaments are also disrupted. (From Rockwood CA Jr, Green DP, Bucholz RW, Heckman JD, eds. *Rockwood and Green's fractures in adults,* 4th ed. Vol. 2. Philadelphia: Lippincott-Raven, 1996:1354, with permission.)

Radiographs demonstrate the distal clavicle superior to the medial border of the acromion; stress views reveal a widened coracoclavicular interspace 25% to 100% greater than the normal side.

- Type IV: type III with the distal clavicle displaced posteriorly into or through the trapezius.
  - Clinically, more pain exists than in type III; the distal clavicle is displaced posteriorly away from the clavicle.
  - Axillary radiograph or computed tomography demonstrates posterior displacement of the distal clavicle.
- Type V: type III with the distal clavicle grossly and severely displaced superiorly.
  - This type is typically associated with tenting of the skin.
  - Radiographs demonstrate the coracoclavicular interspace to be 100% to 300% greater than the normal side.
- Type VI: AC dislocated, with the clavicle displaced inferior to the acromion or the coracoid; the coracoclavicular interspace is decreased compared with normal.
  - The deltoid and trapezius muscles are detached from the distal clavicle.
  - The mechanism of injury is usually a severe direct force onto the superior surface of the distal clavicle, with abduction of the arm and scapula retraction.
  - Clinically, the shoulder has a flat appearance with a prominent acromion; associated clavicle and upper rib fractures and brachial plexus injuries are due to high energy trauma.
  - Radiographs demonstrate one of two types of inferior dislocation: subacromial or subcoracoid.

Treatment

Type I. Rest 7 to 10 days, use ice packs and sling, and refrain from full activity until painless full range of motion is obtained (2 weeks).

Type II. Use a sling for 1 to 2 weeks, start gentle range of motion as soon as possible, and refrain from heavy activity for 6 weeks.

Type III. For inactive, nonlaboring, or recreational athletic patients, especially for the nondominant arm, nonoperative treatment, such as the following, is indicated: sling, early range of motion, strengthening, and acceptance of deformity. Operative treatment is controversial but may be indicated in heavy laborers, especially for those who do overhead work and for patients 20 to 25 years of age.

Type IV. Treatment is open reduction and surgical repair of the coracoclavicular ligaments for vertical stability, especially if the clavicle cannot be manipulated out of the trapezius.

Type V. Treatment is open reduction and surgical repair of the coracoclavicular ligaments for vertical stability.

Type VI. Treatment is open reduction and surgical repair of the coracoclavicular ligaments for vertical stability.

Complications

- Associated fractures and injuries:
  - Fractures: midclavicle, distal clavicle into AC joint, acromion process, coracoid process
  - Type VI: pneumothorax, pulmonary contusion
- Coracoclavicular ossification: not associated with increased disability.
- Distal clavicle osteolysis: associated with chronic dull ache and weakness.

STERNOCLAVICULAR JOINT

Epidemiology

- Injury to the sternoclavicular joint (SC) is rare. Cave and associates reported that of 1,603 shoulder girdle dislocations, only 3% were SC, with 85% glenohumeral and 12% AC dislocations.

Anatomy

- The SC joint is a diarthrodial joint, representing the only true articulation between the clavicle of the upper extremity and the axial skeleton.

- The articular surface of the clavicle is much larger than that of the sternum; both are covered with fibrocartilage. Less than half of the medial clavicle articulates with the sternum; thus, the SC joint has the distinction of having the least amount of bony stability of the major joints of the body.
- Joint integrity is derived from the saddlelike configuration of the joint (convex vertically and concave anteroposteriorly) and from its surrounding ligaments:
  - Intraarticular disk ligament: checkrein against medial displacement of the clavicle.
  - Extraarticular costoclavicular ligament: resists rotation and medial-lateral displacement.
  - Interclavicular ligament: helps to maintain shoulder poise.
  - Capsular ligament (anterior, posterior): prevents superior displacement of the medial clavicle.
- Range of motion is as follows: 35-degree superior elevation, 35 degrees of combined anteroposterior motion, and 50 degrees of rotation around its long axis.
- The medial clavicle epiphysis is the last epiphysis to close. It ossifies at 20 years and fuses with the shaft at 25 to 30 years. Thus, many supposed SC joint dislocations are actually physeal injuries.

Mechanism of Injury

- Direct: Force is applied to the anteromedial aspect of the clavicle, forcing the clavicle posteriorly into the mediastinum to produce posterior dislocation. Such may be the case when an athlete is in the supine position and another falls on him or her, when an individual is run over by a vehicle, or when an individual is pinned against a wall by a vehicle.
- Indirect: Force can be applied indirectly to the SC joint from the anterolateral (producing anterior SC dislocation) or posterolateral (producing posterior SC dislocation) aspects of the shoulder. This is most commonly seen in football "pile-ups," in which an athlete is lying obliquely on the shoulder and force is applied, with the individual unable to change position.

Clinical Evaluation

- The patient typically presents supporting the affected extremity across the trunk with the contralateral uninjured arm. The head may be tilted toward the side of injury to decrease stress across the joint, and the patient may be unwilling to place the affected scapula flat on the examination table.
- Swelling, tenderness, and painful range of motion are usually present, with a variable change of the medial clavicular prominence, depending on the degree and direction of injury.
- Neurovascular integrity must be assessed, as the brachial plexus, trachea, esophagus, and major vascular structures are in the immediate vicinity of the medial clavicle.
- With posterior dislocations, venous engorgement of the ipsilateral extremity, shortness of breath, painful inspiration, difficulty swallowing, and a choking sensation may be present. The chest must be auscultated to ensure bilaterally symmetric breath sounds.

Radiographic Evaluation

- Anteroposterior chest radiographs typically demonstrate asymmetry of the clavicles that should prompt further radiographic evaluation. This view should be scrutinized for the presence of a pneumothorax if the patient presents with breathing complaints.
- The Hobbs view is a 90-degree cephalocaudal lateral view. The patient leans over the plate and the radiographic beam is angled behind the neck.
- The serendipity view is a 40-degree cephalic tilt view, aimed at the manubrium. With an anterior dislocation, the medial clavicle lays above the interclavicular line. With a posterior dislocation, the medial clavicle lays below this line.
- Tomograms are useful to distinguish between dislocation and medial clavicle fracture.

- Computed tomography is the best technique to evaluate injuries to the SC joint, because it can distinguish between fractures of the medial clavicle from dislocation and can delineate minor subluxations that would otherwise go unrecognized.

ANATOMIC CLASSIFICATION (FIG. 10.4)

- Anterior dislocation—more common
- Posterior dislocation

ETIOLOGIC CLASSIFICATION

- Sprain or subluxation
  - Mild: joint stable, ligamentous integrity maintained.
  - Moderate: subluxation, with partial ligamentous disruption.
  - Severe: unstable joint, with complete ligamentous compromise.

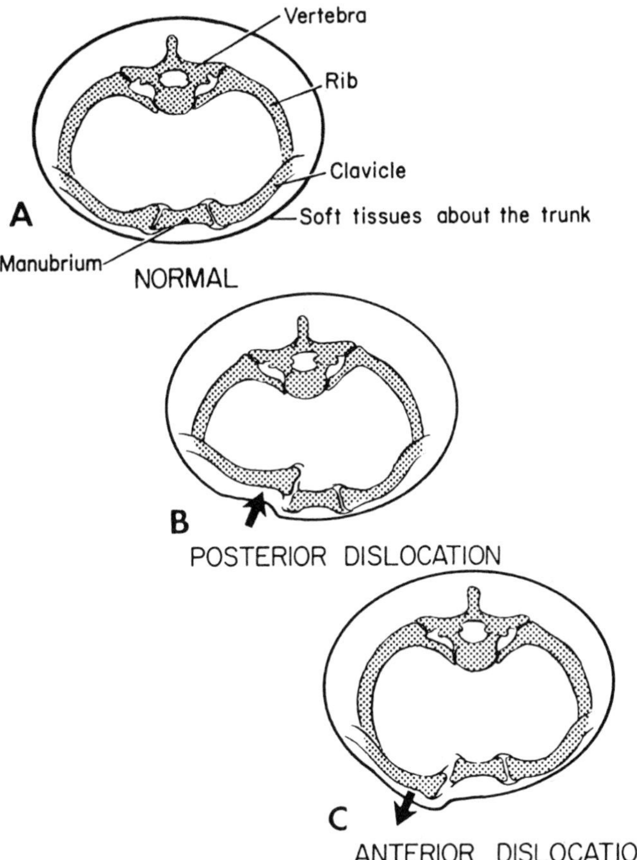

FIG. 10.4. Cross-section through the thorax at the level of the sternoclavicular joint. **A:** Normal anatomic relations. **B:** Posterior dislocation of the sternoclavicular joint. **C:** Anterior dislocation of the sternoclavicular joint. (From Rockwood CA Jr, Green DP, Bucholz RW, Heckman JD, eds. *Rockwood and Green's fractures in adults,* 4th ed. Vol. 2. Philadelphia: Lippincott-Raven, 1996:1422, with permission.)

- Acute dislocation: complete ligamentous disruption with frank translation of the medial clavicle.
- Recurrent dislocation—rare.
- Unreduced dislocation.
- Atraumatic: spontaneous dislocation, developmental (congenital) dislocation, osteoarthritis, condensing osteitis of the medial clavicle, sternoclavicular hyperostosis, or infection.

Treatment

- With a mild sprain, ice for the first 24 hours; immobilize with a sling for 3 to 4 days, with gradual return to normal activities as tolerated.
- With a moderate sprain or subluxation, ice for the first 24 hours; use a clavicle strap, sling and swathe, or figure-of-eight bandage for 1 week and then sling immobilization for 4 to 6 weeks.
- Treat a severe sprain or dislocation as follows:
  Anterior. Nonoperative treatment is common, but whether one should attempt closed reduction is controversal because it is usually unstable. Use a sling for comfort. Closed reduction may be accomplished using general anesthesia or narcotics and muscle relaxants for the stoic patient. The patient is placed supine with a roll between the scapulae. Direct pressure posteriorly usually results in reduction. Postreduction care consists of a clavicle strap, sling and swathe, or figure-of-eight bandage for 4 to 6 weeks. Some advocate a bulky anterior dressing with elastic tape to maintain reduction.
  Posterior. A careful history and physical examination are necessary to rule out associated pulmonary or neurovascular problems. Prompt closed or open reduction is indicated, usually under general anesthesia. The patient is placed supine with a roll between the scapulae. Closed reduction may be obtained using traction with the arm in abduction and extension. Anteriorly directed traction on the clavicle with a towel clip may be required. A clavicle strap, sling and swathe, or figure-of-eight bandage is used for immobilization for 4 to 6 weeks. A general or thoracic surgeon should be available in the event that the major underlying neurovascular structures are inadvertently damaged.
- With a medial physeal injury, closed reduction is usually successful, with postreduction care consisting of a clavicle strap, sling and swathe, or figure-of-eight bandage immobilization for 4 to 6 weeks.
- Operative management of SC dislocation may include fixation of the medial clavicle to the sternum using fascia lata, subclavius tendon, or suture; osteotomy of the medial clavicle; or resection of the medial clavicle. The use of Kirschner wires or Steinmann pins is discouraged because migration of hardware may occur.

Complications

- The major untoward result of an anterior dislocation is cosmetic, with most patients complaining of an enlarged medial prominence.
- Complications are more common with posterior dislocations and reflect the proximity of the medial clavicle to mediastinal and neurovascular structures. The complication rate has been reported to be as high as 25% with posterior dislocations, and complications include the following:
  Pneumothorax;
  Laceration of the superior vena cava;
  Venous congestion in the neck;
  Esophageal rupture;
  Subclavian artery compression;
  Carotid artery compression;
  Voice changes;
  Severe thoracic outlet syndrome.

11. SCAPULA

EPIDEMIOLOGY

- Relatively uncommon injury, representing only 3% to 5% of all shoulder fractures and 0.5% to 1% of all fractures.
- Highest incidence in males between the ages of 30 and 40 years.

ANATOMY

- Flat triangular bone linking the upper extremity to the axial skeleton.
- Protection from impact provided by the large surrounding muscle mass and the mobility of the scapula on the chest wall, further aiding in force dissipation.

MECHANISM OF INJURY

- Injury is usually the result of high energy trauma.
- The presence of a scapular fracture should raise suspicion of associated injuries, because 35% to 98% of scapular fractures occur in the presence of comorbid injuries, including the following:
  - Ipsilateral upper torso injuries—fractured ribs, clavicle, sternum, and shoulder trauma;
  - Pneumothorax—seen in 11% to 55% of scapular fractures;
  - Pulmonary contusion—present in 11% to 54% of scapular fractures;
  - Injuries to neurovascular structures—brachial plexus injuries and vascular avulsions;
  - Spinal column injuries—20% lower cervical spine, 76% thoracic spine and 4% lumbar spine;
  - Concomitant skull fractures, blunt abdominal trauma, pelvic fracture, and lower extremity injuries, all seen with higher incidences in the presence of a scapular fracture.

CLINICAL EVALUATION

- Full trauma evaluation, with attention to airway, breathing, circulation, and disability, should be performed, if indicated.
- Patient typically presents with the upper extremity supported by the contralateral hand in an adducted and immobile position, with painful range of motion, especially with shoulder abduction.
- A careful examination for associated injures should be pursued, with a comprehensive assessment of neurovascular status and an evaluation of breath sounds.
- Compartment syndrome overlying the scapula is uncommon but must be ruled out in the presence of tense swelling overlying the supraspinatus and infraspinatus muscles and with pain out of proportion to the apparent injury.
- *Comolli sign* represents triangular swelling of the posterior thorax overlying the scapula and is suggestive of a hematoma resulting in increased compartmental pressures.

RADIOGRAPHIC EVALUATION

- Initial radiographs should include a trauma series of the shoulder, consisting of a true anteroposterior view, an axillary view, and a scapular-Y view (true scapular lateral). These generally demonstrate most glenoid, scapular neck, body, and acromion fractures.
  - The axillary may be used to delineate further acromial and glenoid rim fractures.
  - An acromial fracture should not be confused with an *os acromiale*, which is a rounded, unfused apophysis at the epiphyseal level and is present in approximately 3% of the population. When present, it is bilateral in 60% of cases.
  - *Glenoid hypoplasia*, or *scapular neck dysplasia*, is an unusual abnormality that may resemble glenoid impaction and that may be associated with humeral head or acromial abnormalities. It has a benign course and is usually noted incidentally.

- Forty-five–degree cephalic tilt (Stryker notch) radiograph may help identify coracoid fractures.
- Tomography or computed tomography may be useful for further characterizing intraarticular glenoid fractures.
- Because of the high incidence of associated injuries, especially to thoracic structures, a chest radiograph is an essential part of the evaluation.

ANATOMIC CLASSIFICATION (ZDRAVKOVIC AND DAMHOLT) (FIG. 11.1)

Type I: scapula body.
Type II: apophyseal fractures, including the acromion and coracoid.
Type III: fractures of the superolateral angle, including the scapular neck and glenoid.

IDEBERG CLASSIFICATION OF INTRAARTICULAR GLENOID FRACTURES (FIG. 11.2)

Type I: avulsion fracture of the anterior margin.
Type IIA: transverse fracture through the glenoid fossa exiting inferiorly.
Type IIB: oblique fracture through the glenoid fossa exiting inferiorly.
Type III: oblique fracture through the glenoid exiting superiorly; often associated with an acromioclavicular joint injury.
Type IV: transverse fracture exiting through the medial border of the scapula.
Type V: combination of a type II and type IV pattern.

ORTHOPAEDIC TRAUMA ASSOCIATION CLASSIFICATION OF SCAPULAR FRACTURES

Type A: scapula, extraarticular
- A1: scapular processes
  - A1.1: acromion, simple
  - A1.2: acromion, multifragmentary
  - A1.3: coracoid process
- A2: scapular body
  - A2.1: simple
  - A2.2: multifragmentary
  - A2.3: glenoid neck

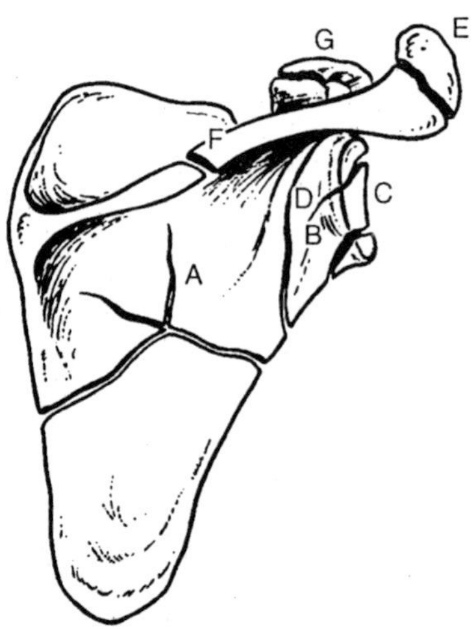

FIG. 11.1. Anatomic classification. **A,** scapula body; **B, C,** glenoid; **D,** scapula neck; **E,** acromion; **F,** scapula spine; **G,** coracoid.

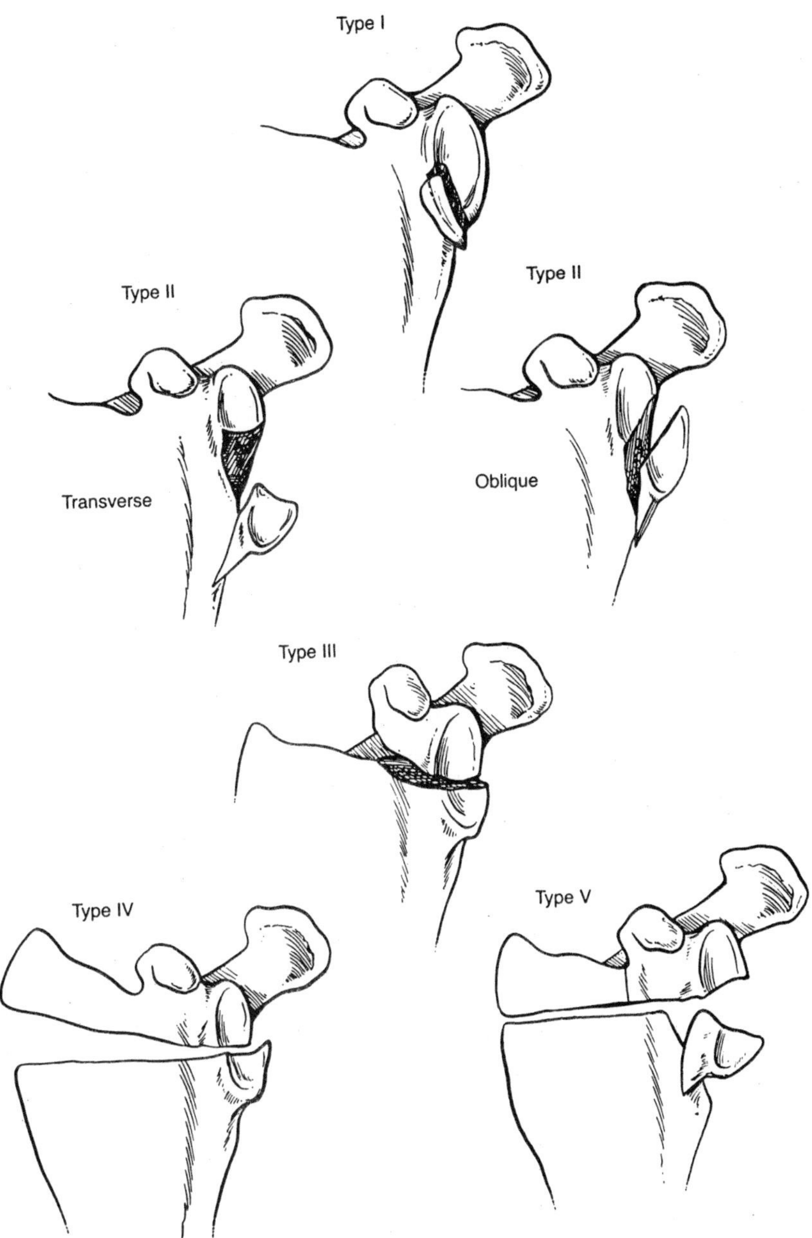

FIG. 11.2. Ideberg classification of intraarticular fracture of the glenoid into five types based on fracture patterns. (From Rockwood CA, Jr, Green DP, Bucholz RW, Heckman JD, eds. *Rockwood and Green's fractures in adults*, 4th ed. Vol. 1. Philadelphia: Lippincott-Raven, 1996:1176, with permission.)

A3: extraarticular, complex
  A3.1: glenoid neck plus body
  A3.2: glenoid neck plus clavicle, simple
  A3.3: glenoid neck plus clavicle, multifragmentary

Type B: scapula, intraarticular glenoid
B1: glenoid impacted
  B1.1: anterior rim
  B1.2: posterior rim
  B1.3: inferior rim
B2: glenoid nonimpacted
  B2.1: anterior rim, free
  B2.2: posterior rim, free
  B2.3: anterior/posterior rim with glenoid neck
B3: glenoid complex
  B3.1: multifragmentary, intraarticular
  B3.2: multifragmentary with glenoid neck and/or body
  B3.3: multifragmentary with associated clavicle fracture

TREATMENT

Nonoperative Treatment

Most scapula fractures are amenable to nonoperative treatment, consisting of sling use and early range of shoulder motion.

Operative Treatment

- Surgical indications are controversial but include the following:
  - Displaced intraarticular fractures involving greater than 25% of the articular surface;
  - Scapular neck fractures with greater than 40-degree angulation or 1 cm medial translation;
  - Scapular neck fractures with associated displaced clavicle fracture;
  - Fractures of the acromion that impinge on the subacromial space;
  - Fractures of the coracoid process that result in a functional acromioclavicular separation;
  - Comminuted fractures of the scapular spine.
- Nondisplaced stellate fractures of the glenoid do not require operative management if the humeral head remains reduced and centered.
- Specific treatment options include the following:
  1. *Intraarticular fractures.*
     - Type I: Fractures involving greater than one-fourth of the glenoid fossa that result in instability may be amenable to open reduction and internal fixation with screw fixation using an anterior (IA) or posterior (IB) approach.
     - Type II: Inferior subluxation of the humeral head may result, necessitating open reduction, especially when associated with a greater than 5 mm articular step-off. An anterior approach typically provides adequate exposure.
     - Type III: Reduction is often difficult and may require superior exposure for superior to inferior screw placement, partial thickness clavicle removal, or distal clavicle resection in addition to anterior exposure for reduction. Additional stabilization of the superior suspensory complex may be necessary.
     - Type IV: Open reduction should be considered for displaced fractures, especially those in which the superior fragment of the glenoid displaces laterally.
     - Type V: Operative management does not necessarily result in improved functional results when compared with nonoperative treatment with early motion but should be considered for an articular step-off greater than 5 mm.
  2. *Scapular body fractures.* Operative fixation is rarely indicated, with nonoperative measures generally proving effective. Open reduction may be considered for cases in which neurovascular compromise is present and exploration is required.
  3. *Glenoid neck fractures.* These generally may be treated symptomatically, with early range-of-motion exercises. If accompanied by a displaced clavicle fracture,

an unstable segment exists, including the glenoid, acromion, and lateral clavicle. Internal fixation of the clavicular fracture generally results in adequate stabilization for healing of the glenoid fracture.

4. *Acromion fractures.* Os acromiale, as well as concomitant rotator cuff injuries, must first be ruled out. Displaced acromion fractures may be stabilized by dorsal tension banding.
5. *Coracoid fractures.* Complete third-degree acromioclavicular separation accompanied by a significantly displaced coracoid fracture is an indication for open reduction and internal fixation of both injuries with transacromioclavicular Steinmann pin fixation, with possible suprascapular nerve exploration.

COMPLICATIONS

- *Associated injuries.* These account for most serious complications due to the high energy nature of these injuries. Increased mortality is associated with concomitant first rib fractures.
- *Malunion.* Fractures of the body generally heal with nonoperative treatment; when malunion occurs it is generally well tolerated but may result in painful scapulothoracic crepitus.
- *Nonunion.* This is extremely rare; but when present and symptomatic, the condition may require open reduction and internal fixation for adequate relief.
- *Suprascapular nerve injury.* This injury may occur in association with body, neck, or coracoid fractures that involve the suprascapular notch. The high association with coracoid fractures prompted Neer to favor early exploration of the suprascapular nerve.

12. PROXIMAL HUMERUS

EPIDEMIOLOGY

- Proximal humerus fractures comprise 4% to 5% of all fractures and represent the most common humeral fractures (45%).
- An increased incidence occurs in the older population and is thought to be related to osteoporosis.
- The occurrence increases in females over males at a ratio of 2:1, which is probably related to issues of bone density.

ANATOMY

- The shoulder has the greatest range of motion of any articulation in the body; this is due to the shallow glenoid fossa that is only 25% of the size of the humeral head and to the fact that the major contributor to stability is not bone but is instead a soft-tissue envelope composed of muscle, capsule, and ligaments.
- The four segments (Neer) are the humeral head, the greater tuberosity, the lesser tuberosity, and the humeral shaft.
- The neurovascular supply comes from the following:
  1. The major supply is from the anterior and posterior humeral circumflex arteries.
  2. The arcuate artery is a continuation of the ascending branch of the anterior humeral circumflex. It enters the bicipital groove and supplies most of the humeral head. Small contributions to the humeral head blood supply arise from the posterior humeral circumflex, reaching the humeral head via tendo-osseous anastomoses through the rotator cuff. Fractures of the anatomic neck are uncommon but portend a poor prognosis due to the precarious vascular supply to the humeral head.
  3. The axillary nerve courses just anteroinferior to the glenohumeral joint, traversing the quadrangular space. It is at particular risk for traction injury due to its relative rigid fixation at the posterior cord and deltoid and because of its proximity to the inferior capsule where it is susceptible to injury during anterior dislocation and anterior fracture-dislocation.
- The forces on the segments are as follows:
  1. The greater tuberosity is displaced superiorly and posteriorly by the supraspinatus and external rotators.
  2. The lesser tuberosity is displaced medially by the subscapularis.
  3. The humeral shaft is displaced medially by the pectoralis major.
  4. The deltoid insertion causes abduction of the proximal fragment.

MECHANISM OF INJURY

- The most common injury is a fall onto an outstretched upper extremity from a standing height, typically seen in an elderly osteoporotic woman.
- Younger patients typically present with proximal humeral fractures following high energy trauma, such as a motor vehicle accident. These usually represent more severe fractures and dislocations with significant associated soft tissue disruption and multiple injuries.
- Less common mechanisms include the following:
  1. Excessive shoulder abduction in an individual with osteoporosis, in which the greater tuberosity prevents further rotation;
  2. Direct trauma, usually associated with greater tuberosity fractures;
  3. Electrical shock or seizure;
  4. Pathologic processes: malignant or benign processes in the proximal humerus.

CLINICAL EVALUATION

- Patients typically present with the upper extremity held closely to the chest wall by the contralateral hand, with pain, swelling, tenderness, painful range of motion, and variable crepitus. Gross instability may be present.

- Chest wall and flank ecchymosis may be present and should be differentiated from thoracic injury.
- A careful neurovascular examination is essential, with particular attention to axillary nerve function. This may be assessed by the presence of sensation in the lateral aspect of the proximal arm overlying the deltoid. Motor testing is usually not possible at this stage due to pain. Inferior translation of the distal fragment may result in deltoid atony; this usually resolves by 4 weeks after fracture but, if persistent, must be differentiated from a true axillary nerve injury.

RADIOGRAPHIC EVALUATION

- A "trauma" series is essential, consisting of anteroposterior, lateral in the scapular plane (Y-view; 40 degrees rotated from the coronal plane), and axillary views (Fig. 12.1).
- An axillary view evaluates the axial plane; it is the best view for glenoid articular fractures and dislocations; however, this view may be difficult to obtain due to pain, or it may result in fracture displacement.
- A Velpeau axillary view is performed if a standard axillary cannot be obtained due to pain or fear of fracture displacement. The patient may be left in the sling and should be leaned obliquely backward 45 degree over the cassette. The beam is directed caudally, orthogonal to the cassette, resulting in an axillary view with magnification.
- Computed tomography is helpful for evaluating articular involvement, degree of displacement, impression fractures, and glenoid rim fractures.
- Magnetic resonance imaging is generally not indicated for fracture management but may be used to assess rotator cuff integrity.

NEER CLASSIFICATION (FIG. 12.2)

- The four parts are the greater and lesser tuberosities, the shaft, and the humeral head.
- A part is displaced if >1 cm of displacement or >45 degree of angulation is seen.
- At least two views of the proximal humerus (anteroposterior and scapular Y views) must be obtained; additionally, the axillary view is very helpful for ruling out dislocation.

ORTHOPAEDIC TRAUMA ASSOCIATION CLASSIFICATION OF PROXIMAL HUMERAL FRACTURES

This system emphasizes the vascular supply to the articular segment.

Type A: extraarticular, unifocal fractures
- A1: avulsion of tuberosity
- A2: impacted metaphysis
- A3: nonimpacted metaphyseal fracture

Type B: extraarticular bifocal fractures
- B1: with metaphyseal impaction
- B2: without metaphyseal impaction
- B3: with glenohumeral dislocation

Type C: articular fractures
- C1: slight displacement, impacted valgus fracture
- C2: marked displacement, impacted
- C3: with glenohumeral dissociation

TREATMENT

Minimally Displaced Fractures

- Sling immobilization is used; a swathe may be required for comfort.
- Early shoulder motion may be instituted at 7 to 10 days if the fracture is stable or impacted.

Two-Part Fractures

- Anatomic neck fractures are rare and are difficult to treat by closed reduction. Open reduction and internal fixation (younger patients) or prosthesis (e.g., shoulder

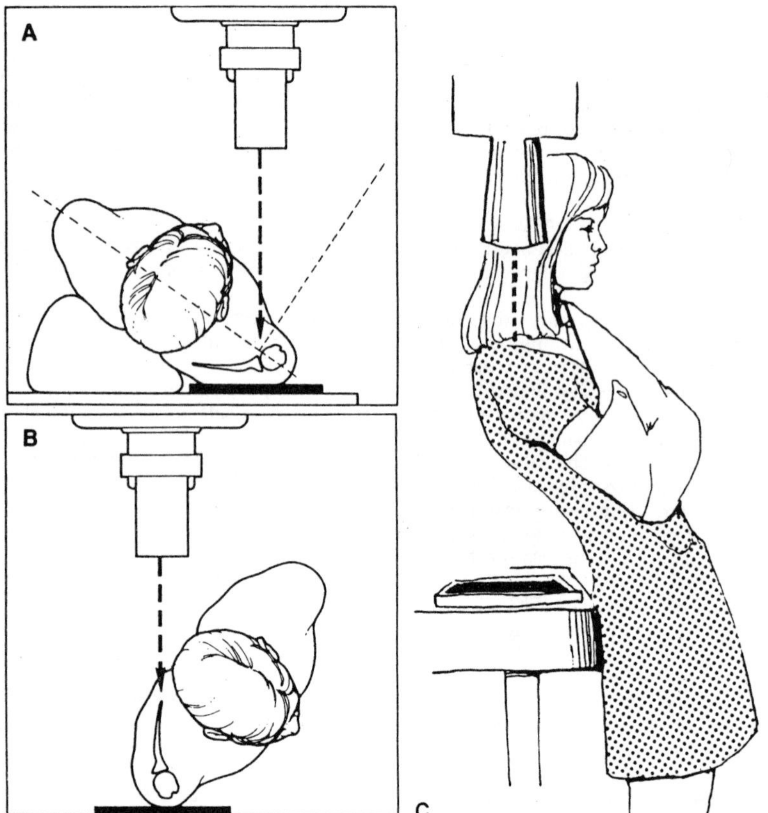

FIG. 12.1. The trauma series consists of anteroposterior and lateral x-rays in the scapular plane and an axillary view. These views may be done sitting, standing, or prone. The lateral is called the tangential or Y-view of the scapula. This series allows evaluation of the fracture in three perpendicular planes so that the fracture-displacement can be accurately assessed. The scapula sits obliquely on the chest wall, and the glenoid surface is tilted 35 to 40 degrees anteriorly. Therefore, the glenohumeral joint is not in the sagittal nor the coronal plane. **A:** For the anteroposterior x-ray in the scapular plane, the posterior aspect of the affected shoulder is placed against the x-ray plate and the opposite shoulder is tilted forward approximately 40 degrees. **B:** For the lateral x-ray in the scapular plane, the anterior aspect of the affected shoulder is placed against the x-ray plate and the other shoulder is tilted forward approximately 40 degrees. The x-ray tube is then placed posteriorly along the scapular spine. **C:** The Velpeau axillary view is preferred after trauma when the patient can be positioned for this view, because it allows the shoulder to remain immobilized and avoids further displacement of the fracture fragments. (From Rockwood CA Jr, Green DP, Bucholz RW, Heckman JD, eds. *Rockwood and Green's fractures in adults,* 4th ed. Vol. 1. Philadelphia: Lippincott-Raven, 1996:1065, with permission.)

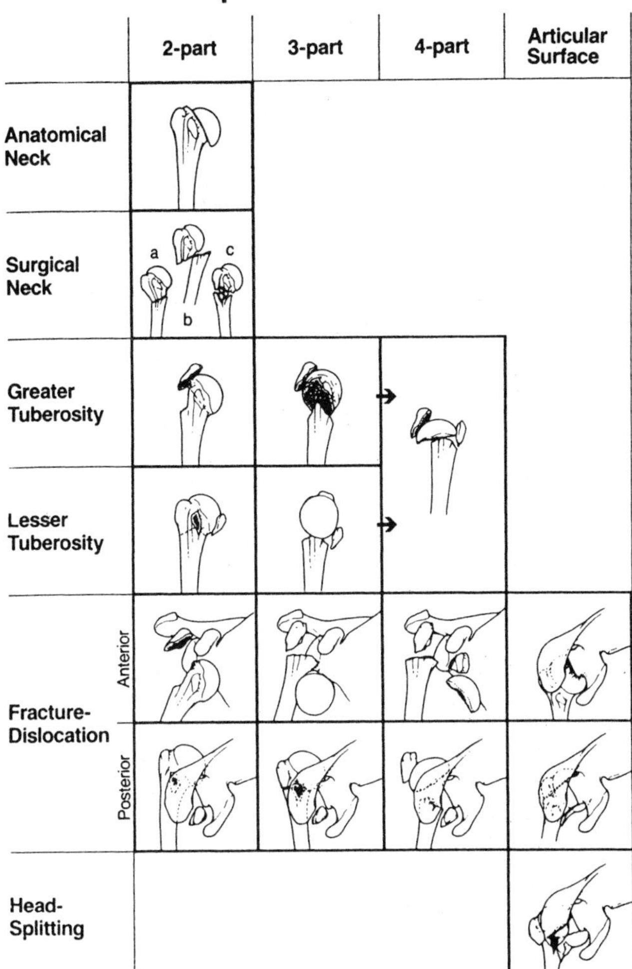

FIG. 12.2. Neer classification. The most commonly used classification at present is the Neer four-part classification. It is a comprehensive system that encompasses anatomy and biomechanical forces that result in the displacement of fracture fragments. It is based on accurate identification of the four major fragments and their relationship to each other. A displaced fracture is either two-part, three-part, or four-part. In addition, fracture-dislocations can be either two-part, three-part, or four-part. Fissure lines or hairline fractures are not considered to be displaced fragments. A fragment is considered displaced when more than 1 cm of separation is seen or a fragment is angulated more than 45 degrees from the other fragments. Impression fractures of the articular surface also occur and are usually associated with an anterior or posterior dislocation. Head-splitting fractures are usually associated with fractures of the tuberosities or surgical neck. (From Neer CS. Displaced proximal humeral fractures. I. Classification and evaluation. *J Bone Joint Surg Am* 1970;52A:1077–1089, with permission.)

hemiarthroplasty) is required. These are associated with a high incidence of osteonecrosis.

- Surgical neck fractures that are impacted with <45-degree angulation that may be treated by sling immobilization with early range-of-motion. Displaced, unstable, or fractures with >45-degree angulation may require closed or open reduction and internal fixation.
- Irreducible fractures (usually interposed soft tissue) require open reduction and internal fixation with either pins, flexible nails with a tension band, or a plate and screws.
- Two-part greater tuberosity fractures are treated in one of two ways. If displaced, open reduction and internal fixation, with or without rotator cuff repair, is required. Otherwise, they may develop nonunion and subacromial impingement. However, a greater tuberosity fracture associated with anterior dislocation may reduce upon relocation of the glenohumeral joint and may be treated nonoperatively.
- Two-part lesser tuberosity fractures may be treated closed unless a displaced fragment blocks internal rotation; consider a posterior dislocation.

Three-Part Fractures

- These are unstable due to opposing muscle forces; as a result, closed reduction and maintenance of reduction is often difficult.
- Displaced fractures require open reduction and internal fixation, except in severely debilitated patients or for those who cannot tolerate surgery.
- Preservation of the vascular supply is of paramount importance; therefore, avoid soft-tissue stripping.
- Older patients may benefit from primary prosthetic replacement (hemiarthroplasty).

Four-Part Fractures

- Closed reduction is difficult to achieve.
- The incidence of osteonecrosis is 13% to 34%.
- Open reduction and internal fixation may be attempted in young patients (<40 years of age) if the humeral head is located within the glenoid fossa and if soft-tissue continuity appears to be present. Fixation may be achieved with multiple Kirschner wires or screw fixation.
- Primary prosthetic replacement of the humeral head (hemiarthroplasty) is the procedure of choice in the elderly.

Fracture-Dislocations

- Two-part fracture-dislocations may be treated closed after reduction unless a residual fracture displacement is found.
- Three- and four-part fracture-dislocations require open reduction and internal fixation in younger individuals (<40 years of age) and hemiarthroplasty in the elderly. The brachial plexus and axillary artery are in proximity to the humeral head fragment with anterior fracture-dislocations.
- Recurrent dislocation is rare following fracture healing.
- Hemiarthroplasty for anatomic neck fracture-dislocation is recommended due to the high incidence of osteonecrosis.
- Fracture-dislocations may be associated with an increased incidence of myositis ossificans with repeated attempts at closed reduction or if open reduction and internal fixation is delayed >5 to 6 days.

Articular Surface Fractures

- These fractures are most often seen with posterior dislocations.
- More than 40% involvement may require hemiarthroplasty; open reduction and internal fixation should initially be considered in patients younger than 40 years of age, if possible.

COMPLICATIONS

- *Vascular injuries.* These are infrequent (5% to 6%), with the axillary artery the most common site (proximal to anterior circumflex artery). An increased incidence is seen in older patients with atherosclerosis due to loss of vessel wall elasticity. The presence of an intact radial pulse does not guarantee the integrity of the axillary artery due to the collateral contribution of the radial artery.

- *Neural injury.* These occur as follows:
  - Brachial plexus injury: infrequent (6%).
  - Axillary nerve injury: especially susceptible in anterior fracture-dislocation because the nerve courses on the inferior capsule and is prone to traction injury or laceration. Complete axillary nerve injuries that do not improve within 2 to 3 months may require exploration.
- *Chest injury.* Intrathoracic dislocation may occur with surgical neck fracture-dislocations; pneumothorax and hemothorax must be ruled out in the appropriate clinical setting.
- *Myositis ossificans.* This is uncommon and is associated with chronic unreduced fracture-dislocations and with repeated attempts at closed reduction.
- *Stiffness.* An aggressive supervised occupational therapy regimen may minimize stiffness, but open lysis of adhesions for recalcitrant cases may be required.
- *Osteonecrosis.* Three percent to 14% of three-part proximal humeral fractures, 13% to 34% of four-part fractures, and a high rate of anatomic neck fractures may be complicated by this condition, leading to posttraumatic osteoarthritis.
- *Nonunion.* This is seen particularly in displaced two-part surgical neck fractures with soft-tissue interposition. Other causes include excessive traction, severe fracture displacement, systemic disease, poor bone quality, inadequate fixation, and infection. It may be addressed with open reduction and internal fixation with or without bone graft, shoulder spica cast immobilization, and electrical stimulation.
- *Malunion.* This can occur after inadequate closed reduction or failed open reduction and internal fixation. It may result in impingement of the greater tuberosity on the acromion, with subsequent restriction of shoulder motion.

13. HUMERAL SHAFT

ANATOMY

- The humeral shaft extends from the pectoralis major insertion to the supracondylar ridge; during this interval, the cross-sectional shape changes from cylindrical to narrow on the anteroposterior view.
- The vascular supply to the humeral diaphysis arises from perforating branches of the brachial artery; the main nutrient artery enters the medial humerus distal to the midshaft.
- The musculotendinous attachments of the humerus result in characteristic fracture displacements as follows:

Position Of Fracture Fragments

Fracture Location	Proximal Fragment	Distal Fragment
Above pectoralis major insertion	Abducted, rotated externally by rotator cuff	Medial, proximal by deltoid and pectoralis major
Between pectoralis major and deltoid tuberosity	Medial by pectoralis, teres major, and latissimus dorsi	Lateral, proximal by deltoid
Distal to deltoid tuberosity	Abducted by deltoid	Medial, proximal by biceps and triceps

MECHANISM OF INJURY

- Direct (most common): direct trauma to humerus from missile projectile or motor vehicle accident; results in transverse or comminuted fractures.
- Indirect: fall on outstretched arm resulting in spiral or oblique fractures, especially in the elderly; rarely, throwing injuries with extreme muscular contraction reported to cause humeral shaft fracture.
- Fracture pattern depends upon type of force applied as follows:
  - Compressive: proximal or distal humeral fracture.
  - Bending: transverse fracture of the humeral shaft.
  - Torsional: spiral fracture of the humeral shaft.
  - Torsional and bending: oblique fracture, often accompanied by a butterfly fragment.

CLINICAL EVALUATION

- Patients with humeral shaft fractures typically present with pain, swelling, deformity, and shortening of the affected arm.
- A careful neurovascular exam with special attention to radial nerve function is essential. In cases of extreme swelling, serial neurovascular examinations with measurement of compartment pressures may be indicated.
- Physical examination frequently reveals gross instability with crepitus on gentle manipulation.
- Soft tissue abrasions and minor lacerations must be differentiated from open fractures.
- Intraarticular extensions of open fractures may be determined by intraarticular injection of saline distant from the wound site and notation of extravasation of fluid from the wound.

RADIOGRAPHIC EVALUATION

- Anteroposterior and lateral radiographs of the humerus should be obtained; the shoulder and elbow joints should be included on each view. To obtain views at 90° from each other, the patient should be rotated because manipulation of the injured extremity will typically result in distal fragment rotation only.
- Traction radiographs may aid in fracture definition in cases of severely displaced or highly comminuted fracture patterns.

- Radiographs of the contralateral humerus may aid in preoperative planning.
- Computed tomography scans, bone scans, and magnetic resonance imaging studies are rarely indicated, except in cases in which a pathologic fracture is suspected.

DESCRIPTIVE CLASSIFICATION

Open versus closed
Location: proximal third, middle third, distal third
Degree: incomplete, complete
Direction and character: transverse, oblique, spiral, segmental, comminuted
Intrinsic condition of the bone
Articular extension

ORTHOPEDIC TRAUMA ASSOCIATION CLASSIFICATION OF HUMERAL DIAPHYSEAL FRACTURES

Type A: simple fracture
- A1: spiral
- A2: oblique (>30°)
- A3: transverse (<30°)

Type B: wedge fracture
- B1: spiral wedge
- B2: bending wedge
- B3: fragmented wedge

Type C: complex fracture
- C1: spiral
- C2: segmental
- C3: irregular (significant comminution)

TREATMENT

- The goal is to establish union with an acceptable humeral alignment in order to restore the patient to his or her preinjury level of function.
- Both patient and fracture characteristics, including patient age, the presence of associated injuries, soft tissue status, and fracture pattern, need to be considered when selecting an appropriate treatment option.

Nonoperative Treatment

- Most humeral shaft fractures (>90%) will heal with nonsurgical management.
- Twenty degrees of anterior angulation, 30° of varus angulation, and up to 3 cm of bayonet apposition are acceptable; they will not compromise function or appearance.
- A hanging cast utilizes dependency traction from the weight of the cast to effect fracture reduction.
  - Indications for use include displaced midshaft humeral fractures with shortening, particularly those with spiral or oblique patterns. Transverse or short oblique fractures represent relative contraindications to use because of the potential for distraction and healing complications.
  - The patient must remain upright or semi-upright at all times with the cast in a dependent position for effectiveness.
  - It is frequently exchanged for functional bracing 1 to 2 weeks postinjury.
  - Greater than 96% union has been reported.
- A coaptation splint utilizes dependency traction to effect fracture reduction but provides greater stabilization and less distraction than a hanging arm cast does. The forearm is suspended in a collar and cuff.
  - It is indicated for the acute treatment of humeral shaft fractures with minimal shortening and for short oblique or transverse fracture patterns that may displace with a hanging arm cast.
  - Disadvantages include axillary irritation, bulkiness, and potential for slippage.
  - The splint is frequently exchanged for functional bracing at 1 to 2 weeks postinjury.

- Thoracobrachial immobilization (Velpeau dressing) is used in elderly patients or children that are unable to tolerate other methods of treatment and where comfort is the primary concern.
  - This technique is indicated for minimally displaced or nondisplaced fractures that do not require reduction.
  - Passive shoulder pendulum exercises may be performed within 1 to 2 weeks postinjury.
  - It may be exchanged for functional bracing at 1 to 2 weeks postinjury.
- The shoulder spica cast has a limited application as operative management is typically performed for the same indications.
  - It is indicated when the fracture pattern necessitates significant abduction and external rotation of the upper extremity.
  - Disadvantages include difficulty of cast application, cast weight and bulkiness, skin irritation, patient discomfort, and the inconvenient upper extremity position.
- Functional bracing utilizes hydrostatic soft tissue compression to effect and maintain fracture alignment while allowing motion of adjacent joints.
  - The bracing is typically applied 1 to 2 weeks postinjury after the patient has been placed in a hanging arm cast or coaptation splint and swelling has subsided.
  - Contraindications include massive soft-tissue injury, an unreliable patient, and an inability to obtain or to maintain acceptable fracture reduction.
  - A collar and cuff may be used to support the forearm; sling application may result in varus angulation.
  - The functional brace is worn for 8 weeks postfracture or until radiographic evidence of union is found.

Operative Treatment

- Associated with increased risk of infection, radial nerve palsy, and nonunion. Indicators for operative treatment include the following:
  - Multiple trauma
  - Inadequate closed reduction position
  - Nonunion
  - Pathologic fracture
  - Associated vascular injury
  - Progressive radial nerve palsy after fracture manipulation
  - "Floating elbow"
  - Segmental fracture
  - Intraarticular extension
  - Bilateral humeral fractures
  - Open fracture
  - Neurologic loss following penetrating trauma
- Surgical approaches to the humeral shaft are as follows:
  - Anterolateral approach: preferred for proximal third humeral shaft fractures; radial nerve identified in the interval between the brachialis and brachioradialis and traced proximally. Can be extended proximally to the shoulder or distally to the elbow.
  - Anterior approach: muscular interval between the biceps and brachialis muscles.
  - Posterior approach: provides excellent exposure to most of the humerus but cannot be extended proximally to the shoulder; muscular interval between the lateral and long heads of the triceps.

Open Reduction and Plate Fixation

- Associated with best functional results.
- Allows direct fracture reduction and stable fixation of the humeral shaft without violation of the rotator cuff.
- Indications for use of plates and screws include the following:
  - Humeri with small medullary canals or preexisting deformity.
  - Proximal and distal humeral shaft fractures.
  - Humerus fractures with intraarticular extension.

Humerus fractures that require exploration for evaluation and treatment of an associated neurologic or vascular lesion.
Humeral nonunions.

- General principles.
  Radiographs of the uninjured, contralateral humerus may be used for preoperative templating.
  Lag screws should be utilized wherever possible.
  Use a 4.5 mm dynamic compression plate with fixation of 8 to 10 cortices proximal and distal to the fracture.

Intramedullary Fixation

- Advantages over plate fixation include the following:
  A closer approximation of the mechanical axis with subsequent smaller bending loads and a decreased likelihood of fatigue failure.
  Less stress-shielding because it is a load-sharing device.
  Lower rate of refracture after implant removal, secondary to fewer stress risers and less cortical osteopenia.
- Indications for use include the following:
  Segmental fractures in which plate placement would require considerable soft tissue dissection.
  Humeral fractures in osteopenic bone.
  Pathologic humeral fractures.
- A high incidence of shoulder pain has been reported following antegrade humeral nailing.
- Flexible intramedullary nails used include Ender nails, Rush rods, and Hackenthal nails.
  Multiple implants; may be inserted in a retrograde or antegrade fashion; disruption of the rotator cuff reported to result in shoulder pain and stiffness.
  Disadvantages: lack of rigid fixation, potential for fracture shortening, and lack of rotational control.
  May require functional bracing as supplementary stabilization.
- Interlocked nails rely on a proximal or distal screw for stability.
  These may be used to stabilize fractures that occur from 2 cm distal to the surgical neck to 3 cm proximal to the olecranon fossa with maintenance of length, alignment, and rotation; they may also be inserted in an antegrade or retrograde fashion.
  Reaming results in increased endosteal surface contact and thus improved stability and in decreased risk of nail incarceration, the ability to place a larger-diameter nail, and the provision of morselized bone chips for autografting.
  Disruption of the endosteal vascular supply is a result of reaming; precautions must be taken to maintain the periosteal vascular supply.
  With antegrade insertion, the proximal aspect of the nail should be countersunk to prevent subacromial impingement.
  The axillary nerve is at risk for injury during insertion of the proximal locking screw.

External Fixation

- Indicated for the following:
  Infected nonunion
  Bone defect or loss
  Burn patients with fractures
  Open fractures with extensive soft tissue injury
- Complications: pin tract infection, neurovascular injuries, nonunion, bulky frame.

POSTOPERATIVE REHABILITATION

Range-of-motion exercises for the hand and wrist should be started immediately postoperatively. Shoulder and elbow range-of-motion exercises should be instituted as pain subsides.

COMPLICATIONS

- Radial nerve injury: as high as 18%.
  - Most common with middle third fractures, although it is best known for its association with the Holstein-Lewis type distal third fracture, which may entrap or lacerate the nerve as it passes through the intermuscular septum.
  - Injuries generally neuropraxias or axonotmesis; function returns within 3 to 4 months; laceration more common in open fractures or gunshot injuries.
  - Progressive nerve palsy after closed reduction may be an indication for early exploration; delayed surgical exploration should be done after 3 to 4 months if no evidence of recovery seen by electromyography or nerve conduction velocity studies.
- Vascular injury: uncommon; may be associated with fractures of the humeral shaft lacerating or impaling the brachial artery or with penetrating trauma.
  - Constitutes true orthopedic emergency; arteriogram controversial as may prolong time to definitive treatment for an ischemic limb.
  - May necessitate vascular repair and/or graft; ideally, total ischemic time should not exceed 6 hours.
- Nonunion: as high as 15%; defined as a lack of healing by 4 months postinjury.
  - Risk factors include fracture at the proximal or distal third of the humerus, transverse fracture pattern, fracture distraction, soft tissue interposition, and inadequate immobilization.
  - May necessitate open reduction and internal fixation with bone grafting and possible postoperative electrical stimulation.
- Malunion: may be functionally inconsequential; arm musculature and shoulder, elbow, and trunk range of motion can compensate for angular, rotational, and shortening deformities (see above).

14. DISTAL HUMERUS

EPIDEMIOLOGY

- Intercondylar fractures of the distal humerus are the most common fracture pattern.
- Extension-type supracondylar fractures of the distal humerus account for >80% of all supracondylar fractures in adults.
- Flexion-type supracondylar fractures account for 2% to 4% of all supracondylar fractures in adults.
- Fractures of the capitellum account for only 0.5% to 1% of all elbow injuries.
- Fractures of a single condyle of the distal humerus account for 5% of all fractures of the distal humerus, involving the lateral condyle more often than the medial.

ANATOMY

- The distal humerus may be conceptualized into medial and lateral "columns," each of which is roughly triangular and is composed of an *epicondyle*, or the nonarticulating terminus of the supracondylar ridge, and a *condyle*, which is the articulating unit of the distal humerus.
- Displacement is common when a condyle loses continuity from its supporting column because no muscles are attached to the condyles to oppose those attached to the epicondyles.
- The articulating surface of the capitellum and trochlea projects distally and anteriorly at an angle of approximately 45 degrees. The centers of the arcs of rotation of the articular surfaces of each condyle lie on the same horizontal axis; thus, malalignment of the relationships of the condyles to each other changes their arcs of rotation, limiting flexion and extension.

ORTHOPAEDIC TRAUMA ASSOCIATION (OTA) CLASSIFICATION OF FRACTURES OF THE DISTAL HUMERUS

Type A: extraarticular fracture
- A1: apophyseal avulsion
- A2: metaphyseal simple
- A3: metaphyseal multifragmentary

Type B: partial articular
- B1: lateral sagittal
- B2: medial sagittal
- B3: frontal

Type C: complete articular
- C1: articular simple, metaphyseal simple
- C2: articular simple, metaphyseal multifragmentary
- C3: articular, metaphyseal multifragmentary

SUPRACONDYLAR FRACTURES

Extension-Type Supracondylar Fractures

- Extraarticular by definition; if the joint is involved, the fracture should be classified as transcondylar or intercondylar with proximal extension.

Mechanism of Injury

- Fall on outstretched hand with or without an abduction or adduction force.

Clinical Evaluation

- Signs and symptoms vary with the degree of swelling and displacement; considerable swelling frequently occurs, rendering landmarks difficult to palpate. However, the normal relationship of the olecranon, medial, and lateral condyles should be maintained, roughly delineating an equilateral triangle.
- Crepitus with range of motion and gross instability may be present; although this is highly suggestive of fracture, no attempt should be made to elicit it because neurovascular compromise may result.

- A careful neurovascular evaluation is essential because the sharp fractured end of the proximal fragment may impale or contuse the brachial artery, median nerve, or radial nerve.
- Serial neurovascular examinations with compartment pressure monitoring may be necessary with massive swelling because cubital fossa swelling may result in vascular impairment or in the development of a volar compartment syndrome resulting in Volkmann ischemia.
- Open fractures are rare and tend to occur with direct trauma to the elbow.

Radiographic Evaluation

- Standard anteroposterior and lateral views of the elbow should be obtained. Oblique radiographs may also be obtained for further fracture definition.
- Traction radiographs may better delineate the fracture pattern and may be useful for preoperative planning.
- For nondisplaced fractures, an anterior or posterior "fat pad sign" may be present on the lateral radiograph, representing displacement of the adipose layer overlying the joint capsule in the presence of effusion or hemarthrosis.
- Minimally displaced fractures may result in a decrease in the normal condylar shaft angle of 45 degrees.
- In extension-type supracondylar fractures, the fracture line runs obliquely from anterodistal to posteroproximal on the lateral radiograph.
- Because intercondylar fractures are much more common in adults than are supracondylar fractures, the anteroposterior (or oblique) radiograph should be scrutinized for evidence of a vertical split in the intercondylar region of the distal humerus.

Treatment

Nonoperative treatment is as follows:

- It is indicated for nondisplaced or minimally displaced fractures and for severely comminuted fractures in elderly patients with limited functional capacity.
- Posterior long arm splint in at least 90 degrees of elbow flexion is used if swelling and neurovascular status permits, with the forearm in neutral.
- Posterior splint immobilization or functional bracing is continued for 1 to 2 weeks, after which range-of-motion exercises are initiated. The splint may be discontinued after approximately 6 weeks, when radiographic evidence of healing is present.
- Up to a 20-degree loss of condylar-shaft angle may be accepted without compromising motion.
- For traction, an olecranon pin may be used initially in cases of severe swelling or open fracture.

Operative treatment is as follows:

- It is indicated for displaced fractures, vascular injury, and open fractures.
- Percutaneous pinning does not provide rigid fixation, and closed reduction may be difficult in the severely swollen elbow. Closed reduction requires postoperative casting, and does not allow early range of motion.
- Open reduction with internal fixation, with one plate on each column, either in parallel or set at 90 degrees, is the procedure of choice because it allows rapid mobilization.
- Total elbow replacement may be considered in elderly patients who otherwise are active with good preinjury function and in whom a severely comminuted fracture of the distal humerus is deemed unreconstructable. In these patients, total elbow replacement provides a reliable return to function.
- The medial triceps-sparing approach may be used, rather than an olecranon osteotomy, for exposure of the elbow articulation.
- Range-of-motion exercises should be initiated as soon as the patient is able to tolerate therapy.

Complications

- *Volkmann ischemic contracture.* This may result from unrecognized compartment syndrome with subsequent neurovascular compromise, from plaster immobilization

with elbow flexion further exacerbating swelling in the antecubital fossa, or post-operatively, especially with the use of regional anesthesia. A high index of suspicion accompanied by aggressive elevation (with traction, if necessary) and serial neurovascular examinations with or without compartment pressure monitoring must be maintained.
- *Stiffness.* Up to a 20-degree decrease in the condylar shaft angle may be tolerated due to compensatory motion of the shoulder.

Flexion-Type Supracondylar Fractures
- This is an uncommon injury, frequently associated with open lesions because the sharp proximal fragment pierces the triceps tendon and overlying skin.
- Associated vascular injuries are rare, accounting for 2% to 4% of supracondylar fractures.

Mechanism of Injury
- Force directed against the posterior aspect of a flexed elbow.

Clinical Evaluation
- The patient typically presents with the elbow held in the flexed position, with resistance encountered on attempted elbow extension.
- The olecranon, medial, and lateral epicondyles maintain their normal spatial relationship, but the triangular plane is shifted anterior to the humeral shaft.
- The posterior aspect of the arm should be inspected for presence of lesions, which may indicate open fracture.

Radiographic Evaluation
- Standard anteroposterior and lateral views of the elbow reveal a fracture line running obliquely from anteroproximal to posterodistal.
- The distal fragment is displaced anteriorly and flexed (apex posterior angulation).

Treatment
Nonoperative treatment is as follows:

- Nondisplaced or minimally displaced fractures may be immobilized in a posterior elbow splint in relative extension. Elbow flexion may result in fracture displacement.
- Alternatively, a long-arm cast may be placed in stages (Soltanpur), enabling the elbow to be immobilized in a flexed position for 6 weeks, after which aggressive range-of-motion exercises are instituted.

Operative treatment is as follows:

- Open reduction and internal fixation, with one 3.5-mm reconstruction plate on each column, either in parallel or set at 90 degrees is performed.
- Range-of-motion exercises should be initiated as soon as the patient is able to tolerate therapy.

Complications
An open fracture requires debridement; partial laceration of the triceps tendon typically does not require repair.

TRANSCONDYLAR FRACTURES
- Occur primarily in elderly patients with osteopenic bone.
- Include fractures that traverse both condyles but are within the joint capsule.

Mechanism of Injury
Mechanisms that produce supracondylar fractures may also result in transcondylar fractures: a fall onto an outstretched hand with or without an abduction or adduction component or a force applied to a flexed elbow.

Clinical Evaluation

- The patient typically presents with the elbow held in flexion, with variable crepitus and gross instability.
- A neurovascular examination must be performed because swelling may result in neurovascular compromise in the cubital fossa or in compartment syndrome.

Radiographic Evaluation

- Standard anteroposterior and lateral radiographs of the elbow should be obtained. Oblique views may be obtained for further fracture definition.
- The fracture line passes proximal to the articular surface and the old epiphyseal line, traversing the coronoid and olecranon fossae.
- A *posadas fracture* is a transcondylar fracture with anterior displacement of the distal fragment accompanied by dislocation of the radial head and proximal ulna from the fragment.

Treatment

Nonoperative Treatment

Nonoperative treatment may be pursued for patients with nondisplaced or minimally displaced fractures, with posterior splinting for 3 to 5 weeks followed by range-of-motion exercises.

Operative Treatment

- Operative treatment should be undertaken for open fractures, unstable fractures, or displaced fractures.
- Fractures with gross displacement should be reduced in the emergency setting, with placement of a posterior splint for provisional stabilization. This is done to minimize traction injury to neurovascular structures or direct laceration by sharp fracture ends. A careful neurovascular examination should be performed after reduction, and postreduction radiographs are essential.
- Operative management may range from closed reduction and percutaneous pinning to open reduction and plate fixation, depending on the fracture pattern.
- The normal condylar shaft angle of 45 degrees should be restored to maintain the functional arc of elbow motion.
- Fixation of the small distal articular fragment may be difficult or impossible; total elbow arthroplasty (semiconstrained) may be considered in the elderly patient with good preinjury functional status if fixation cannot be obtained.

Complications

- Because the fracture lies within the coronoid and olecranon fossae, excessive callus production can result in loss of motion.
- Unrecognized dislocation of the radius and ulna from the articular fragment may result in pseudarthrosis or ankylosis.

INTERCONDYLAR FRACTURES

- Most common distal humeral fracture.
- Comminution common.
- Fracture fragments often displaced by unopposed muscle pull at the medial (flexor mass) and lateral (extensor mass) epicondyles, which rotates the articular surfaces proximally.

Mechanism of Injury

Force directed against the posterior aspect of an elbow flexed >90 degrees, driving the ulna into the trochlea.

Clinical Evaluation

- The patient typically presents with the elbow flexed and the forearm held in pronation, with the arm appreciably foreshortened.
- Crepitus is often appreciated with range of motion, and independent mobility of individual medial and lateral condyles can be elicited.

- The normal spatial relationship between the olecranon, medial, and lateral condyles is typically distorted.

Radiographic Evaluation

- Standard anteroposterior, lateral, and oblique views of the elbow should be obtained.
- Traction radiographs may better delineate the fracture pattern and may be useful for preoperative planning.
- Comminution is often more significant than that appreciated on plain radiographs. Polytomography or computed tomography may be used to delineate fracture fragments further.

RISEBOROUGH AND RADIN CLASSIFICATION (FIG. 14.1)

See also the OTA Classification above.

Type I: nondisplaced
Type II: slight displacement with no rotation between the condylar fragments in the frontal plane
Type III: displacement with rotation
Type IV: severe comminution of the articular surface

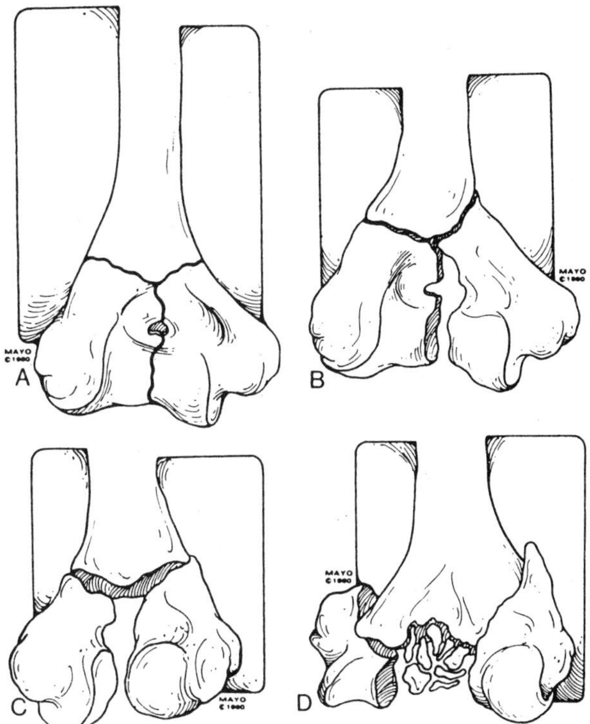

FIG. 14.1. A. Type I undisplaced condylar fracture of the elbow. **B.** Type II displaced but not rotated T-condylar fracture. **C.** Type III displaced and rotated T-condylar fracture. **D.** Type IV displaced, rotated, and comminuted condylar fracture. (From Bryan RS. Fractures about the elbow in adults. *AAOS Instr Course Lect* 1981;30:200–223, with permission.)

Treatment

- Treatment must be individualized according to the patient's age, bone quality, and degree of comminution.

Nonoperative Treatment

This was recommended before the 1960s; today it is indicated for elderly patients with severe osteopenia and comminution or for patients with significant comorbid conditions precluding operative management. Options include the following:

- Cast immobilization: few advocates; represents the "worst of both worlds"—inadequate reduction and prolonged immobilization.
- Traction: olecranon pin—overhead to reduce swelling; problematic in that longitudinal traction alone will not derotate the intercondylar fragments in the axial plane, which leads to malunion.
- "Bag of bones": arm placed in collar and cuff with as much flexion as possible after initial reduction is attempted; gravity traction affects reduction.

Operative Treatment

- Open reduction and internal fixation:
  - Goals of fixation are to restore articular congruity and to secure supracondylar component.
  - Methods of fixation are interfragmentary screws and dual-plate fixation: one plate is placed medially and another plate posterolaterally, 90 degrees from the medial plate. This offers the most stable and fatigue-resistant construct.
- Total elbow arthroplasty (semiconstrained): may be considered in markedly comminuted fractures and in fractures with osteoporotic bone. Surgical exposures include the following:
  - Tongue of triceps: does not allow full exposure of joint and deters early active motion for fear of triceps rupture.
  - Olecranon osteotomy: intraarticular; chevron to give rotational stability.
  - Triceps-sparing extensile posterior approach (Bryan and Morrey).
- Postoperative care: early range of motion of the elbow is essential unless fixation is tenuous.

Complications

- Posttraumatic arthritis: results from articular injury at the time of trauma and from a failure to restore articular congruity.
- Failure of fixation: postoperative collapse of fixation is related to the degree of comminution, the stability of fixation, and the protection of the construct during the postoperative course.
- Loss of motion (extension): increased with prolonged periods of immobilization. Range-of-motion exercises should be instituted as soon as the patient is able to tolerate therapy, unless fixation is tenuous.

CONDYLAR FRACTURES

- Rare in adults; much more common in the pediatric age group.
- Less than 5% of all distal humerus fractures; lateral are more common than medial.
- Medial condyle fractures: include trochlea and medial epicondyle; less common than medial epicondylar fractures.
- Lateral condyle fractures: include capitellum and lateral epicondyle.

Mechanism of Injury

Abduction or adduction of the forearm with elbow extension.

Clinical Evaluation

- Patients typically present with painful range of motion with variable crepitus, swelling, and loss of normal carrying angle of the elbow.

- Independent motion of either the medial or lateral condyle of the humerus may be appreciated.

Radiographic Evaluation

- Standard anteroposterior and lateral radiographs of the elbow should be obtained.
- Condylar fracture lines extend from the articular surface of the distal humerus proximally to the supracondylar ridge, including both articular and nonarticular components.

MILCH CLASSIFICATION (FIG. 14.2)

See also the OTA Classification above.
Two types for medial and lateral; the key is the lateral trochlear ridge.

Type I: Lateral trochlear ridge is left intact.
Type II: Lateral trochlear ridge is part of the condylar fragment (medial or lateral).

- Less stable.
- May allow for radioulnar translocation if capsuloligamentous disruption occurs on the contralateral side.

JUPITER CLASSIFICATION

Low or high, based on proximal extension of fracture line to the supracondylar region:

Low: equivalent to Milch type I fracture
High: equivalent to Milch type II fracture

Treatment

Anatomic restoration of articular congruity is essential to maintain the normal elbow arc of motion and to minimize posttraumatic arthritis.

Nonoperative Treatment

- Indicated for nondisplaced or minimally displaced fractures.
- Consists of posterior splinting with the elbow flexed to 90 degrees and the forearm in supination or pronation for lateral or medial condylar fractures, respectively.

Operative Treatment

- Indicated for open or displaced fractures.
- Consists of screw fixation with or without collateral ligament repair if necessary, with attention to restoration of the rotational axes.
- Prognosis dependent on degree of comminution, accuracy of reduction, and stability of internal fixation.
- Range-of-motion exercises instituted as soon as the patient can tolerate therapy.

Complications

- *Lateral condyle fractures.* Improper reduction or failure of fixation may result in cubitus valgus. This risk is greater with an associated capitellar fracture with fragment excision; it may result in tardy ulnar nerve palsy requiring nerve transposition.
- *Medial condyle fractures.* Residual incongruity is more problematic because of involvement of the trochlear groove and may result in the following:
  - Posttraumatic arthritis, especially with fractures involving the trochlear groove;
  - Ulnar nerve symptoms with excess callus formation or malunion;
  - Cubitus varus with inadequate reduction or failure of fixation.

CAPITELLUM FRACTURES

- Represent <1% of all elbow fractures.
- Occur in the coronal plane with shear fracture, parallel to the anterior humerus.
- Little or no soft-tissue attachments—results from free articular fragment that may displace.

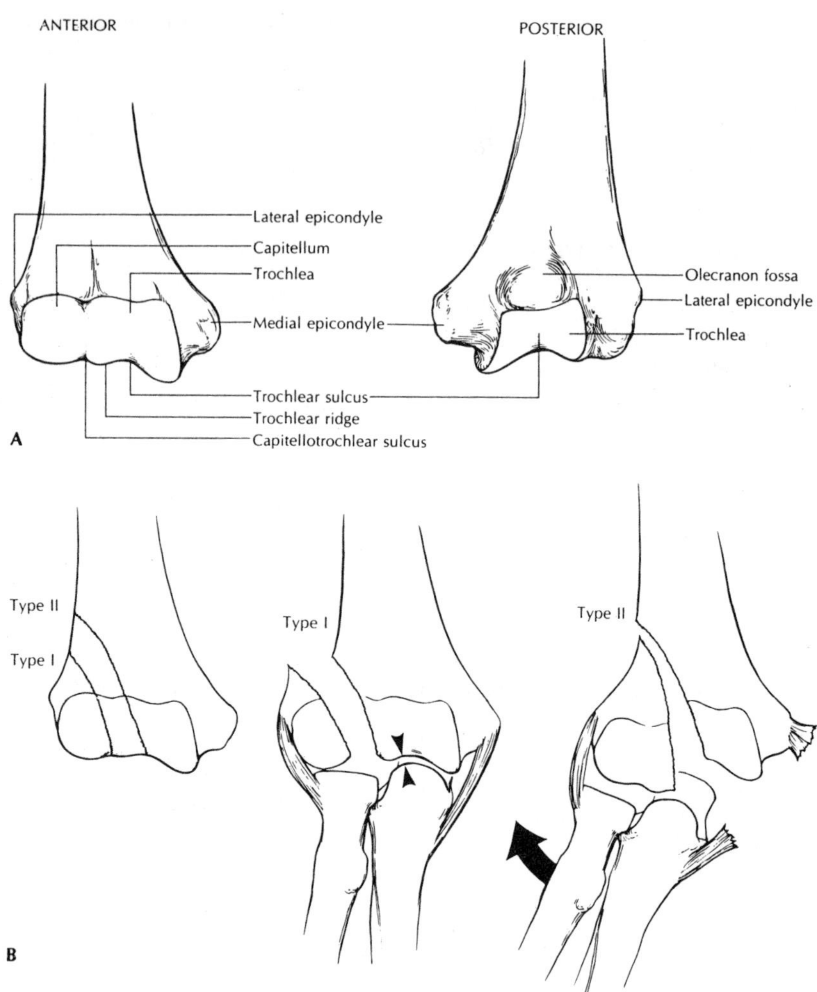

FIG. 14.2. Classification of condylar fractures according to Milch and the location of the common fracture lines seen in type I and II fractures of the lateral (B) and medial (C) condyles. **A.** Anterior view of the anatomy of the distal articular surface of the humerus. The capitellotrochlear sulcus divides the capitellar and trochlear articular surfaces. The lateral trochlear ridge is the key to analyzing humeral condyle fractures. In type I fractures, the lateral trochlear ridge remains with the intact condyle, providing medial to lateral elbow stability. In type II fractures, the lateral trochlear ridge is a part of the fractured condyle, which may allow the radius and ulna to translocate in a medial to lateral direction with respect to the long axis of the humerus. **B.** Fractures of the lateral condyle. In type I fractures, the lateral trochlear ridge remains intact, therefore preventing dislocation of the radius and ulna. In type II fractures, the lateral trochlear ridge is a part of the fractured lateral condyle. With capsuloligamentous disruption medially, the radius and ulna may dislocate.

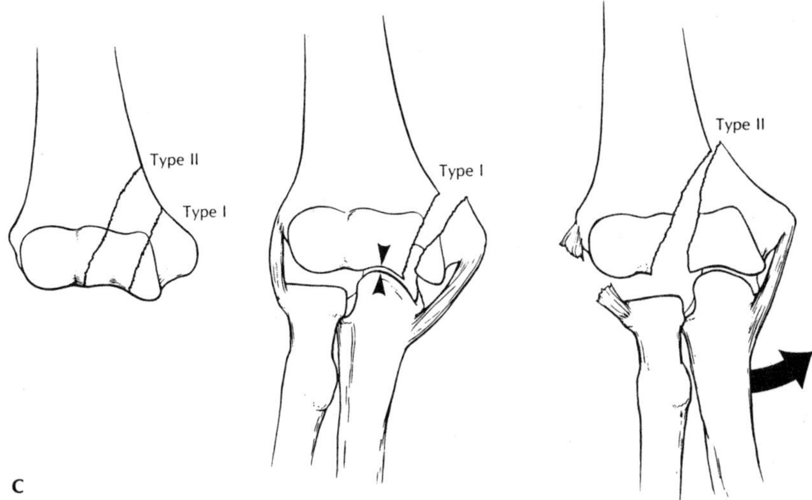

FIG. 14.2. *Continued.* **C.** Fractures of the medial condyle. In type I fractures, the lateral trochlear ridge remains intact to provide medial-to-lateral stability of the radius and ulna. In type II fractures, the lateral trochlear ridge is a part of the fractured medial condyle. With lateral capsuloligamentous disruption, the radius and ulna may dislocate medially on the humerus. (From Rockwood DA Jr, Green DP, Bucholz RW, Heckman JD, eds. *Rockwood and Green's fractures in adults,* 4th ed. Vol. 1. Philadelphia: Lippincott-Raven, 1996:954-955, with permission.)

Mechanism of Injury

- Fall on outstretched hand with elbow in varying degrees of flexion; force transmitted through the radial head into the capitellum.
- Occasionally associated with radial head fractures.

Clinical Evaluation

- The patient typically presents with limited range of motion of the elbow with variable crepitus and joint effusion and/or hemarthrosis.
- Anterior displacement of the articular fragment into the coronoid or radial fossae may result in a block to flexion; posterior displacement of the fragment does not typically present as a bony block but may result in a functional block because severe pain is elicited by abutment of the fragment on the posterior capsule.

Radiographic Evaluation

- Standard anteroposterior and lateral radiographs of the elbow should be obtained. A true lateral is essential in making the diagnosis of capitellar fracture.
- Radiographs must be scrutinized for associated trochlear involvement and radial head fracture.
- Plain radiographs typically underestimate the size of the fragment due to the cartilaginous cap; computed tomography or arthrogram may be used to evaluate the fracture pattern further.

CLASSIFICATION (FIG. 14.3)

Type I: Hahn-Steinthal fragment. Large osseous component of capitellum, sometimes with trochlear involvement

Type II: Kocher-Lorenz fragment. Articular cartilage with minimal subchondral bone attached—"uncapping of the condyle"

Type III: Markedly comminuted

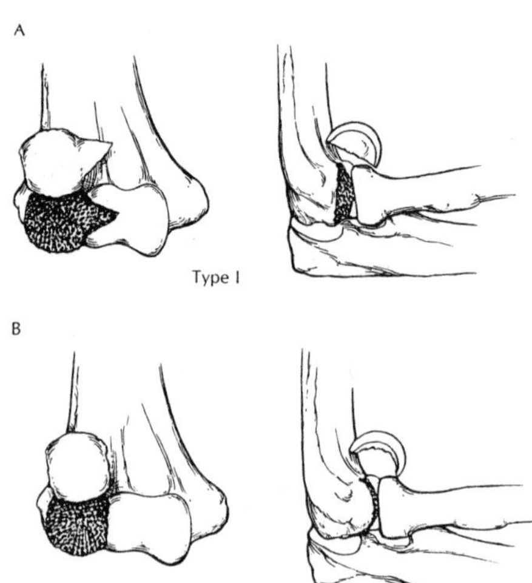

FIG. 14.3. A. Type I (Hahn-Steinthal) capitellar fracture. A portion of the trochlea may be involved in this fracture. **B.** Type II (Kocher-Lorenz) capitellar fracture. Very little subchondral bone is attached to the capitellar fragment. (From Rockwood DA Jr, Green DP, Bucholz RW, Heckman JD, eds. *Rockwood and Green's fractures in adults,* 4th ed. Vol. 1. Philadelphia: Lippincott-Raven, 1996:960, with permission.)

Treatment

Nonoperative Treatment

- Primarily for nondisplaced fractures.
- Consists of immobilization in a posterior splint for 3 weeks.

Operative Treatment

- The goal is anatomic restoration.
- Open reduction with internal fixation is done as follows:
    - This treatment is indicated for displaced type I fractures.
    - Screws may be placed via a posterolateral or posterior approach from a posterior to anterior direction; alternatively, headless screws (e.g., Herbert, Acutrac) may be placed from anterior to posterior.
    - Fixation should be stable enough to allow early range of elbow motion.
- Excision is used as follows:
    - Indicated for severely comminuted type I fractures and most type II fractures.
    - Proximal migration of radius with distal radioulnar joint pain uncommon.
    - Relatively contraindicated in the presence of associated elbow fractures due to compromise of elbow stability.
    - Allows for early mobilization and less morbidity.
    - Recommended treatment in old missed fractures with limited range of motion.

Complications

- *Osteonecrosis.* Despite complete severance from the vascular supply at the time of fracture, osteonecrosis and collapse are relatively uncommon, with revascularization of subchondral bone by creeping substitution. This may be due to the load across the radiocapitellar articulation, which is insufficient to cause subchondral collapse during the remodeling process.
- *Posttraumatic arthritis.* This is increased with failure to restore articular congruity and with excision of the articular fragment.

- *Cubital valgus.* This may result after excision of the articular fragment or with associated lateral condylar or radial head fracture. It is associated with tardy ulnar nerve palsy.
- *Loss of motion (flexion).* This is associated with retained chondral or osseous fragments that may become entrapped in the coronoid or radial fossae.

TROCHLEA FRACTURES (LAUGIER FRACTURE)

- Extremely rare.
- Associated with elbow dislocation.

Mechanism of Injury

Tangential shearing force produced during dislocation.

Clinical Evaluation

Patients present with nonspecific findings of effusion, pain, restricted range of elbow motion, and crepitus.

Radiographic Evaluation

Standard anteroposterior and lateral views of the elbow typically reveal a fragment on the medial aspect of the elbow just distal to the medial epicondyle and variably involving the distal epicondyle.

Treatment

- Nondisplaced fractures may be managed with posterior splinting for 3 weeks, followed by aggressive range-of-motion exercises.
- Displaced fractures should receive open reduction and internal fixation with Kirschner wire or screw fixation.
- Fragments not amenable to internal fixation should be excised.

Complications

- Posttraumatic arthritis may result with retained osseous fragments within the elbow joint or from incongruity of the articular surface.
- Restricted range of motion may occur due to malunion of the trochlear fragment.

LATERAL EPICONDYLAR FRACTURES

Extremely rare.

Mechanism of Injury

- Direct trauma is the cause in adults.
- Prepubescent patients may experience avulsion fractures.

Clinical Evaluation

Patients present with swelling and tenderness about the lateral epicondyle, with painful range of elbow motion and resisted wrist extension.

Radiographic Evaluation

Standard anteroposterior and lateral views of the elbow demonstrate a fracture of the lateral epicondyle, occasionally extending to the capitellum.

Treatment

Symptomatic immobilization followed by early motion.

Complications

Nonunion may result in continued symptoms of pain that are exacerbated by wrist or elbow range of motion, necessitating excision for relief.

MEDIAL EPICONDYLAR FRACTURES

- Fusion of medial epicondylar ossification center does not occur until approximately 20 years of age. However, in some it may never fuse, thus setting the stage for either a misread fracture or an actual avulsion.
- This fracture is more common than lateral epicondylar fractures due to the relative prominence of the epicondyle on the medial side of the elbow.

Mechanism of Injury

- In children and adolescents, the medial epicondyle may be avulsed during a posterior elbow dislocation.
- In adults it is most commonly due to direct trauma, although it can occur as an isolated fracture or in association with elbow dislocation.

Clinical Evaluation

- Patients typically present with local tenderness, swelling, and crepitus over the medial epicondyle.
- A careful neurovascular examination is important, because the fragment may entrap the ulnar nerve.
- Pain is increased with active flexion of the wrist and forearm pronation.
- Range of motion may be limited by fragment incarceration within the elbow articulation.

Radiographic Evaluation

- Standard anteroposterior and lateral views of the elbow demonstrate a fracture of the medial epicondyle, occasionally extending to the condylar region, with the fragment pulled anterior and distal by the forearm flexors.
- Uncommonly, the fragment may become incarcerated within the elbow joint.

Treatment

- Nondisplaced or minimally displaced fractures may be managed by short-term immobilization for 10 to 14 days in a posterior splint with the forearm pronated and the wrist and elbow flexed.
- Displaced fragments may be managed in one of three ways:
  1. Manipulation and immobilization: may result in fibrous union but does not result in forearm weakness or loss of elbow function, even if the fragment remains displaced.
  2. Open reduction and internal fixation: indications for screw or Kirschner wire fixation include the presence of ulnar nerve symptoms, elbow instability to valgus stress, wrist flexor weakness, or symptomatic nonunion of the displaced fragment.
  3. Excision: indicated for fragments not amenable to internal fixation that may become incarcerated within the joint space.

Complications

- Posttraumatic arthritis: may result from osseous fragments retained within the joint space, with possible pain, restricted range of motion, and third body articular wear.
- Weakness of the flexor mass: may result from nonunion of the fragment or malunion with severe distal displacement.

FRACTURES OF THE SUPRACONDYLAR PROCESS

- The supracondylar process is a congenital osseous or cartilaginous projection that arises from the anteromedial surface of the distal humerus.
- The ligament of Struthers is a fibrous arch connecting the supracondylar process with the medial epicondyle, from which fibers of the pronator teres or the coracobrachialis may arise.
- The median nerve and the brachial artery traverse through this arch.
- Fractures are rare, with reported incidences between 0.6% and 2.7%, but may result in significant pain and median nerve or brachial artery compression.

Mechanism of Injury

Direct trauma to the anterior aspect of the distal humerus.

Clinical Evaluation

- Patients present with local tenderness and swelling along the anterior aspect of the distal humerus associated with an often palpable osseous projection proximal to the elbow.
- Active extension of the elbow with pronation or supination may heighten the pain.
- Neurovascular examination is essential, because compression of the brachial artery or median nerve may be present and may be accentuated by elbow range of motion.

Radiographic Evaluation

- Standard anteroposterior and lateral radiographs of the elbow and distal humerus should be obtained.
- Because of the small size and location on the anteromedial aspect of the distal humerus, the process is often not visualized; in such cases, oblique radiographs may demonstrate the presence of the fractured process.

Treatment

- Most fractures are amenable to nonoperative treatment with symptomatic immobilization in a posterior elbow splint in relative flexion until pain-free, followed by early range-of-motion and strengthening exercises.
- Median nerve or brachial artery compression may require surgical exploration and release.

Complications

- Myositis ossificans: increased risk with surgical exploration, thus emphasizing the role of primary immobilization as the first line of treatment.
- Recurrent spur formation: may result in recurrent symptoms of neurovascular compression, necessitating surgical exploration and release, with excision of the periosteum and attached muscle fibers to prevent recurrence.

15. GLENOHUMERAL DISLOCATION

EPIDEMIOLOGY

- The shoulder is the most commonly dislocated major joint of the body, accounting for up to 45% of dislocations.
- Most shoulder dislocations are anterior, occurring between eight and nine times more frequently than posterior dislocation—the second most common direction of dislocation.
- Inferior and superior shoulder dislocations are rare.

ANATOMY

Glenohumeral stability depends on various passive and active mechanisms. Passive mechanisms include the following:

1. Joint conformity;
2. Vacuum effect of limited joint volume;
3. Adhesion and cohesion due to the presence of synovial fluid;
4. Scapular inclination—for >90% of shoulders, the critical angle of scapular inclination is between 0 and 30 degrees, below which the glenohumeral joint is considered unstable and prone to inferior dislocation;
5. Ligamentous and capsular restraints as follows:
   - *Joint capsule.* Redundancy prevents significant restraint, except at terminal ranges of motion. The anteroinferior capsule limits anterior subluxation of the abducted shoulder. The posterior capsule and teres minor limit internal rotation. The anterior capsule and lower subscapularis restrain abduction and external rotation.
   - *Superior glenohumeral ligament.* Restraint is primary to inferior translation of the adducted shoulder.
   - *Middle glenohumeral ligament.* This is variable, poorly defined, or absent in 30% of individuals. It limits external rotation at 45 degrees of abduction.
   - *Inferior glenohumeral ligament.* Three bands, the superior of which is of primary importance to prevent anterior dislocation of the shoulder, are found. This ligament limits external rotation at 45 to 90 degrees of abduction.
6. Glenoid labrum;
7. Bony restraints—acromion, coracoid, glenoid fossa.

Active mechanisms include the following:

1. Biceps, long-head;
2. Rotator cuff.

Coordinated shoulder motion involves the following:

1. Glenohumeral motion;
2. Scapulothoracic motion;
3. Clavicular and sternoclavicular motion;
4. Acromioclavicular motion.

ANTERIOR DISLOCATION

Incidence

- The shoulder is the most commonly dislocated major joint in the body, accounting for up to 45% of dislocations.
- In one series of 394 shoulder dislocations, 84% were anterior glenohumeral dislocations.

Mechanism of Injury

Anterior glenohumeral dislocation may occur as a result of either direct or indirect trauma.

- An anteriorly directed impact to the posterior shoulder may produce an anterior dislocation.
- Indirect trauma to the upper extremity with the shoulder in abduction, extension, and external rotation is the most common mechanism.
- Convulsive mechanisms or electrical shock typically produce posterior shoulder dislocations but may also result in anterior dislocation.
- Recurrent instability related to congenital or acquired laxity or to volitional mechanisms may result in anterior dislocation with minimal trauma.

Clinical Evaluation

- Determining the nature of the trauma, the chronicity of the dislocation, the pattern of recurrence with inciting events, and the presence of laxity or history of instability in the contralateral shoulder is helpful.
- The patient typically presents with the affected shoulder held in slight abduction and external rotation. The acutely dislocated shoulder is painful, with muscular spasm.
- Examination typically reveals squaring of the shoulder due to a relative prominence of the acromion, a relative hollow beneath the acromion posteriorly, and a palpable mass anteriorly.
- A careful neurovascular examination with attention to axillary nerve integrity is important. Deltoid muscle testing is usually not possible, but sensation over the deltoid may be assessed. Deltoid atony may be present and should not be confused with axillary nerve injury. Musculocutaneous nerve integrity can be assessed by the presence of sensation on the anterolateral forearm.
- Patients may present after spontaneous reduction or reduction in the field. If the patient is not acutely in pain, examination may reveal a positive *apprehension test*, in which passive placement of the shoulder in the provocative position (abduction, extension, and external rotation) reproduces the patient's sense of instability and pain. Posteriorly directed counterpressure over the anterior shoulder may mitigate the sensation of instability.

Radiographic Evaluation

- A trauma series of the affected shoulder should be obtained in the anteroposterior, scapular-Y, and axillary views (Figs. 15.1 and 15.2).
- A Velpeau axillary view is performed if a standard axillary cannot be obtained due to pain; the patient may be left in a sling and leaned obliquely backward 45 degrees over the cassette. The beam is directed caudally, orthogonal to the cassette, resulting in an axillary view with magnification (Fig. 15.3).
- A Hill-Sachs lesion is a posterolateral head defect caused by an impression fracture on the glenoid rim, which is seen in 27% of acute anterior dislocations and in 74% of recurrent anterior dislocations, although it can be visualized in only 50% of anteroposterior radiographs.
- The following special views can be obtained:
  1. West Point axillary: taken with the patient prone and with the beam directed cephalad to the axilla 25 degrees from the horizontal and 25 degrees medial; provides tangential view of the anteroinferior glenoid rim (Fig. 15.4).
  2. Hill-Sachs view: anteroposterior radiograph taken with shoulder in maximal internal rotation to visualize a posterolateral defect.
  3. Stryker notch view: patient is supine with ipsilateral palm on the crown of his or her head and the elbow pointing straight up. X-ray beam directed 10 degrees cephalad, aimed at the coracoid. Able to visualize 90% of posterolateral humeral head defects (Fig. 15.5).
- Computed tomography may be useful in defining humeral head or glenoid impression fractures, loose bodies, and anterior labral bony injuries (bony Bankart lesion).
- Single or double contrast arthrography may be used to evaluate rotator cuff pathology.
- Magnetic resonance imaging may be used to identify rotator cuff, capsular, and glenoid labral (Bankart lesion) pathology.

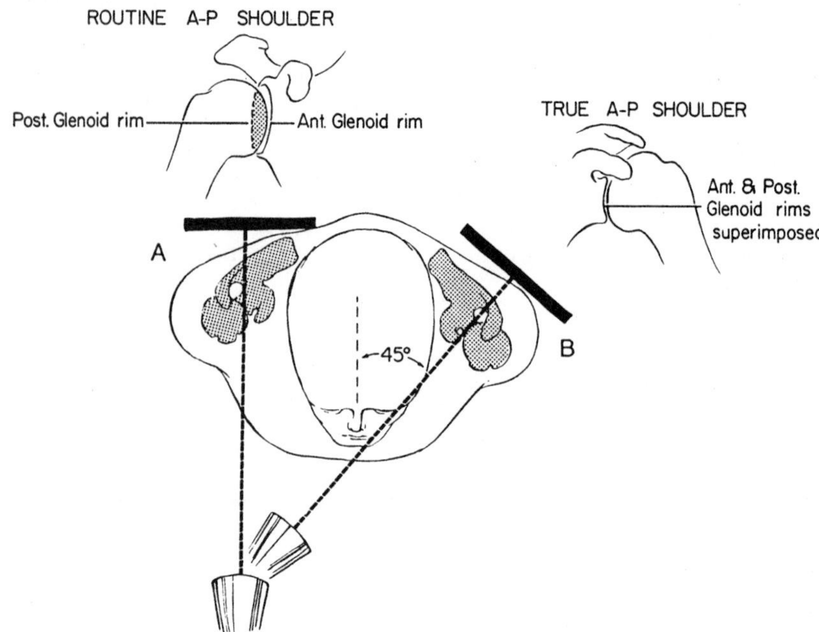

FIG. 15.1. A: Positioning of the patient for a routine anteroposterior (AP) shoulder x-ray and **B:** a true AP shoulder radiograph. (From Rockwood CA, Szalay EA, Curtis RJ, et al. X-ray evaluation of shoulder problems. In: Rockwood CA, Matsen FA III, eds. *The shoulder*. Philadelphia: W.B. Saunders, 1990:201, with permission.)

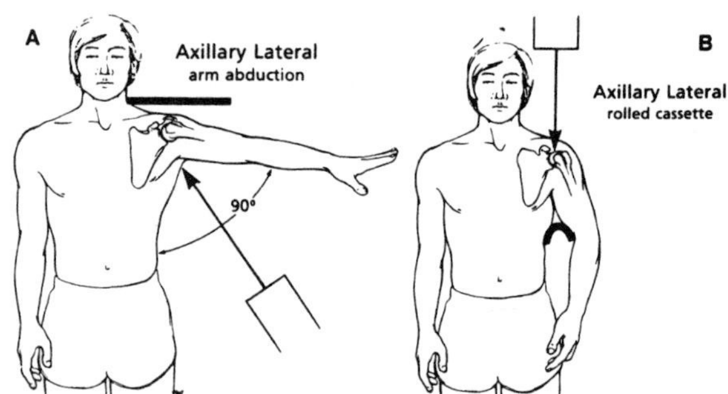

FIG. 15.2. A: The axillary lateral x-ray view. Ideally, the arm is abducted 70° to 90° and the beam is directed superiorly up to the x-ray cassette. **B:** When the patient cannot fully abduct the arm, a curved cassette can be placed in the axilla and the beam can be directed inferiorly through the glenohumeral joint into the cassette. (From Rockwood CA, Szalay EA, Curtis RS, et al. X-ray evaluation of shoulder problems. In: Rockwood CA, Matsen FA III, eds. *The shoulder*. Philadelphia: W.B. Saunders, 1990, with permission.)

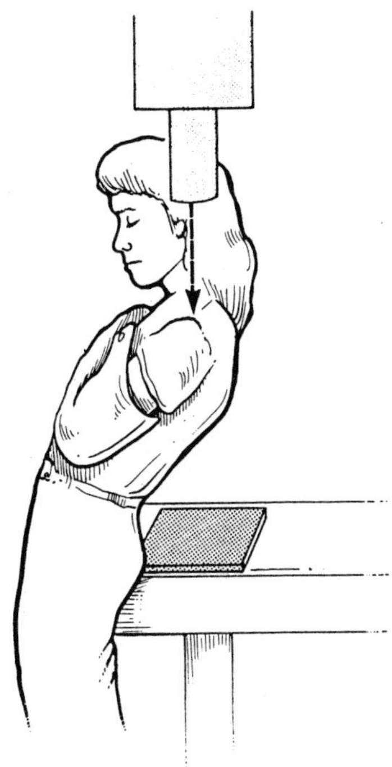

FIG. 15.3. Positioning of the patient for the Velpeau axillary lateral x-ray view, as described by Bloom and Obata. (Modified from Bloom MR, Obata WG. Diagnosis of posterior dislocation of the shoulder with use of the Velpeau axillary and angled up radiographic views. *J Bone Joint Surg Am* 1967;49A:943–949, with permission.)

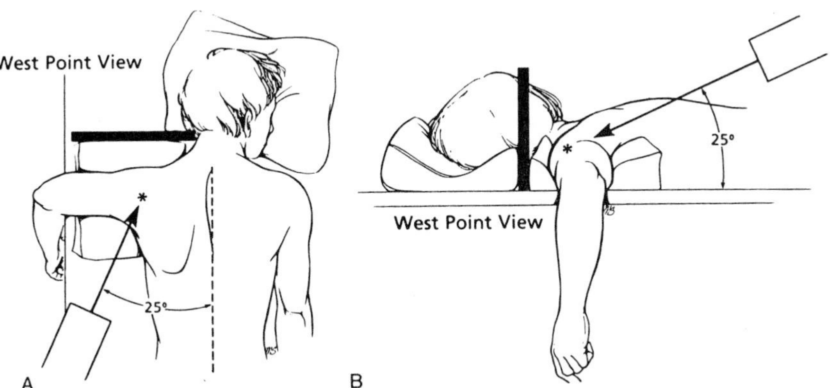

FIG. 15.4. A and B. Positioning of the patient for the West Point x-ray view to visualize the anteroinferior glenoid rim of the shoulder. (Modified from Rokous JR, Feagin JA, Abbott HG. Modified axillary roentgenogram. *Clin Orthop* 1972;82:84–86, with permission.)

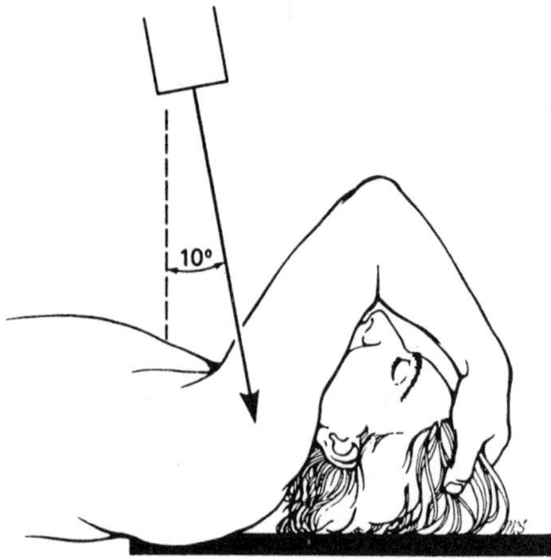

FIG. 15.5. The position of the patient for the Stryker notch view. The patient is supine with the cassette posterior to the shoulder. The humerus is flexed approximately 120 degrees so that the hand can be placed on top of the patient's head. Note that the angle of the x-ray tube is 10 degrees superior. (From Heckman JD, Bucholz RW, eds. *Rockwood, Green, and Wilkin's fractures in adults,* 5th ed. Vol. 2. Philadelphia: Lippincott Williams & Wilkins, 2000:1235, with permission.)

CLASSIFICATION

- Degree of instability: dislocation versus subluxation
- Chronology/Type
  - Congenital
  - Acute versus chronic
  - Locked (fixed)
  - Recurrent
  - Acquired: generally from repeated minor injuries (e.g., from swimming, gymnastics, weights); labrum often intact; capsular laxity; increased glenohumeral joint volume; subluxation is common
- Force
  - Atraumatic: usually due to congenital laxity; no injury; often asymptomatic; self-reducing
  - Traumatic: etiology usually due to one major injury; anterior/inferior labrum may be detached (Bankart lesion); unidirectional; generally requires assistance for reduction
- Patient contribution: voluntary versus involuntary
- Direction
  - Subcoracoid
  - Subglenoid
  - Intrathoracic

Treatment

Nonoperative Treatment

- Older individuals and those with high-energy mechanisms of injury should have an associated fracture of the shoulder girdle ruled out before closed reduction.
- Closed reduction should be performed after adequate clinical evaluation and administration of analgesics and/or sedation. Described techniques include the following:
  - *Traction-countertraction.*
  - *Hippocratic technique.* This technique is effective with only one person performing reduction, with one foot placed across the axillary folds and onto the chest wall; use gentle internal and external rotation with axial traction on the affected upper extremity.
  - *Stimson technique.* After administration of analgesics and/or sedatives, the patient is placed prone on the stretcher with the affected upper extremity hanging

free. Gentle manual traction or 5 pounds of weight is applied to the wrist, with reduction effected over 15 to 20 minutes.

Milch technique. With the patient supine and the upper extremity abducted and externally rotated, thumb pressure is applied by the physician to push the humeral head into place.

Kocher maneuver. The humeral head is levered on the anterior glenoid to effect reduction; this is not recommended due to an increased rate of fracture.

- Postreduction care includes immobilization for 2 to 5 weeks; a shorter period of immobilization may be pursued for patients older than 40 years of age because stiffness of the ipsilateral hand, wrist, elbow, and shoulder tend to complicate treatment. Younger patients with a history of recurrent dislocation may require longer periods of immobilization for adequate treatment.
- Aggressive occupational therapy should be instituted after immobilization, including increasing degrees of shoulder external rotation, flexion, and abduction as time progresses, accompanied by full active range of motion to the hand, wrist, and elbow.
- Irreducible acute anterior dislocation (rare) is usually due to interposed soft-tissue and requires open reduction.

Operative Treatment

- Indications for surgery include the following:
  - Soft-tissue interposition;
  - Displaced greater tuberosity fracture;
  - Glenoid rim fracture >5 mm in size;
  - Selective repair in the acute period (e.g., in young athletes): arthroscopic stabilization, which is controversial.
- Surgical options for stabilization include repair of the anterior labrum, capsular shifts, capsulorraphy, muscle/tendon transfers, and bony transfers. Recent developments include the use of arthroscopy for diagnostic and therapeutic purposes (e.g., arthroscopic anterior labral repair) and thermal capsulorraphy. Anatomic considerations during surgery include the following:
  - Anteriorly, the deltopectoral interval provides access to the glenohumeral articulation. Retraction of the cephalic vein laterally preserves the venous drainage of the deltoid muscle. Anterior cutaneous branches of the axillary nerve may course as proximal as 2 cm distal to the acromion.
  - Posteriorly, access to the glenohumeral joint requires splitting of the deltoid at the junction of the middle and posterior thirds. This ensures that the surgical field is away from the posterior exit of the axillary nerve through the quadrangular space, which is inferior to the field of exposure.
  - Medial to the lateral border of the coracobrachialis muscle lies the musculocutaneous nerve and vascular anastomoses. Surgical dissection should thus be limited to the "safe side," lateral to the lateral border of the coracobrachialis.
  - Inferior to the glenohumeral joint capsule traverses the axillary nerve; it is thus at risk for traction injuries or laceration with dislocations, fractures, or fracture-dislocation.
- Postoperative management typically includes the use of a shoulder immobilizer for 3 weeks in patients <30 years old, for 2 weeks with patients aged 30 to 50 years, and for 1 to 2 weeks in patients over 50 years of age, depending on the integrity of the surgical stabilization. The patients are allowed to remove the immobilizer two to four times per day for shoulder, wrist, and hand range of motion. Occupational therapy is aimed at active and passive range of motion and at regaining upper extremity strength.

Complications

- Recurrent anterior dislocation: related to ligament and capsular changes.
  - The most common complication after dislocation is recurrent dislocation, with an incidence of 80% to 92% (lower in nonathletes) at age 20, 60% at age 30, and 10% to 15% at age 40.
  - Most recurrences occur within the first 2 years, most often in men.

  Prognosis is most affected by the patient's age at the time of initial dislocation.
  Incidence is unrelated to the type or length of immobilization.
- Osseous lesions
  - Hill-Sachs lesion
  - Glenoid lip fracture ("bony Bankart lesion")
  - Greater tuberosity fracture
  - Fracture of the acromion or coracoid
  - Posttraumatic degenerative changes
- Soft-tissue injuries
  - Rotator cuff tear (older patients)
  - Capsular or subscapularis tendon tears
- Vascular injuries: typically occur in the elderly with atherosclerosis; usually axillary artery.
- May occur at the time of open or closed reduction.
- Nerve injuries: particularly to the musculocutaneous and axillary nerves, usually in elderly individuals; neuropraxia almost always heals, but if persistent beyond 3 months following injury, this condition requires further evaluation with possible exploration.

POSTERIOR GLENOHUMERAL DISLOCATION

Incidence
- These dislocations represent 10% of shoulder dislocations and 2% of shoulder injuries.
- They are often unrecognized by primary care and emergency physicians, with 60% to 79% missed on initial examination.

Mechanism of Injury
- Direct trauma: results from force application to the anterior shoulder, resulting in posterior translation of the humeral head.
- Indirect trauma: most common mechanism.
  - Shoulder typically in the position of adduction, flexion, and internal rotation at the time of injury.
  - Electric shock or convulsive mechanisms may produce posterior dislocations due to the greater muscular force of the external rotators of the shoulder (infraspinatus and teres minor muscles) compared with the internal rotators (latissimus dorsi, pectoralis major, and subscapularis muscles).

Clinical Evaluation
- Clinically, a posterior glenohumeral dislocation does not present with striking deformity; the injured upper extremity is typically held in the traditional sling position of shoulder internal rotation and adduction.
- A careful neurovascular examination is important to rule out axillary nerve injury, although this is much less common than with anterior glenohumeral dislocation.
- On examination, limited external rotation (often <0 degrees) and limited anterior forward elevation (often <90 degrees) may be appreciated.
- A palpable mass posterior to the shoulder, flattening of the anterior shoulder, and coracoid prominence may be observed.

Radiographic Evaluation
- The trauma series of the affected shoulder includes anteroposterior, scapular-Y, and axillary views. A Velpeau axillary view (see above) may be obtained if the patient is unable to position the shoulder for a standard axillary view.
- On a standard anteroposterior view of the shoulder, "classic signs" suggestive of a posterior glenohumeral dislocation include the following:
  - Absence of the normal elliptical overlap of the humeral head on the glenoid;
  - Vacant glenoid sign: glenoid appears partially vacant (space between anterior rim and humeral head >6 mm);
  - Trough sign: impaction fracture of anterior humeral head caused by the posterior rim of glenoid (reverse Hill-Sachs lesion), reported to be present in 75% of cases;

  - Loss of profile of the neck of the humerus: humerus is in full internal rotation;
  - Void in the superior/inferior glenoid fossa, due to inferior/superior displacement of the dislocated humeral head.
- Glenohumeral dislocations are most readily recognized on the axillary view; this view may also demonstrate the reverse Hill-Sachs defect.
- Computed tomography is valuable in assessing the percentage of the humeral head involved with an impaction fracture.

ETIOLOGIC CLASSIFICATION

Traumatic: sprain, subluxation, dislocation, recurrent, fixed (unreduced)
Atraumatic: voluntary, congenital, acquired (due to repeated microtrauma)

ANATOMIC CLASSIFICATION

Subacromial (98%). Articular surface directed posteriorly with no gross displacement of the humeral head as in anterior dislocation; the lesser tuberosity typically occupies the glenoid fossa; often associated with an impaction fracture on the anterior humeral head.

Subglenoid (very rare). Humeral head posterior and inferior to the glenoid.

Subspinous (very rare). Humeral head medial to the acromion and inferior to the spine of the scapula.

Treatment

Nonoperative Treatment

- Closed reduction requires full muscle relaxation, sedation, and analgesia.
  - The pain from an acute traumatic posterior glenohumeral dislocation is usually greater than with an anterior dislocation and may require general anesthesia for reduction.
  - With the patient supine, traction should be applied to the adducted arm in the line of deformity with gentle lifting of the humeral head into the glenoid fossa.
  - The shoulder should not be forced into external rotation because this may result in a humeral head fracture if an impaction fracture is locked on the posterior glenoid rim.
  - If prereduction radiographs demonstrate an impaction fracture locked on the glenoid rim, axial traction should be accompanied by lateral traction on the upper arm to unlock the humeral head.
- Postreduction care should consist of a sling and swathe if the shoulder is stable. If the shoulder subluxes or redislocates in the sling and swathe, a shoulder spica cast should be placed with the amount of external rotation determined by the position of stability. Immobilization is continued for 3 to 6 weeks, depending on the age of the patient and the stability of the shoulder.
  - With a large anteromedial head defect, better stability may be achieved with immobilization in external rotation.
  - External rotation and deltoid isometric exercises may be performed during the period of immobilization.
  - After discontinuation of immobilization, an aggressive internal and external rotator strengthening program is instituted.

Operative Treatment

- Indications for surgery include the following:
  - Major displacement of an associated lesser tuberosity fracture;
  - Large posterior glenoid fragment;
  - Irreducible dislocation or impaction fracture on the posterior glenoid, preventing reduction;
  - Open dislocation;
  - Anteromedial humeral impaction fracture (reverse Hill-Sachs lesion) as follows:
    - Twenty percent to 40% humeral head involvement: transfer the lesser tuberosity with attached subscapularis into the defect (modified McLaughlin procedure).

Greater than 40% humeral head involvement: hemiarthroplasty with neutral version.

- Surgical options include open reduction, infraspinatus muscle/tendon plication (reverse Putti-Platt procedure), long head of the biceps tendon transfer to the posterior glenoid margin (Boyd-Sisk procedure), humeral and glenoid osteotomies, and capsulorraphy.
- Voluntary dislocators should be treated nonoperatively with counseling and strengthening exercises.

Complications

- Fracture: includes fractures of the posterior glenoid rim, humeral shaft, lesser and greater tuberosities, and the humeral head.
- Recurrent dislocation: increased incidence with atraumatic posterior glenohumeral dislocations, large anteromedial humeral head defects resulting from impaction fractures on the glenoid rim, and large posterior glenoid rim fractures. May require surgical stabilization to prevent recurrence.
- Neurovascular injury: much less common in posterior versus anterior dislocation but may include injury to the axillary nerve as it exits the quadrangular space or to the nerve to the infraspinatus (branch of the suprascapular nerve) as it traverses the spinoglenoid notch.
- Anterior subluxation: may result from "overtightening" posterior structures, forcing the humeral head anteriorly. May also result in limited flexion, adduction, and internal rotation.

INFERIOR GLENOHUMERAL DISLOCATION (LUXATIO ERECTA)

Very rare injury; more common in elderly individuals.

Mechanism of Injury

- This injury results from a hyperabduction force causing impingement of the neck of the humerus on the acromion, which levers the humeral head out inferiorly.
- Superior aspect of the articular surface is directed inferiorly and is not in contact with the inferior glenoid rim, with the humeral shaft directed superiorly.
- Severe soft-tissue injury or fracture of the proximal humerus may occur, with possible open dislocation. Rotator cuff avulsion and tear, pectoralis injury, proximal humeral fracture, and injury to the axillary artery or brachial plexus are common.

Clinical Evaluation

- Patients typically present in the characteristic "salute" fashion, with the humerus locked in 110 to 160 degrees of abduction and forward elevation. Pain is usually severe.
- The humeral head is typically palpable on the lateral chest wall and axilla.
- A careful neurovascular examination is essential because neurovascular compromise almost always complicates these dislocations.

Radiographic Evaluation

- A trauma series of the affected shoulder includes anteroposterior, scapular-Y, and axillary views.
- The anteroposterior radiograph is typically diagnostic, with inferior dislocation of the humeral head and superior direction of the humeral shaft along the glenoid margin.
- The radiograph must be carefully scrutinized for associated fractures, which are common and which may not be clinically detected due to a diffusely painful shoulder.

Treatment

Nonoperative Treatment

- Reduction may be accomplished by the use of traction-countertraction maneuvers.
- Axial traction should be performed in line with the humeral position (superolaterally), with a gradual decrease in shoulder abduction. Countertraction should be applied with a sheet around the patient, in line with, but opposite to, the traction vector.

- The patient should be immobilized in a sling for 3 to 6 weeks, depending on the age of the patient. Older patients may be immobilized for shorter periods of time to avoid stiffness.

Operative Treatment
Occasionally, the dislocated humeral head "buttonholes" through the inferior capsule and soft-tissue envelope, preventing closed reduction. Open reduction is then indicated with enlargement of the capsular defect and repair of the damaged structures.

Complications
Neurovascular compromise: complicates nearly all cases of inferior glenohumeral dislocation; usually recovers after reduction.

SUPERIOR GLENOHUMERAL DISLOCATION
Very rare injury; less common than inferior glenohumeral dislocation.

Mechanism of Injury
- Extreme anterior and superior force applied to the adducted upper extremity, such as a fall from a height onto the upper extremity, forcing the humeral head superiorly from the glenoid fossa.
- Associated with fractures of the acromion, clavicle, coracoid, and humeral tuberosities and with injury to the acromioclavicular joint.
- Typically accompanied by soft-tissue injury to the rotator cuff, glenohumeral capsule, biceps tendon, and surrounding musculature.

Clinical Evaluation
- The patient typically presents with a foreshortened upper extremity held in adduction.
- Neurovascular injuries are common and must be ruled out.
- Clinical examination typically reveals a palpable humeral head above the level of the acromion.

Radiographic Evaluation
- Trauma series of the affected shoulder includes anteroposterior, scapular-Y, and axillary views.
- The anteroposterior radiograph is typically diagnostic, with dislocation of the humeral head superior to the acromion process.
- The radiograph must be carefully scrutinized for associated fractures, which are common and which may not be clinically detected due to a diffusely painful shoulder.

Treatment
- Closed reduction should be attempted with the use of analgesics and sedatives.
- Axial traction with countertraction may be applied in an inferior direction while lateral traction is applied to the upper arm to facilitate reduction.
- As with inferior dislocations, soft-tissue injury and associated fractures are common; irreducible dislocations may require open reduction.

Complications
Neurovascular complications are usually present and typically represent traction injuries that resolve with reduction.

16. ELBOW

DISLOCATION

Epidemiology

- Accounts for 11% to 28% of injuries to the elbow.
- Posterior dislocation most common.
- Highest incidence in the 10- to 20-year age group; associated with sports injuries, although recurrent dislocation is uncommon.

Anatomy

- "Modified hinge" joint (ginglymotrochoid) with a high degree of intrinsic stability due to joint congruity, opposing tension of the triceps and flexors, and ligamentous constraints.
- Three separate articulations:
  - Ulnohumeral (hinge);
  - Radiohumeral (rotation);
  - Proximal radioulnar (rotation).
- Stability
  - Anterior/posterior: trochlea/olecranon fossa (extension); coronoid fossa, radiocapitellar joint, biceps/triceps/brachialis (flexion).
  - Valgus: medial collateral ligament (MCL) complex—the anterior bundle is the primary stabilizer in flexion and extension; anterior capsule and radiocapitellar joint (extension).
  - Varus: ulnohumeral articulation, lateral ulnar collateral ligament (static); anconeus muscle (dynamic).
- Range of motion: 0 to 150 degrees of flexion, 85 degrees of supination, 80 degrees of pronation; functionally require 30 to 130 degrees of flexion, 50 degrees of supination, 50 degrees of pronation.

Mechanism of Injury

- Most commonly due to a fall onto an outstretched hand or elbow, resulting in a levering force to unlock the olecranon from the trochlea and combining with translation of the articular surfaces to produce the dislocation.
- Posterior dislocation following a combination of elbow hyperextension, valgus stress, arm abduction, and forearm supination with resultant soft tissue injuries to the capsule, collateral ligaments (especially medial), and musculature.
- Anterior dislocation ensuing from a direct force striking the posterior forearm with the elbow in a flexed position.

Clinical Evaluation

- Patients typically present guarding the injured upper extremity with variable gross instability and massive swelling.
- A careful neurovascular examination is crucial and should be performed *immediately,* before radiographs or manipulation.
- After manipulation or reduction, repeat neurovascular examinations should be performed to monitor neurovascular status.
- Serial neurovascular examinations should be performed in cases in which massive antecubital swelling exists or in which the patient is believed to be at risk for compartment syndrome.
- Angiography may be necessary to evaluate vascular compromise.
- After reduction, if arterial flow is not reestablished and the hand remains poorly perfused, the patient should be prepared for arterial reconstruction with saphenous vein grafting.
- Angiography should be performed in the operating room and should never delay operative intervention when vascular compromise is present.
- Noting that the radial pulse may be present with brachial artery compromise as a result of collateral circulation is important.

Radiographic Evaluation

- Standard anteroposterior and lateral radiographs of the elbow should be obtained.
- Radiographs should be evaluated for associated fractures about the elbow.

CLASSIFICATION

Chronologic: acute, chronic (unreduced), recurrent

Descriptive: based on relationship of radius/ulna to the distal humerus (Fig. 16.1), as follows:

- Posterior
    - Posterolateral: >90% dislocations
    - Posteromedial
- Anterior
- Lateral
- Medial
- Divergent (rare)

Fracture Dislocations: Elbow Dislocation with Associated Fracture About the Elbow

- Radial head (5% to 11%).
- Medial or lateral epicondyle (12% to 34%): may result in mechanical block after closed reduction due to entrapment of the fragment.
- Coronoid process (5% to 10%): secondary to avulsion by brachialis muscle; most common with posterior dislocation.
    - Types I, II, and III based on size of fragment (Regan and Morrey; see figure).
    - Large fragment: associated with recurrent dislocation (type III).

Instability Scale (Morrey)

Type I: posterolateral rotatory instability; positive pivot shift test; lateral ulnar collateral ligament disrupted.

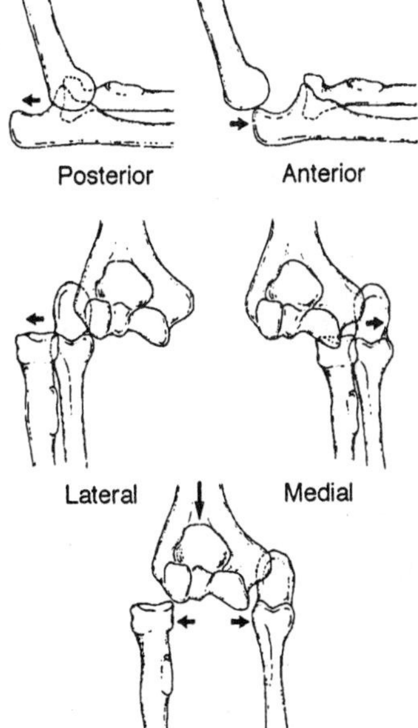

FIG. 16.1. Elbow dislocations. (From Browner BD, Jupiter JB, Levine AM, eds. *Skeletal trauma*. Philadelphia: W.B. Saunders, 1992: 1142, with permission.)

Type II: perched condyles; varus instability; lateral ulnar collateral ligament, anterior and posterior capsule disrupted.
Type IIIa: posterior dislocation; valgus instability; lateral ulnar collateral ligament, anterior and posterior capsule, and posterior medial collateral ligament disrupted.
Type IIIb: posterior dislocation; grossly unstable; lateral ulnar collateral ligament, anterior and posterior capsule, anterior and posterior medial collateral ligament disrupted.

TREATMENT

Posterior Dislocation

Nonoperative Treatment

- Acute posterior elbow dislocations should be managed initially with closed reduction under sedation and analgesia. Alternatively, general or regional anesthesia may be used.
- Reduction should be performed with the elbow flexed while providing distal traction. Reduction with the elbow hyperextended may be associated with median nerve entrapment and increased soft-tissue trauma.
- Neurovascular status should be reassessed, followed by the evaluation of stable range of elbow motion.
- Postreduction radiographs are essential.
- Postreduction management should consist of a posterior splint at 90 degrees with loose circumferential wraps and elevation. Attention should be paid to antecubital and forearm swelling.
- Early, gentle, active range of elbow motion is associated with better long-term results. Forced passive range of motion should be avoided because redislocation may occur. Prolonged immobilization is associated with unsatisfactory results and greater flexion contractures.
- A hinged elbow brace through a stable arc of motion may be indicated in cases of instability without associated fracture.
- Recovery of motion and strength may require from 3 to 6 months.

Operative Treatment

- Surgery is indicated for cases of soft-tissue and/or bony entrapment in which closed reduction is not possible.
- A large, displaced coronoid fragment (type III) requires open reduction and internal fixation to prevent recurrent instability.
- Lateral ligamentous reconstruction in cases of recurrent instability and dislocation is usually unnecessary.
- The chronically dislocated elbow requires open reduction combined with various reconstructive approaches.
- The Morrey dynamic external fixator for grossly unstable dislocations (with disruption of the medial collateral ligament) may be required as a salvage procedure.

Anterior Dislocation

- Acute anterior dislocation of the elbow may initially be managed with closed reduction under sedation/analgesia.
- Initial distal traction is applied to the flexed forearm to relax the forearm musculature, followed by dorsally directed pressure on the volar forearm coupled with anteriorly directed pressure on the distal humerus.
- Triceps function should be assessed after reduction, because avulsion of the triceps tendon from its olecranon insertion may occur.
- Associated olecranon fractures usually require open reduction and internal fixation.

Medial/Lateral Dislocation

- Lateral dislocation may be unrecognized because limited flexion/extension may be possible due to ulnar articulation with the capitulotrochlear sulcus.

- Closed reduction of acute dislocation with sedation/analgesia may be performed by distal forearm traction, arm countertraction, and straight medial or lateral forearm pressure.
- Lateral dislocations are associated with greater soft-tissue injury.
- Interposition of the anconeus muscle may prevent closed reduction.

Divergent Dislocation
Rare injury, presenting with two types as follows:

- Anterior-posterior type (ulna posterior, radial head anterior): more common; reduction achieved in the same manner as a posterior dislocation concomitant with posteriorly directed pressure over the anterior radial head.
- Mediolateral (transverse) type (distal humerus wedged between radius lateral and ulna medial): extremely rare; reduction by direct distal traction on extended elbow with pressure on the proximal radius and ulna to converge them.

COMPLICATIONS

- *Loss of motion (extension).* This is associated with prolonged immobilization with initially unstable injuries. Some authors recommend posterior splint immobilization for 3 to 4 weeks, although recent trends have been to begin early (1 week) supervised range of elbow motion.
- *Neurologic compromise.* Sustained neurologic deficits at the time of injury should be observed.
  - Spontaneous recovery usually occurs; a decline in nerve function (especially after manipulation) or severe pain in nerve distribution should be explored and decompressed.
  - Exploration is recommended if no recovery is seen after 3 months following electromyography and serial clinical examinations.
- *Vascular injury.* Brachial artery is most commonly disrupted during injury.
  - Prompt recognition of vascular injury is essential, with closed reduction to reestablish perfusion.
  - If after reduction perfusion is not reestablished, angiography is indicated to identify the lesion, with arterial reconstruction when indicated.
- *Compartment syndrome (Volkmann contracture).* This may result from massive swelling due to soft-tissue injury. Postreduction care must include elevation and avoidance of hyperflexion of the elbow. Serial neurovascular examinations and compartment pressure monitoring may be necessary, with forearm fasciotomy when indicated.
- *Instability / redislocation.* This is rare after isolated traumatic posterior elbow dislocation; incidence increases in the presence of associated coronoid process and radial head fracture (*terrible triad of the elbow*). It may necessitate hinged external fixation, capsuloligamentous reconstruction, internal fixation, or prosthetic replacement of the radial head.
- *Heterotopic bone / myositis ossificans.* Occurrence is as follows:
  - Anteriorly forms between the brachialis muscle and the capsule; posteriorly may form medially or laterally between the triceps and the capsule.
  - Risk increased with greater degree of soft-tissue trauma or presence of associated fractures.
  - May result in significant loss of function.
  - Forcible manipulation or passive stretching—soft-tissue trauma increased; should be avoided.
  - Indocin or local radiation therapy recommended for prophylaxis postoperatively and in the presence of significant soft-tissue injury and/or associated fractures.

17. OLECRANON

EPIDEMIOLOGY

A bimodal distribution of olecranon fractures occurs, with a younger age peak sustaining olecranon fractures as a result of high energy trauma and an older age peak sustaining olecranon fractures as a result of falls.

ANATOMY

- The coronoid process delineates the distal border of the greater sigmoid (semilunar) notch of the ulna, which articulates with the trochlea. This articulation allows rotational motion only about the flexion-extension axis, providing intrinsic stability to the elbow joint.
- The articular cartilage surface is interrupted by a transverse ridge known as the "bare area."
- Posteriorly, the triceps tendon envelops the articular capsule before it is inserted onto the olecranon. A fracture of the olecranon with displacement represents a functional disruption of the triceps mechanism, resulting in loss of active extension of the elbow.
- The ossification center for the olecranon appears at 10 years and fuses by about the age of 16. Persistent epiphyseal plates can be found in adults; these are usually bilateral and demonstrate familial inheritance.
- The patella cubiti is a true accessory ossicle located in the triceps tendon at its insertion into the olecranon.
- The subcutaneous position of the olecranon makes it vulnerable to direct trauma.

MECHANISM OF INJURY

- Two common mechanisms exist, each resulting in a predictable fracture pattern:
  - *Direct.* Fall on the point of the elbow or direct trauma to the olecranon typically results in a comminuted olecranon fracture.
  - *Indirect.* Fall on the outstretched upper extremity accompanied by a strong sudden contraction of the triceps typically results in a transverse or oblique fracture.
- An intact triceps aponeurosis may limit the degree of fragment displacement. A combination of the above may produce displaced comminuted fractures or, in cases of extreme violence, fracture-dislocation with anterior displacement of the distal ulnar fragment and radial head.

CLINICAL EVALUATION

- Patients typically present with the upper extremity supported by the contralateral hand so that the elbow is in relative flexion. Abrasions over the olecranon or hand are indicative of the mechanism of injury. Effusions of the elbow joint are invariably present because all fractures of the olecranon process have an intraarticular component.
- Physical examination may demonstrate a palpable defect at the fracture site. An inability to extend the elbow actively against gravity indicates discontinuity of the triceps mechanism.
- A careful neurosensory evaluation should be performed because associated ulnar nerve injuries are possible, especially with comminuted fractures resulting from high energy injuries.

RADIOGRAPHIC EVALUATION

- Standard anteroposterior and lateral radiographs of the elbow should be obtained. A true lateral x-ray is imperative because this will demonstrate the extent of the fracture, degree of comminution, degree of articular surface involvement in the semilunar notch, and displacement of the radial head, if present.
- The anteroposterior view should be evaluated to exclude associated fractures or dislocations. The distal humerus may obscure osseous details of the olecranon fracture.

SCHATZKER CLASSIFICATION (FIG. 17.1)

- Transverse: occurs at the apex of the sigmoid notch; represents avulsion fracture from a sudden violent pull of both triceps and brachialis and uncommonly from direct trauma.
- Transverse-impacted: direct force leading to comminution and depression of articular surface.
- Oblique: results from hyperextension injury; begins at the midpoint of the sigmoid notch and runs distally.
- Comminuted fractures and associated injuries: result from direct high energy trauma; fractures of the coronoid process may lead to instability, especially with fracture types II through IV.
- Oblique-distal: fractures extending distal to the coronoid; compromise elbow stability.
- Fracture-dislocation: usually associated with severe trauma.

COLTON CLASSIFICATION

- Nondisplaced fractures
  - Less than 2 mm
  - No increase with 90-degree flexion
  - Able to extend actively against gravity
- Displaced fractures
  - Avulsion fractures
  - Common in the elderly
  - Indirect trauma
- Oblique and transverse fractures—indirect trauma
- Comminuted fractures—direct trauma
- Fracture-dislocations—severe injury

ORTHOPAEDIC TRAUMA ASSOCIATION CLASSIFICATION OF PROXIMAL RADIUS/ULNA FRACTURES

Type A: extraarticular
- A1: ulna only
- A2: radius only
- A3: radius and ulna

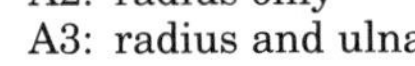

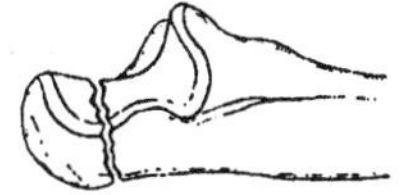

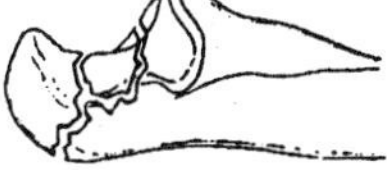

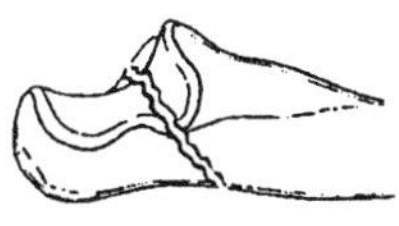

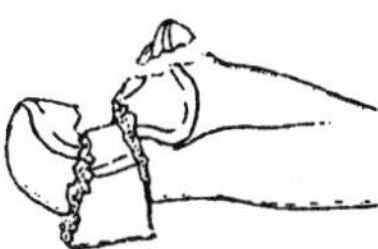

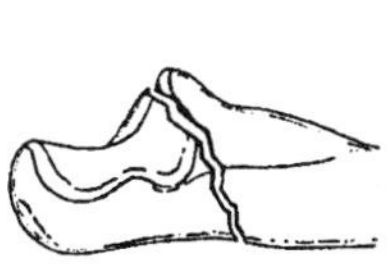

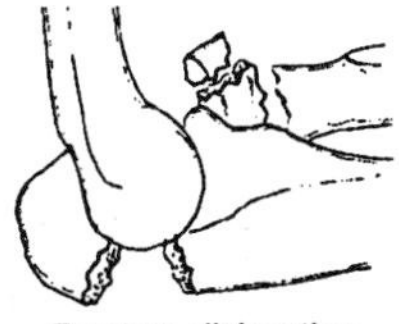

FIG. 17.1. Schatzker classification of olecranon fractures. (From Browner BD, Jupiter JB, Levine AM, eds. *Skeletal trauma*. Philadelphia: W.B. Saunders, 1992:1137, with permission.)

Type B: articular involvement of either radius or ulna
- B1: ulna fractured, radius intact
- B2: radius fractured, ulna intact
- B3: articular fracture of radius or ulna with extraarticular fracture of the other

Type C: articular involvement of both the radius and ulna
- C1: simple fracture of radius and ulna
- C2: simple fracture of radius or ulna, multifragmentary fracture of the other
- C3: multifragmentary fracture of radius and ulna

TREATMENT

Nonoperative Treatment

- Nonoperative treatment is indicated for nondisplaced fractures.
- Immobilization in a long arm cast with the elbow in 45- to 90-degree flexion is favored by many authors, although in reliable patients, a posterior splint or orthosis with gradual initiation of range of motion after 5 to 7 days may be used.
- Follow-up radiographs should be obtained within 5 to 7 days after cast application to rule out displacement. Osseous union is usually not complete until 6 to 8 weeks.
- In general, adequate stability exists at 3 weeks to remove the cast and allow protected range-of-motion exercises, avoiding flexion past 90 degrees.

Operative Treatment

- Displaced fractures (>2 mm) are an indication for open reduction and internal fixation or excision.
- The goals of operative fixation include the following:
  - Maintenance of power of elbow extension;
  - Restoration of articular congruity;
  - Preservation of elbow stability;
  - Maintenance of elbow range of motion.
- Types of operative treatment include the following:
  - Internal suture: using fascia, wire, catgut, or nonabsorbable suture; in general, does not provide adequate fixation and is not recommended.
  - Intramedullary fixation: 6.5-mm cancellous lag screw fixation; must be of sufficient length to engage the distal intramedullary canal for adequate fixation. May be used in conjunction with tension band wiring (described below).
  - Bicortical screw fixation: indicated for transverse or oblique fractures of the olecranon at the level of the coronoid process.
  - Tension band wiring in combination with two parallel Kirschner wires: counteracts the tensile forces and converts them to compressive forces; indicated for avulsion-type olecranon fractures (Fig. 17.2).
  - Plate and screw fixation: for comminuted or longitudinal oblique fractures and for fractures that extend distal to the coronoid.
  - Excision (with repair of the triceps tendon): indicated for nonunited fractures, extensively comminuted fractures, fractures in elderly patients with severe osteopenia and low functional requirements, and extraarticular fractures.
    - Wolfgang et al. demonstrated that excision of as much as 50% of the olecranon is effective in treating comminuted fractures.
    - Morrey et al. demonstrated decreasing elbow stability with increasingly larger excisions.
    - Excision is contraindicated in fracture-dislocations of the elbow or in fractures of the radial head, because it results in compromised elbow stability.
- Postoperatively, the patient should be placed in a posterior elbow splint at 45 degrees, with early range-of-motion exercises.

COMPLICATIONS

- Decreased range of motion: may complicate up to 50% of cases, particularly loss of extension, although only 3% of the patients noted functional limitation (Eriksson); may be minimized by stable internal fixation and early range of motion. A displaced fragment in the olecranon fossa may result in a loss of full extension.

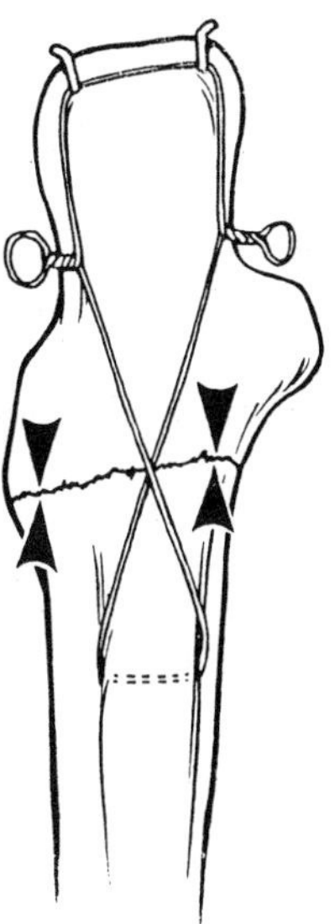

FIG. 17.2. Anteroposterior view demonstrating a modification of the tension band wiring technique in which both limbs of the figure-of-eight wire are twisted. This permits the wire to be tightened on both sides of the fracture to achieve equal compression (note the *arrows*). (From Rockwood CA Jr, Green DP, Bucholz RW, Heckman JD, eds. *Rockwood and Green's fractures in adults*, 4th ed. Vol. 1. Philadelphia: Lippincott-Raven, 1996:990, with permission.)

- Posttraumatic arthritis: especially with >2 mm step-off in articular surface. With articular cartilage and bone loss, the use of cancellous grafting in the defect may provide a fibrocartilaginous surface after revascularization.
- Nonunion (5%): type of treatment dependent on age and functional requirements—younger active patients may require excision of the pseudarthrosis with tension-band fixation or plate fixation with bone grafting. Older patients may be treated with excision of the nonunited fragment with repair of the triceps mechanism.
- Ulnar nerve symptoms (10%): may be secondary to injury from the initial trauma or after surgical fixation; usually resolves spontaneously without definitive treatment.
- Decreased power of extension: secondary to healing of the fracture in an elongated position, resulting in shortening of the triceps mechanism.

18. RADIAL HEAD

EPIDEMIOLOGY

- Frequently associated with injury to the ligamentous structures of the elbow.
- Less commonly associated with fracture of the capitellum.

ANATOMY

- The radial head is intraarticular; the capitellum and the radial head are reciprocally curved.
- Force transmission across the radiocapitellar articulation takes place at all angles of elbow flexion, the greatest occurring in extension (Morrey).
- Full rotation of the head of the radius requires accurate anatomic positioning in the lesser sigmoid notch.
- The radial head plays a role in valgus stability of the elbow, but the degree of conferred stability remains disputed.

MECHANISM OF INJURY

- *Indirect trauma.* This occurs from a fall on an outstretched hand with longitudinal impact of the radius against the capitellum.
- *Direct trauma.* Direct or indirect mechanisms that produce elbow dislocations may result in secondary trauma to the radial head, resulting in dislocation or fracture.

CLINICAL EVALUATION

- Patients typically present with limited elbow and forearm motion (supination/pronation, flexion/extension), painful passive rotation of the forearm with variable crepitus, and pain and swelling of the lateral elbow.
- On clinical examination, well-localized tenderness overlying the radial head may be present, as well as an elbow effusion.
- The ipsilateral forearm and wrist should be examined; tenderness to palpation or stress may indicate the presence of an Essex-Lopresti lesion (radial head fracture-dislocation with associated interosseous ligament disruption).
- Medial collateral ligament competence should be tested, especially with type IV radial head fractures in which valgus instability may result.
- Aspiration of the hemarthrosis through a direct lateral approach with injection of lidocaine will decrease acute pain and will allow evaluation of passive range of motion. This will help identify a mechanical block to motion (Fig. 18.1).

RADIOGRAPHIC EVALUATION

- Standard anteroposterior and lateral radiographs of the elbow should be obtained, with oblique views (Greenspan view) for further fracture definition or in cases in which fracture is suspected but is not apparent on anteroposterior and lateral views.
- A Greenspan view is taken with the forearm in neutral rotation and with the radiographic beam angled 45 degrees cephalad; this view provides visualization of the radiocapitellar articulation.
- Nondisplaced fractures may not be readily appreciable but may be suggested by a positive fat pad sign (posterior more sensitive than anterior) on the lateral radiograph, especially if they are clinically suspected.
- Posterior elbow dislocation or capitellar fracture should heighten suspicion of a radial head fracture.
- Complaints of forearm or wrist pain should be followed with radiographic evaluation.
- Computed tomography may be used for further fracture definition for preoperative planning, especially in cases of comminution or fragment displacement.

MASON CLASSIFICATION (FIG. 18.2)

Type I: nondisplaced fractures
Type II: marginal fractures with displacement (impaction, depression, angulation)

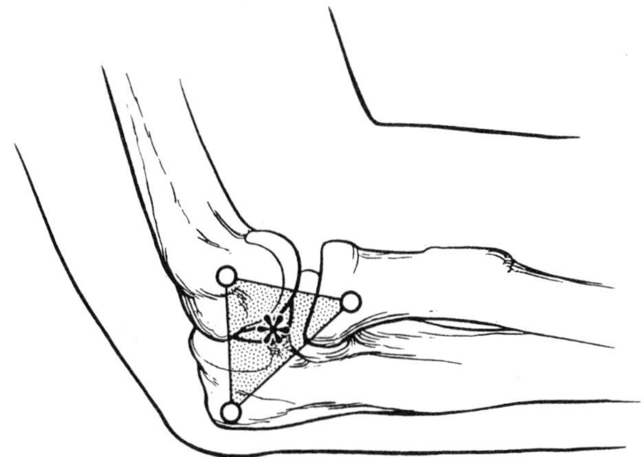

FIG. 18.1. The landmarks for aspiration of the elbow joint are the radial head, lateral epicondyle, and tip of the olecranon. A needle inserted into the center of the triangle (*asterisk*) penetrates only the anconeus muscle and capsule before entering the joint. (From Rockwood CA Jr, Green DP, Bucholz RW, Heckman JD, eds. *Rockwood and Green's fractures in adults*, 4th ed. Vol. 1. Philadelphia: Lippincott-Raven, 1996:1008, with permission.)

Type III: comminuted fractures involving the entire head
Type IV: associated with dislocation of the elbow (Johnston)

SCHATZKER

Type I: wedge fracture—simple wedge fragment, displaced or nondisplaced
Type II: impaction fracture—part of the head and neck remain intact; variable degree of comminution
Type III: severely comminuted fracture—no portion of the head or neck remains in continuity

ORTHOPAEDIC TRAUMA ASSOCIATION CLASSIFICATION OF PROXIMAL RADIUS/ULNA FRACTURES

Type A: extraarticular
- A1: ulna only
- A2: radius only
- A3: radius and ulna

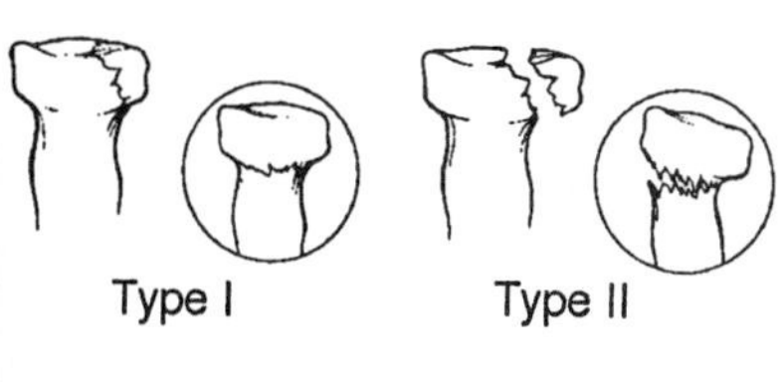

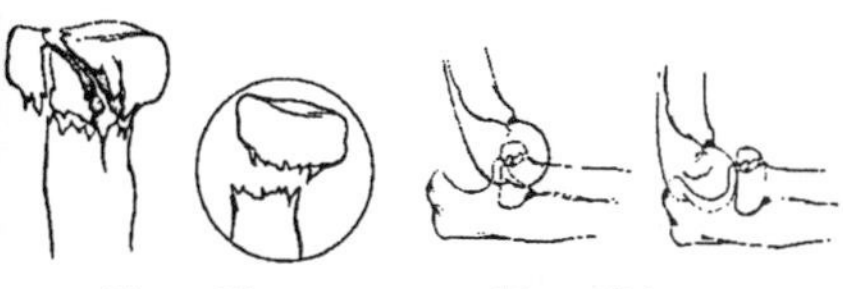

FIG. 18.2. Mason classification of radial head and neck fractures. (From Broberg MA, Morrey BF. Results of treatment of fracture-dislocations to the elbow. *Clin Orthop Rel Res* 1987; 216:109, with permission.)

Type B: articular involvement of either the radius or ulna
- B1: ulna fractured, radius intact
- B2: radius fractured, ulna intact
- B3: articular fracture of radius or ulna with extraarticular fracture of the other

Type C: articular involvement of both the radius and ulna
- C1: simple fracture of the radius and ulna
- C2: simple fracture of the radius or ulna, multifragmentary fracture of the other
- C3: multifragmentary fracture of the radius and ulna

TREATMENT

Mason Type I

- Symptomatic management consists of a sling and early range of motion 24 to 48 hours after injury as pain subsides.
- Aspiration of the joint with or without injection of local anesthesia is advocated by some.
- Persistent pain, contracture, and inflammation may represent capitellar fracture (possibly osteochondral) that was not appreciated on radiographs.

Mason Type II

- If supination and pronation are limited, aspiration of the hemarthrosis should be performed, followed by injection with lidocaine to assess mechanical block.
  - No mechanical block: temporarily protect with sling immobilization and start early range-of-motion exercises as symptoms subside.
  - Mechanical block: open reduction and internal fixation versus excision of the radial head.
- Operative indications are controversial, with some authors advocating nonoperative treatment of Mason type II fractures with early motion, even with comminution and displacement.
- Mason concluded that any displacement or tilt of the radial head involving >25% of the radial head should be treated with excision.
- Most authors favor open reduction and internal fixation of displaced (>2 mm) radial head fractures with Kirschner wires or headless screws (e.g., Herbert or Acutrac) countersunk beneath the articular surface.
- At least 50% of the radial head is needed for stable fixation.

Mason Type III

- Excision of the radial head may be performed if a mechanical block to motion exists.
- The distal radioulnar joint or interosseous ligament must be repaired, if involved, because excision of the radial head may lead to proximal migration.
- Medial collateral ligament integrity must be confirmed because excision may result in instability of the elbow to valgus stressing. Repair or reconstruction of the medial collateral ligament may be necessary.

Mason Type IV

- Perform excision if comminuted fracture; retain it if open reduction with internal fixation is possible.
- Medial collateral ligament and distal radioulnar joint injuries must be addressed at the time of treatment. Some recommend prosthetic replacement if the radial head is excised and wrist pain is present.

Postoperative Care

With stable fixation, beginning early active flexion-extension and pronation-supination exercises is essential.

Radial Head Excision

- The level of excision should be just proximal to the annular ligament. Medial collateral ligament and interosseous ligament injuries must be addressed.
- A direct lateral approach is preferred; however, the posterior interosseous nerve is at risk with this approach.

- Patients generally have few complaints, mild occasional pain, and nearly normal range of motion; the distal radioulnar joint is rarely symptomatic, with proximal migration averaging 2 mm (except with associated Essex-Lopresti lesion). Symptomatic migration of the radius may necessitate radioulnar synostosis.
- Late excision for Mason types II and III fractures has produced good to excellent results in 80% of cases.

Radial Head Prosthesis

- Rationale for use is the prevention of proximal migration of the radius.
- Long-term studies of fracture-dislocations and Essex-Lopresti lesions demonstrated poor function with silicone implants. Metallic (titanium, vitallium) radial head implants have been used with increasing frequency and are the prosthetic implants of choice in the unstable elbow.
- The disrupted interosseous ligament or medial collateral ligament must be repaired.
- Late excision of a symptomatic or fractured prosthesis has yielded good results.

COMPLICATIONS

- Contracture may occur with prolonged immobilization or in cases with unremitting pain, swelling, and inflammation, even after seemingly minimal trauma. These may represent unrecognized capitellar osteochondral injuries. After a brief period of immobilization, the patient should be encouraged to pursue flexion/extension and supination/pronation exercises. Outcome may be maximized by a formal supervised therapy regimen.
- Chronic wrist pain may represent an unrecognized interosseous ligament, distal radioulnar joint, or triangular fibrocartilage complex injury. Recognition of such injuries is important, especially in Mason types III or IV fractures in which radial head excision is considered. Proximal migration of the radius may require radioulnar synostosis to prevent progressive migration.
- Posttraumatic osteoarthritis may occur, especially in the presence of articular incongruity or with free osteochondral fragments.
- Reflex sympathetic dystrophy may occur after surgical management of radial head fractures.
- Unrecognized fracture-dislocation of the elbow may result in a late dislocation due to a failure to address associated ligamentous injuries.

19. FOREARM

EPIDEMIOLOGY

- The ratio of open fractures to closed fractures is higher for the forearm bones than for any other bone except the tibia.
- Forearm fractures are more common in males than in females; this is accounted for by the higher incidence of trauma for males in motor vehicle accidents, contact athletic participation, altercations, and falls from a height.

ANATOMY

- The forearm, like the pelvis, acts as a ring; thus a fracture that shortens either the radius or the ulna results either in a fracture or a dislocation of the other forearm bone at the proximal or distal radioulnar joint. Nightstick injuries are an exception.
- The ulna, which is relatively straight, acts as an axis around which the laterally bowed radius rotates in supination and pronation. A loss of supination and pronation may thus result from radial shaft fractures in which the lateral curvature is not restored.
- The interosseous membrane occupies the space between the radius and ulna. The central band is approximately 3.5 cm thick running obliquely from its proximal origin on the radius to its distal insertion on the ulna. Sectioning of the central band alone reduces stability by 71% (Hotchkiss). Fracture location dictates deforming forces as follows:
  - Radial fractures distal to the supinator muscle insertion but proximal to the pronator teres insertion tend to result in supination of the proximal fragment due to unopposed pull of the supinator and biceps brachii muscles.
  - Radial fractures distal to the supinator and pronator teres muscles tend to result in neutral rotational alignment of the proximal fragment.

FRACTURES OF BOTH THE RADIAL AND ULNAR DIAPHYSES

Mechanism of Injury

- These injuries are most commonly associated with vehicular trauma, although they are also commonly caused by direct trauma (while protecting one's head), missile projectiles, and falls either from a height or during athletic competition.
- Pathologic fractures are uncommon.

Clinical Evaluation

- Patients typically present with gross deformity of the involved forearm, pain, swelling, and loss of hand and forearm function.
- A careful neurovascular examination is essential, with assessment of radial and ulnar pulses and of median, radial, and ulnar nerve function.
- Excruciating unremitting pain, tense forearm compartments, or pain on passive stretch of the fingers should raise suspicions of impending or present compartment syndrome. Compartment pressure monitoring should be undertaken, with emergent fasciotomy indicated for diagnosed compartment syndrome (compartment pressure >30 to 40 mm Hg or more than diastolic blood pressure – 30 mm Hg).

Radiographic Evaluation

- Anteroposterior and lateral views of the forearm should be obtained; oblique views should be obtained as necessary for further fracture definition.
- Radiographic evaluation should also include the ipsilateral wrist and forearm to rule out the presence of associated fracture or dislocation, which may impact prognosis and treatment heavily.
- A *tuberosity view* may be obtained to ascertain rotational deformity of the proximal radius; this is taken with the beam tilted 20 degrees toward the olecranon with the subcutaneous border of the ulna flat on the cassette (Fig. 19.1).

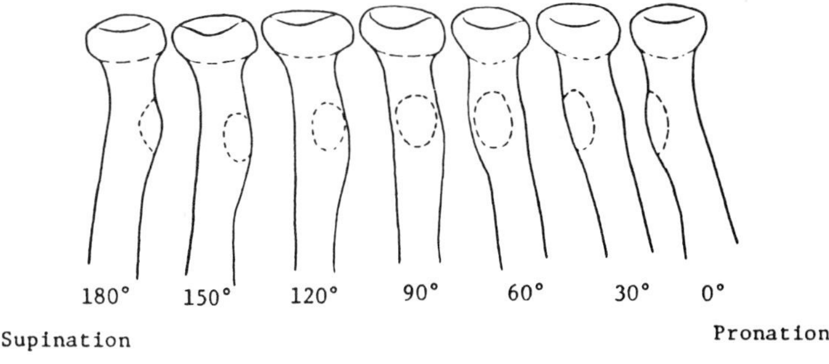

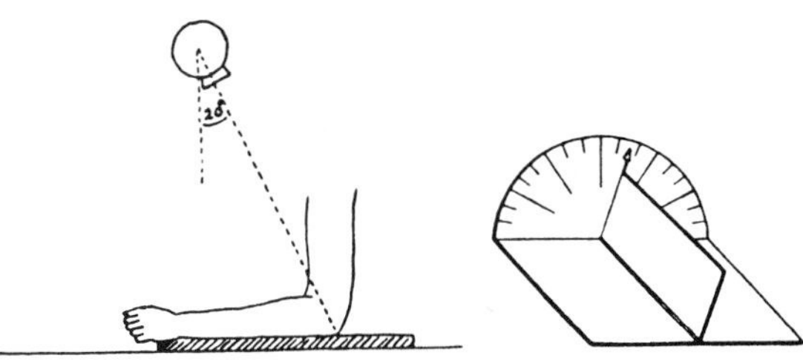

FIG. 19.1. The tuberosity view. The position of the humeral condyles should be at equal distance from the x-ray film. The appearance of the bicipital tuberosity of the radius is shown at the top in different degrees of pronation and supination. The protractor for measuring rotation is shown at the bottom right. The hand is laid against the vertical plate, and the degree of rotation is read from the calibrated scale. (From Evans EM. Rotational deformity in the treatment of fractures of both bones of the forearm. *J Bone Joint Surg* 1945;27:373–379, with permission.)

DESCRIPTIVE CLASSIFICATION

- Closed versus open
- Location
- Comminuted, segmental, or multifragmented
- Displacement
- Angulation
- Rotational alignment

ORTHOPAEDIC TRAUMA ASSOCIATION (OTA) CLASSIFICATION OF FRACTURES OF THE RADIAL AND ULNAR DIAPHYSES

Type A: simple, diaphyseal
- A1: ulna simple, radius intact
- A2: radius simple, ulna intact
- A3: radius and ulna, simple

Type B: wedge fracture, diaphyseal
- B1: ulnar wedge, radius intact
- B2: radial wedge, ulna intact
- B3: wedge of radius or ulna, simple or wedge of other

Type C: complex, diaphyseal
- C1: ulna complex, simple or wedge of radius
- C2: radial complex, simple or wedge of ulna
- C3: complex of both radius and ulna

Treatment

Nonoperative Treatment

- The rare nondisplaced fracture of both the radius and the ulna may be treated with a well-molded long-arm cast in neutral rotation with the elbow flexed to 90 degrees.
- The patient should be followed radiographically at weekly or biweekly intervals to ensure that loss of reduction does not occur.
- Closed reduction and casting is not recommended for displaced fractures because almost all studies demonstrate unsatisfactory results. Functional bracing has been described by Sarmiento with good results, although this has not been reproduced in the literature.

Operative Treatment

- Open reduction with internal fixation is the procedure of choice for displaced forearm fractures involving the radius and ulna in adults.
- Osteosynthesis may be achieved using compression plating (3.5-mm dynamic compression plate [DCP]), with or without autogenous bone grafting.
- A volar Henry approach may be used for fixation of the distal one-third of the radius with plate placement on the flat volar aspect. Midshaft fractures may be approached and stabilized via a dorsal or volar approach.
- The ulna may be plated on either the volar or dorsal aspect, depending on the location of the fragments and contour of the ulna surrounding the fracture site. Using two separate incisions decreases the incidence of radioulnar synostosis.
- Any malreduction will cause a loss of pronation and supination. Radial bow and length must be restored.
- Open fractures may receive primary open reduction and internal fixation after meticulous irrigation and debridement, except in severe Gustilo type IIIB or IIIC open injuries. This restores stability, limits dead space, and improves wound care. Bone grafting of open fractures can be performed at the time of delayed primary closure.
- External fixation may be used in cases with severe bone or soft-tissue loss or gross contamination, with infected nonunions, or with open elbow fracture-dislocations with soft tissue loss.
- Intramedullary fixation has been described for fracture stabilization. Technical considerations include the following:
  - The use of a nail of appropriate length to stabilize the fracture sufficiently without penetration of the bone end.
  - The use of triangular or diamond-shaped nails or of locked intramedullary nails to control length and rotation.
  - Adequate restoration of the radial bow with the use of pre-bent nails.

Complications

- Nonunion and malunion is uncommon and is most often related to infection and errors of technique. If infected, this may require debridement, removal of hardware, intravenous antibiotics, bone grafting, and reosteosynthesis.
- Infection has an incidence of only 3.1% with open reduction and internal fixation, even with open fractures with massive crush injuries. It necessitates surgical drainage, debridement, copious irrigation, wound cultures, and antibiotics. If internal fixation is found to be stable, it does not necessarily need to be removed because most fractures will heal even in the face of infection. Massive infections with severe soft-tissue and osseous compromise may necessitate external fixation with wounds left open and serial debridements.
- Neurovascular injury is uncommon and is associated with missile projectile injury or iatrogenic causes. Nerve palsies can generally be observed for 3 months, with surgical exploration indicated for failure of return of nerve function after this time. Injuries to the radial or ulnar arteries may be addressed with simple ligation if the other vessel is patent.
- Volkmann ischemia is a devastating complication after compartment syndrome. Clinical suspicion must be followed by compartment pressure monitoring with emergent fasciotomy if a compartment syndrome is diagnosed.

- Posttraumatic radioulnar synostosis is uncommon (3% to 9.4% incidence); risk increases with massive crush injuries or closed head injury. Surgical excision may be necessary if functional limitations of supination and pronation result, although a nonarticular synostosis excision is rarely successful in the proximal forearm. Postoperative low dose radiation may decrease the incidence.

FRACTURES OF THE ULNAR DIAPHYSIS

- These include *nightstick* and *Monteggia* fractures and stress fractures in athletes.
- A *Monteggia* lesion denotes a fracture of the proximal ulna accompanied by radial head dislocation.

Mechanism of Injury

- Nightstick fractures occur from direct trauma to the ulna along its subcutaneous border, classically as a victim attempts to protect his or her head from assault with a hard object.
- Monteggia fractures are produced by various mechanisms as follows:
  Type I: forced pronation of the forearm;
  Type II: axial loading of the forearm with a flexed elbow;
  Type III: forced abduction of the elbow;
  Type IV: type I mechanism in which the radial shaft additionally fails.

Clinical Evaluation

- Patients with a nightstick fracture typically relate a history of altercation or trauma in which the forearm was struck along the subcutaneous border of the ulna. The patient presents with focal swelling, pain, tenderness, and variable abrasions at the site of trauma.
- Patients with Monteggia fractures present with elbow swelling, deformity, crepitus, and a painful range of elbow motion, especially supination and pronation. Often the radial head is palpable.
- A careful neurovascular examination is essential because nerve injuries, especially to the radial or posterior interosseous nerve, are common. Most nerve injuries have been described with type II injuries.

Radiographic Evaluation

- Anteroposterior and true lateral views of the elbow and forearm should be obtained.
- Oblique views may aid in fracture definition.

BADO CLASSIFICATION OF MONTEGGIA FRACTURES (FIG. 19.2)

See above for classification of ulnar diaphyseal fractures.

Type I: anterior dislocation of the radial head with fracture of the ulnar diaphysis at any level with anterior angulation

Type II: posterior/posterolateral dislocation of the radial head with fracture of the ulnar diaphysis with posterior angulation

Type III: lateral/anterolateral dislocation of the radial head with fracture of the ulnar metaphysis

Type IV: anterior dislocation of the radial head with fractures of both the radius and ulna within proximal third at the same level

Treatment

Nightstick Fractures

- Nondisplaced or minimally displaced fractures may be treated with plaster immobilization in a sugar-tong splint for 7 to 10 days. Depending on the patient's symptoms and the surgeon's preference, this may be followed by functional bracing for 8 weeks with active range-of-motion exercises for the elbow, wrist, and hand or by simple immobilization in a sling with a compression wrap. This is indicated only for fractures with <10-degree angulation without associated neurovascular compromise.

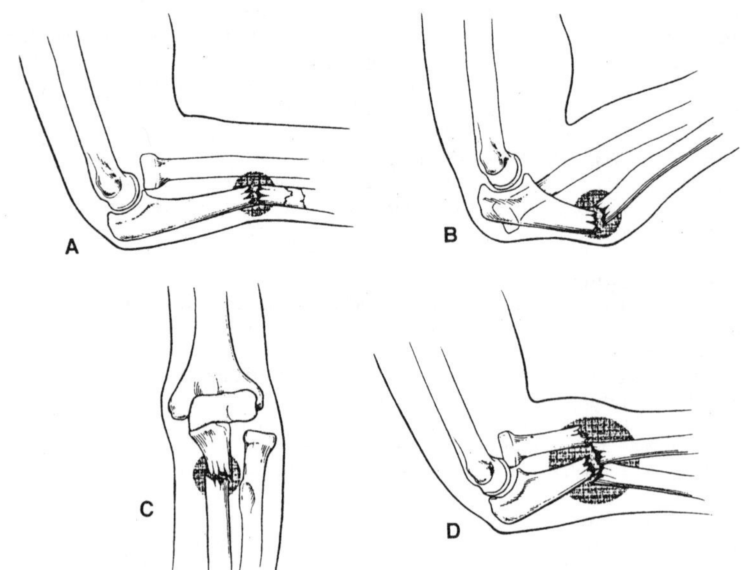

FIG. 19.2. Bado's classification of Monteggia fractures. **A.** Type I. An anterior dislocation of the radial head with associated anteriorly angulated fracture of the ulna shaft. **B.** Type II. Posterior dislocation of the radial head with a posteriorly angulated fracture of the ulna. **C.** Type III. A lateral or anterolateral dislocation of the radial head with a fracture of the ulnar metaphysis. **D.** Type IV. Anterior dislocation of the radial head with a fracture of the radius and ulna. (From Bado JL. The Monteggia lesion. *Clin Orthop* 1967;50:70–86, with permission.)

- Displaced fractures (>10-degree angulation in any plane or >50% displacement of the shaft) should be treated with open reduction and internal fixation using a 3.5-mm dynamic compression plate.

Monteggia Fractures

- Closed reduction and casting of Monteggia fractures should be reserved only for the pediatric population.
- Monteggia fractures require timely operative fixation, with closed reduction of the radial head under anesthesia and open reduction and internal fixation of the ulnar fracture with a 3.5-mm dynamic compression plate or a 3.5-mm pelvic reconstruction plate.
- Postoperatively, the patient is placed in a posterior elbow splint for 5 to 7 days and with stable fixation may be put on a supervised physical therapy regimen of active flexion/extension and supination/pronation exercises. If fixation or radial head stability is questionable, the patient may be placed in a long-arm cast with serial radiographic evaluation to determine healing, followed by a supervised physical therapy regimen as above.

Complications

- Nerve injury: most commonly associated with Bado types II and III injuries involving the radial and median nerves and their respective terminal branches, the posterior and anterior interosseous nerves. These may also complicate open reduction due to overzealous traction or reduction maneuvers. Surgical exploration is indicated for failure of nerve palsy recovery after a 3-month period of observation.

- Radial head instability: uncommon after anatomic reduction. If redislocation occurs <6 weeks postoperatively with a nonanatomic reduction of the ulnar, replating of the ulna with an open reduction of the radial head may be considered. Dislocation of the radial head >6 weeks postoperatively is best managed by radial head excision.

FRACTURES OF THE RADIAL DIAPHYSIS

- Fractures of the proximal two-thirds of the radius without associated injuries may be considered to be truly isolated. However, radial fractures involving the distal third involve the distal radioulnar joint until proven otherwise.
- A *Galeazzi* or *Piedmont fracture* refers to a fracture of the radial diaphysis at the junction of the middle and distal thirds with associated disruption of the distal radioulnar joint. It has also been referred to as the "fracture of necessity," because it requires open reduction and internal fixation to achieve a good result. This lesion is approximately three times as common as Monteggia fractures.
- Four major deforming forces contribute to a loss of reduction if treated by nonoperative means:
  1. Weight of the hand: results in dorsal angulation of the fracture and subluxation of the distal radioulnar joint.
  2. Pronator quadratus insertion: tends to pronate the distal fragment with proximal and volar displacement.
  3. Brachioradialis: tends to cause proximal displacement and shortening.
  4. Thumb extensors and abductors: result in shortening and relaxation of the radial collateral ligament, thus allowing displacement of the fracture despite immobilization of the wrist in ulnar deviation.
- A *reverse Galeazzi fracture* denotes a fracture of the distal ulna with associated disruption of the distal radioulnar joint.

Mechanism of Injury

- Radial diaphyseal fractures may be caused by direct trauma or indirect trauma, such as a fall onto an outstretched hand.
- The radial shaft in the proximal two-thirds is well padded by the extensor musculature; thus, most injuries severe enough to result in proximal radial shaft fractures typically result in ulna fractures as well. Also, the anatomic position of the radius in most functional activities renders it less vulnerable to direct trauma than the ulna.
- Galeazzi fractures may result from direct trauma to the wrist, typically on the dorsolateral aspect, or from a fall onto an outstretched hand with forearm pronation.
- Reverse Galeazzi fractures may result from a fall onto an outstretched hand with forearm supination.

Clinical Evaluation

- Patient presentation is variable and is related to the severity of the injury and to the degree of fracture displacement. Pain, swelling, and point tenderness over the fracture site are typically present.
- Elbow range of motion, including supination and pronation, should be assessed; rarely, limited forearm rotation may suggest a radial head dislocation in addition to the diaphyseal fracture.
- Galeazzi fractures typically present with wrist pain or midline forearm pain that is exacerbated by stressing of the distal radioulnar joint in addition to the radial shaft fracture.
- Neurovascular injury is rare.

Radiographic Evaluation

- Anteroposterior and lateral radiographs of the forearm, elbow, and wrist are essential.
- The direction of the radial tuberosity on the anteroposterior forearm radiograph is the key in determining the position of the proximal fragment:

  Supination: tuberosity directed medial (ulnar).

  Pronation: tuberosity directed lateral (radial).

CLASSIFICATION

See above for classification of radial diaphyseal fractures.

Treatment

Proximal Radius

- Nondisplaced or minimally displaced fractures may be managed in a long-arm cast with the forearm in neutral to full supination, depending on the fracture site in relation to the pronator teres insertion and the resulting rotational displacement as outlined above. The cast is continued until radiographic evidence of healing is found.
- Displaced fractures are best managed by open reduction and plate fixation.

Galeazzi Fractures

- Open reduction and internal fixation should be performed as closed treatment is associated with a 92% failure rate.
- Plate and screw fixation is the treatment of choice; intramedullary nailing does not provide adequate rotational control of the fracture and may additionally result in medial offset of the distal fragment and in shortening of the radius.
- An anterior Henry approach typically provides adequate exposure of the radial fracture, with plate fixation on the flat volar surface of the radius.
- The distal radioulnar joint injury typically results in dorsal instability; thus, a dorsal capsulotomy may be used to gain access to the distal radioulnar joint. After inspection of the joint and the triangular fibrocartilage complex, appropriate repairs or debridement may be accomplished, with closure including dorsal capsulorraphy to imbricate the injured dorsal structures. Kirschner wire fixation may be necessary to maintain reduction of the distal radioulnar joint. However, if the distal radioulnar joint is believed to be stable, postoperative plaster immobilization may suffice.
- Postoperatively, the wrist is immobilized with a sugar-tong splint in supination to minimize tension on the dorsal repair for 10 to 14 days. At this time a removable splint with the elbow at 90 degrees in full supination is placed. At 4 weeks, active forearm rotation is begun. Night splinting is continued for a total of 12 weeks to ensure complete healing of the distal radioulnar joint.

Complications

- *Malunion.* Nonanatomic reduction of the radius fracture with a failure to restore rotational alignment or lateral bow may result in a loss of supination and pronation and painful range of motion. This may require osteotomy or distal ulnar shortening for cases in which symptomatic shortening of the radius results in ulnocarpal impaction. In such cases, care must be taken to preserve the ulnar collateral ligament complex.
- *Nonunion.* This is uncommon with stable fixation but may require bone grafting.
- *Compartment syndrome.* Clinical suspicion must be followed by compartment pressure monitoring with emergent fasciotomy if a compartment syndrome is diagnosed.
- *Radioulnar synostosis.* This is uncommon (3% to 9.4% incidence); risk increases with crush injuries or closed head injury. It may necessitate surgical excision if functional limitations of supination and pronation result.
- *Recurrent dislocation.* This may arise as a result of radial malreduction and emphasizes the need for anatomic restoration of the radial fracture to ensure adequate healing and biomechanical function of the distal radioulnar joint.

20. DISTAL RADIUS

EPIDEMIOLOGY

- Distal radius fractures are among the most common fractures of the upper extremity.
- Common injuries in younger patients include falls from a height, motor vehicle accidents, or injuries sustained during athletic participation. In elderly patients, distal radial injuries may arise from low energy mechanisms, such as a simple fall from standing.
- The incidence of distal radius fractures in the elderly correlates with osteopenia and rises in incidence with increasing age, nearly in parallel with the increased incidence of hip fractures.

ANATOMY

- The metaphysis of the distal radius is composed primarily of cancellous bone. The articular surface has a biconcave surface for articulation with the proximal carpal row (scaphoid and lunate fossae) and a notch for articulation with the distal ulna.
- Eighty percent of axial load is supported by the distal radius and 20% by the ulna and the triangular fibrocartilage complex.
- Reversal of the normal palmar tilt results in load transfer onto the ulna and triangular fibrocartilage complex; the remaining load is then borne eccentrically by the distal radius and is concentrated on the dorsal aspect of the scaphoid fossa.
- Numerous ligamentous attachments to the distal radius exist; these often remain intact during distal radius fractures, facilitating reduction through "ligamentotaxis."
- The volar ligaments are stronger and confer more stability to the radiocarpal articulation than do the dorsal ligaments.

MECHANISM OF INJURY

- The most common mechanism of injury is a fall onto an outstretched hand with the wrist in dorsiflexion.
- Fractures of the distal radius are produced when the dorsiflexion of the wrist varies between 40 and 90 degrees, with lesser degrees of force required at smaller angles.
- The radius initially fails in tension on the volar aspect, with the fracture propagating dorsally where bending forces induce compression stresses, resulting in dorsal comminution. Cancellous impaction of the metaphysis further compromises dorsal stability. Additionally, shearing forces influence the injury pattern, often resulting in articular surface involvement.
- High energy injuries (i.e., vehicular trauma) may result in significantly displaced or highly comminuted, highly unstable fractures to the distal radius.

CLINICAL EVALUATION

- Patients typically present with gross deformity of the wrist and variable displacement of the hand in relation to the wrist (dorsal in Colles fractures; volar in Smith-type fractures). The wrist is typically swollen with ecchymosis, tenderness, and a painful range of motion.
- The ipsilateral elbow and shoulder should be examined for associated injuries.
- A careful neurovascular assessment should be performed, with particular attention to median nerve function because carpal tunnel compression symptoms are common (13% to 23%) due to traction during forced hyperextension of the wrist, direct trauma from fracture fragments, hematoma formation, or increased compartment pressure.

RADIOGRAPHIC EVALUATION

- Anteroposterior and lateral views of the wrist should be obtained, with oblique views for further fracture definition, if necessary. Shoulder or elbow symptoms should be evaluated radiographically.
- Normal radiographic relationships are as follows:
  Radial inclination: averages 23 degrees (range, 13 to 30 degrees);

Radial length: averages 13 mm (range, 8 to 18 mm);
Volar tilt: averages 11 degrees (range, 1 to 21 degrees).

DESCRIPTIVE CLASSIFICATION

- Open versus closed
- Displacement
- Angulation
- Comminution
- Loss of radial length

MELONE CLASSIFICATION OF INTRAARTICULAR FRACTURES (FIG. 20.1)

Based on a consistent mechanism (lunate impaction injury).

Type I: stable, without comminution
Type II: unstable die-punch, dorsal or volar
  IIA: reducible
  IIB: irreducible
Type III: spike fracture; contuses volar structures
Type IV: split fracture; medial complex fractured with dorsal and palmar fragments displaced separately
Type V: explosion fracture; severe comminution with major soft-tissue injury

ORTHOPAEDIC TRAUMA ASSOCIATION (OTA) CLASSIFICATION OF FRACTURES OF THE DISTAL RADIUS AND ULNA

Based on severity of the bony and articular lesion.

Type A: extraarticular
  A1: extraarticular ulna, radius intact
  A2: extraarticular radius, ulna intact
  A3: extraarticular, multifragmentary radius fracture

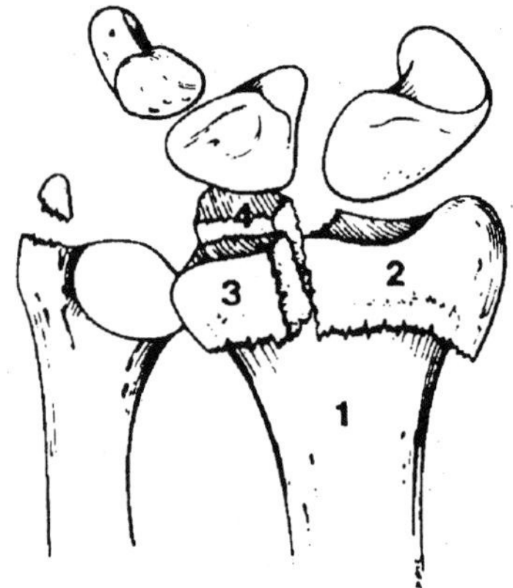

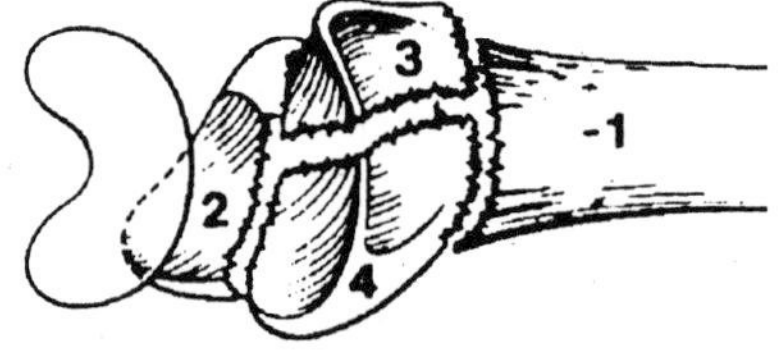

FIG. 20.1. Intraarticular distal radius fractures. (From Melone CP Jr. Open treatment for displaced articular fractures of the distal radius. *Clin Orthop Rel Res* 1986;202:103, with permission.)

Type B: partial articular fracture of the radius
- B1: sagittal
- B2: dorsal rim (Barton)
- B3: volar rim (reverse Barton)

Type C: complete articular fracture of the radius
- C1: simple articular and metaphysis
- C2: simple articular and metaphyseal multifragmentary
- C3: multifragmentary articular

JENKINS CLASSIFICATION

Based on comminution.

Type 1: no radiographically visible comminution
Type 2: comminution of the dorsal radial cortex without comminution of the fracture fragment
Type 3: comminution of the fracture fragment without significant involvement of the dorsal cortex
Type 4: comminution of both the distal fragment and the dorsal cortex

Because the fracture line involves the distal fracture fragment in types 3 and 4, intraarticular involvement is very common within these groups; such involvement is not inevitable, however, nor does it affect the fracture's placement within the classification.

CLASSIFICATION OF INTRAARTICULAR FRACTURES BASED ON THE NUMBER OF FRACTURE PARTS

Two part: opposite portion of the radiocarpal joint remains intact (i.e., dorsal/volar Barton fracture).
Three part: lunate and scaphoid facets separate from each other and proximal radius.
Four part: same as three part except lunate facet is further fractured into dorsal and volar fragments.
Five (+) part: a wide variety of comminuted fragments seen.

EPONYMS

Colles Fracture

- The original description was for extraarticular fractures; the present usage of eponym includes both extra- and intraarticular distal radius fractures demonstrating various combinations of dorsal angulation (apex volar), dorsal displacement, radial shift, and radial shortening.
- More than 90% of distal radius fractures are of this pattern.
- The mechanism of injury is a fall on a hyperextended, radially deviated wrist with the forearm in pronation.
- Intraarticular fractures are generally seen in the younger age group secondary to higher energy forces; concomitant injuries (i.e., to nerve, carpus, and distal ulna) are more frequent, as is involvement of both the radiocarpal and distal radioulnar joints.
- The Frykman classification of Colles fractures (Fig. 20.2) is based on the pattern of intraarticular involvement (Table 20.1).

Smith Fracture (Reverse Colles Fracture)

- Describes fractures with volar angulation (apex dorsal) of the distal radius with a "garden spade" deformity or volar displacement of the hand and distal radius.
- Mechanism of injury: fall on a flexed wrist with forearm fixed in supination.
- Notoriously unstable fracture pattern; often requires open reduction with internal fixation because of the difficulty maintaining adequate closed reduction.

Barton Fracture

- This fracture is a fracture-dislocation or subluxation of the wrist in which the dorsal or volar rim of the distal radius is displaced with the hand and carpus. Volar involvement is more common.

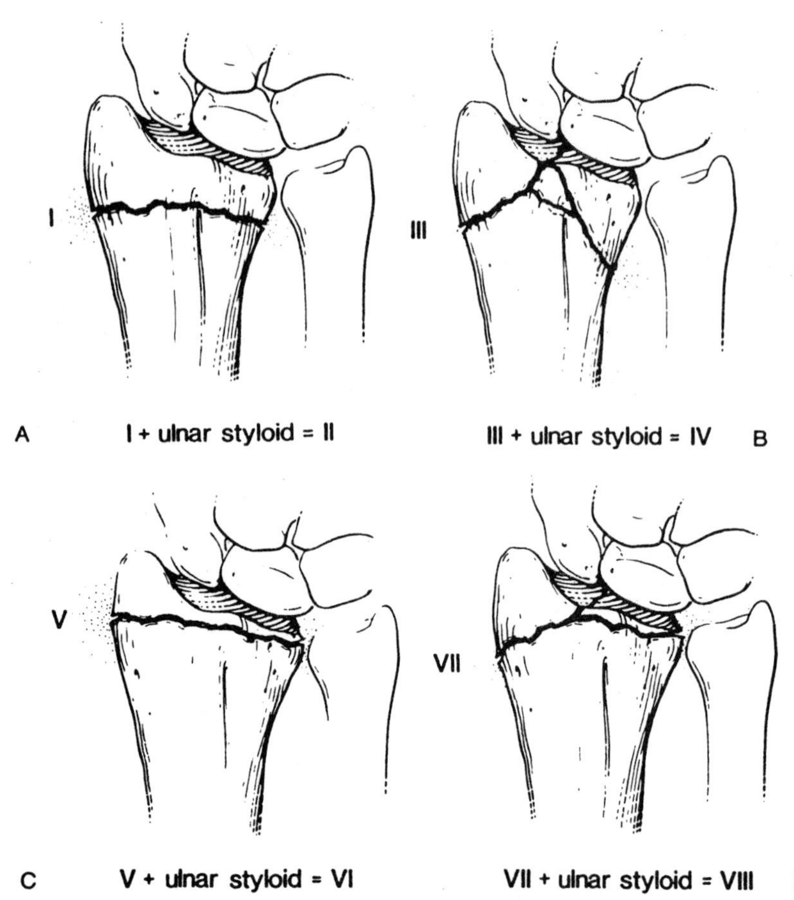

FIG. 20.2. Frykman classification of distal radius fractures. **A.** Frykman type I/II, extraarticular. **B.** Frykman type III/IV, intraarticular radiocarpal joint. **C.** Frykman type V/VI, intraarticular distal radioulnar joint. **D.** Frykman type VII/VIII, intraarticular radiocarpal and distal radioulnar joints. (From Rockwood CA Jr, Green DP, Bucholz RW, Heckman JD, eds. *Rockwood and Green's fractures in adults,* 4th ed. Vol. 1. Philadelphia: Lippincott-Raven, 1996:771, with permission.)

Table 20.1 Intraarticular involvement and classification of Colles fractures

Fracture	Distal ulnar fracture	
	Absent	Present
Extraarticular	I	II
Intraarticular involving radiocarpal joint	III	IV
Intraarticular involving distal radioulnar joint	V	VI
Intraarticular involving radiocarpal and distal radioulnar joint	VII	VIII

- The mechanism of injury is a fall on a dorsiflexed wrist with forearm fixed in pronation.
- Most are unstable and require open reduction and internal fixation with a buttress plate to achieve stable anatomic reduction.

Radial Styloid Fracture ("Chauffeur Fracture," "Backfire Fracture," Hutchinson Fracture)

- Avulsion fracture with extrinsic ligaments remaining attached to the styloid fragment.
- Mechanism of injury: compression of scaphoid against styloid with wrist in dorsiflexion and ulnar deviation.
- May involve the entire styloid or only the dorsal or volar portion.
- Often associated with intercarpal ligamentous injuries (i.e., scapholunate dissociation, perilunate dislocation).
- Open reduction and internal fixation often necessary.

TREATMENT

Factors affecting treatment are as follows:

- Fracture pattern;
- Local factors, such as bone quality, soft-tissue injury, associated comminution, extent of displacement, and energy of injury;
- Patient factors, such as physiologic age, life-style, occupation, dominance, associated medical conditions, associated injuries, and compliance.

Nonoperative Treatment

- Stable nondisplaced or minimally displaced fractures may be amenable to closed reduction and plaster immobilization. This is the treatment of choice for 75% to 80% of distal radius fractures.
- The patient may initially be placed in a sugar-tong splint. Once swelling has subsided, he or she may be changed to a well-molded cast with the wrist in 20-degree volar flexion and ulnar deviation.
- The ideal forearm position, duration of immobilization, and need for a long-arm cast remain controversial; no prospective study has demonstrated the superiority of one method over another.
- Extreme wrist flexion should be avoided because it increases carpal canal pressure (and thus median nerve compression) and digital stiffness. Reductions that require maintenance of extreme wrist flexion may require operative fixation.
- The cast should be worn for approximately 6 weeks or until radiographic evidence of union is found, at which time the patient may be switched to a molded splint for 2 to 3 weeks. The patient should be instituted on a supervised therapy regimen of active-assisted wrist motion exercises.

Operative Treatment

- Unstable or displaced fractures may require operative fixation after closed or open reduction.
- Percutaneous pinning is primarily used for extraarticular fractures or with two-part intraarticular fractures.
  - May be accomplished using two or three Kirschner wires placed across the fracture site; generally placed from the radial styloid proximally and from the dorsoulnar side of the distal radial fragment proximally. Alternatively, transulnar pinning with multiple pins has been described.
  - Generally used to supplement short-arm casting or external fixation. The pins may be removed 3 to 4 weeks postoperatively, with the cast maintained as above.
- External fixation has grown in popularity based on studies yielding relatively low complication rates. Secondary external fixation may be indicated when a loss of reduction occurs with cast immobilization.
  - Ligamentotaxis can restore radial length and radial inclination but rarely restores palmar tilt.

Frame configuration is not critical; quadrilateral frame design is probably unnecessary.
Overdistraction should be avoided and may be recognized by increased intercarpal distance on intraoperative fluoroscopy.
External fixation may be supplemented with percutaneous pinning of comminuted or articular fragments that require pin fixation for further stabilization.
Pins may be removed at 3 to 4 weeks, although most authorities recommend 6 to 8 weeks of external fixation.

- Limited open reduction is used as follows:
  It is useful in fractures with persistent intraarticular (>2 mm) incongruity despite closed reduction and traction; this often involves the displaced lunate facet.
  Restoration of the articular surface may then be followed by Kirschner wire fixation and a bone graft with external fixation.
- Open reduction and internal fixation are used as follows:
  Primary indication is with articular fragment displacement in fracture patterns not amenable to closed or limited open procedures, especially of the shear variety (frequently dorsal and volar Barton fractures and unstable Smith fractures).
  Some complex articular fractures may also be treated with open reduction and internal fixation with careful preoperative planning.
  Provisional application of an external fixator is often helpful for visualizing and aiding in obtaining a reduction.
  A buttress plate with or without Kirschner wires is used to stabilize the articular fragments.

COMPLICATIONS

Reported complication rates are approximately 30% but vary from series to series.

- Median nerve dysfunction management is controversial, although general agreement is found on the following points:
  A complete median nerve lesion with no improvement after reduction requires surgical exploration.
  A nerve lesion developing postreduction mandates release of the splint and positioning of the wrist in neutral position; if no improvement occurs, exploration and release should be considered.
  An incomplete lesion in a fracture requiring operative intervention is a relative indication for carpal tunnel release.
- Malunion or nonunion typically results from inadequate reduction or immobilization and may require open reduction and internal fixation with bone graft.
- Complications of external fixation include reflex sympathetic dystrophy, pin tract infection, wrist stiffness, fracture through pin sites, and radial sensory neuritis; some of these can be avoided by open pin placement to allow visualization of radial sensory branches and central placement of the pins.
- Posttraumatic osteoarthritis occurs as a consequence of radiocarpal and radioulnar articular injury, thus emphasizing the need for anatomic restoration of the articular surface.
- Digital, wrist, and elbow stiffness may occur, especially with prolonged immobilization in a cast or with external fixation. Aggressive occupational therapy is needed to mobilize the digits and elbow while wrist immobilization is in place, as well as a supervised therapy regimen once immobilization has been discontinued.
- Tendon rupture, most commonly the extensor pollicis longus, may occur as a late complication of distal radius fractures, even in cases of minimally displaced injuries in which degeneration of the tendon due to vascular disruption of the tendon sheath and mechanical impingement upon the callus results in the attrition of tendon integrity.
- Midcarpal instability (i.e., dorsal or volar intercalated segmental instability) may be a result of a radiocarpal ligamentous injury or a dorsal or volar rim distal radius disruption (Barton).

21. WRIST

EPIDEMIOLOGY

Although wrist injuries are fairly common, especially with athletic participation, the true incidence is unknown due to a failure to recognize carpal injuries in the presence of associated more obvious injuries (e.g., metacarpal fractures, forearm fractures, etc.), the variety of health care personnel treating such fractures, and the tendency of such personnel to dismiss such injuries as wrist "sprains."

ANATOMY

- The distal radius has two articular facets separated by a ridge for articulation with the scaphoid and lunate. The sigmoid notch articulates with the distal ulna.
- The distal ulna articulates with the sigmoid notch of the distal radius. The styloid process serves as the attachment for the triangular fibrocartilage complex (TFCC).
- The carpal bones are as follows:
  - Distal row: trapezium, trapezoid, capitate, and hamate, connected to one another and to the base of the metacarpals by strong ligaments, making the distal row relatively immobile.
  - Proximal row: scaphoid (an oblique strut that spans both rows), lunate, triquetrum, and pisiform.
- The joints are the distal radioulnar, radiocarpal, and midcarpal.
- Normal anatomic relationships are as follows:
  - 10-degree volar tilt of distal radius;
  - 20-degree radial inclination;
  - 12 mm from radial styloid to articular surface of the radius;
  - 0-degree capitolunate angle—a straight line drawn down the third metacarpal shaft, capitate, lunate, and shaft of radius when the wrist is in its neutral position;
  - 47-degree scapholunate angle (normal range, 30 to 70 degrees); less than 2 mm scapholunate space.
- Wrist ligaments are as follows:
  - Extrinsic ligaments connect the radius to the carpus and the carpus to the metacarpals.
  - Intrinsic ligaments connect carpal bone to carpal bone (e.g., scapholunate and lunotriquetral ligaments).
  - In general, the dorsal ligaments are weaker than the volar ligaments.
  - Important volar ligaments include the following:
    - Radioscaphocapitate (guides scaphoid kinematics);
    - Radioscapholunate (stabilizes scapholunate articulation);
    - Radiolunate;
    - Radiolunotriquetral (supports proximal row, stabilizes radiolunate and lunotriquetral joints).
  - The Space of Poirier is a ligament-free area in the capitolunate space—an area of potential weakness.
  - TFCC is a major stabilizer of the ulnar carpus and distal radioulnar joint.
    - The TFCC absorbs about 20% of the axial load across the wrist joint.
    - The TFCC consists of several components, including the radiotriquetral ligament (meniscal homologue), articular disk, ulnolunate ligament, and ulnar collateral ligament.
- The vascular supply is as follows:
  - The radial, ulnar, and anterior interosseous arteries combine to form a network of transverse arterial arches both dorsal and volar to the carpus.
  - The blood supply to the scaphoid is derived primarily from the radial artery, both dorsally and volarly. The volar scaphoid branches supply the distal 20% to 30% of the scaphoid, whereas branches entering the dorsal ridge supply the proximal 70% to 80%.
  - The lunate receives blood supply from both its volar and dorsal surfaces in most individuals (80%). About 20% have only a volar blood supply.

- Wrist kinematics are as follows:
  - Due to its complex articulations and ligamentous interconnections, the motion of the wrist's components is complicated.
  - The scaphoid rests on the radioscaphocapitate ligament at its waist. Using the ligament as an axis, it rotates from a volar flexed perpendicular position to a dorsiflexed longitudinal position.
- Pathomechanics are as follows:
  - Classically, the radius, lunate, and capitate have been described as a central "link" that is colinear in the sagittal plane.
  - The scaphoid serves as a connecting strut. Any flexion moment transmitted across the scaphoid is balanced by an extension moment at the triquetrum.
  - When the scaphoid is destabilized by fracture or ligament disruption, the lunate and triquetrum assume a position of excessive dorsiflexion (dorsal intercalated segmental instability) and the scapholunate angle becomes abnormally high (>70 degrees) (Figs. 21.1 and 21.2).
  - When the triquetrum is destabilized (usually by disruption of the lunotriquetral ligament complex), the opposite pattern (volar intercalated segmental instability) is seen as the intercalated lunate segment volarflexes.

MECHANISM OF INJURY

- The most common mechanism of carpal injury is a fall on the outstretched hand, resulting in an axial compressive force with the wrist in hyperextension. The volar ligaments are thus placed under tension with compression and shear forces applied dorsally, especially when the wrist is extended beyond its physiologic limits.
- In addition, ulnar deviation and intercarpal supination result in a predictable pattern of injury, progressing from the radial side of the carpus to the midcarpus and finally to the ulnar carpus.

CLINICAL EVALUATION

- The clinical presentation of individual carpal injuries is variable, but in general, the most consistent sign of carpal injury is well-localized tenderness.

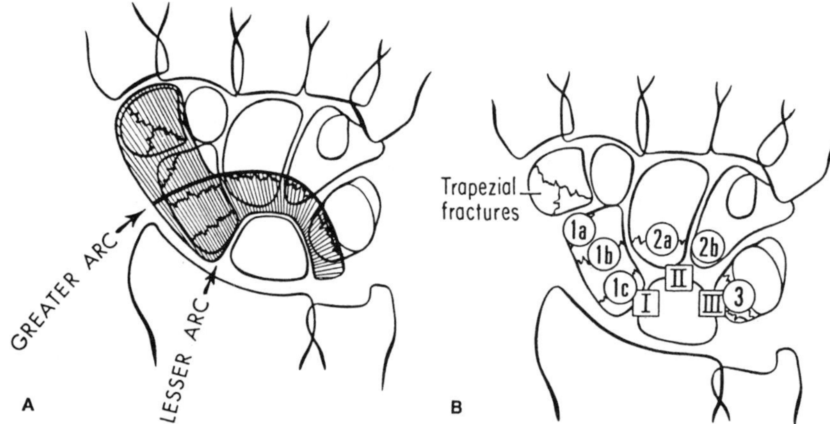

FIG. 21.1. Vulnerable zones of the carpus. **A.** A lesser arc injury follows a curved path through the radial styloid, midcarpal joint, and lunatotriquetral space. A greater arc injury passes through the scaphoid, capitate, and triquetrum. **B.** Lesser and greater arc injuries can be considered as three stages of perilunate fracture or ligament instabilities. (From Johnson RP. The acutely injured wrist and its residuals. *Clin Orthop* 1980;149:33–44, with permission.)

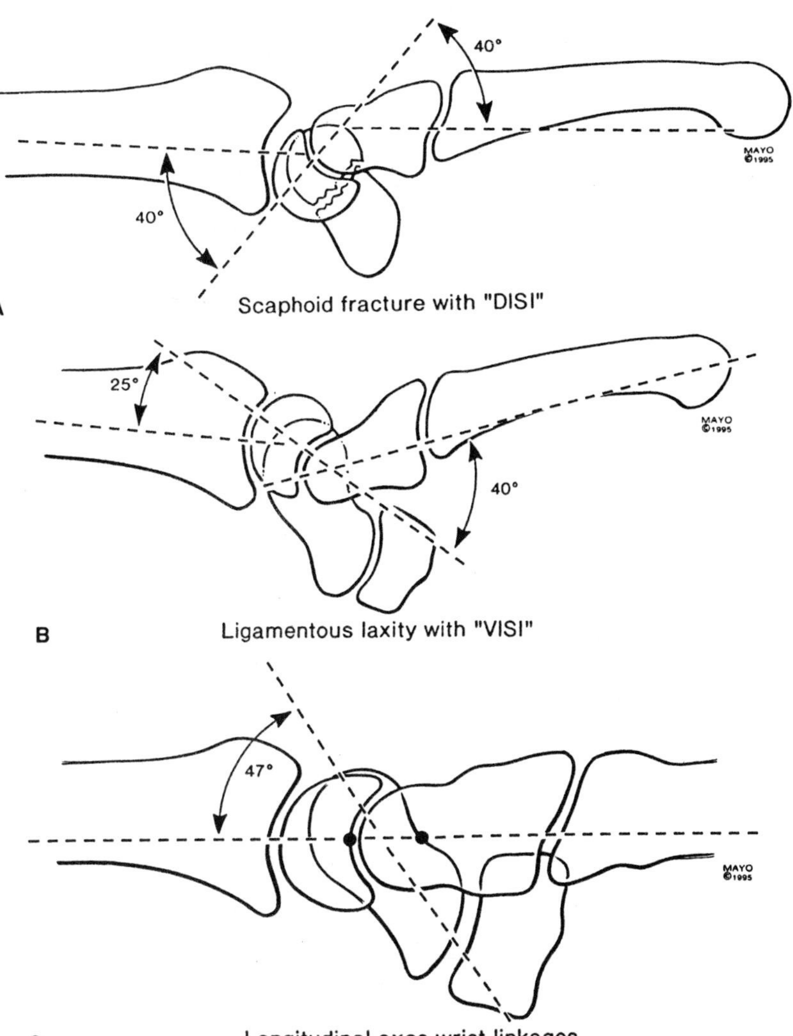

FIG. 21.2. Diagrammatic representation of carpal instability. **A.** Dorsal intercalated segmental instability (DISI) deformity is associated with scapholunate ligament disruption or a displaced scaphoid fracture. **B.** Volar intercalated segmental instability (VISI) deformity is usually associated with disruption of the lunatotriquetral ligament complex. **C.** Normal longitudinal alignment of the carpal bones with the scaphoid axis at a 47-degree angle to the axes of the capitate, lunate, and radius. (From Rockwood CA Jr, Green DP, Bucholz RW, Heckman JD, eds. *Rockwood and Green's fractures in adults,* 4th ed. Vol. 1. Philadelphia: Lippincott-Raven, 1996: 760, with permission.)

- Gross deformity may be present, ranging from displacement of the carpus to prominence of individual carpal bones.
- Provocative tests may reproduce or exacerbate pain, crepitus, or displacement indicative of individual carpal injuries (*see specific carpal injury*).

RADIOGRAPHIC EVALUATION

- Anteroposterior and lateral views of the wrist should be obtained.
- In cases in which specific carpal injuries are suspected, special or stress views should be obtained to evaluate the area of interest (*see specific carpal injury under Specific Fractures below*).

ORTHOPAEDIC TRAUMA ASSOCIATION (OTA) CLASSIFICATION OF CARPAL FRACTURES AND FRACTURE-DISLOCATIONS

Type A: common carpal fracture-dislocation
- A1.1: transscaphoid perilunate dislocation
- A1.2: transscaphoid perilunate dislocation with associated other carpal fractures
- A1.3: perilunate dislocation with associated other carpal fractures except scaphoid

Type B: carpal fractures
- B1: vertical
- B2: oblique
- B3: transverse

Type C: scaphoid fractures, isolated
- C1: avulsions
- C2: horizontal, transverse, oblique
  - C2.1: distal third
  - C2.2: middle third
  - C2.3: proximal third
- C3: vertical/multifragmentary

SPECIFIC FRACTURES

Scaphoid (Fig. 21.3)

- The scaphoid is the most commonly fractured carpal bone.
- Anatomically, the scaphoid is divided into proximal and distal poles, a tubercle, and the waist. Eighty percent of the scaphoid is covered with articular cartilage.
- Ligamentous attachments to the scaphoid include the radioscaphocapitate ligament, which variably attaches to the ulnar aspect of the scaphoid waist, and the dorsal intercarpal ligament, which provides the primary vascular supply to the scaphoid.
- The major vascular supply is derived from scaphoid branches of the radial artery entering the dorsal ridge and supplying 70% to 80% of the scaphoid, including the proximal pole. The remaining distal aspect is supplied through branches entering the tubercle. Thus, fractures at the scaphoid waist or proximal third depend on fracture union for revascularization (Gelberman).
- The most common mechanism is a fall on the outstretched hand that imposes a force of dorsiflexion, ulnar deviation, and intercarpal supination.
- Patients present with wrist pain and swelling, with tenderness to deep palpation overlying the scaphoid and in the anatomic snuffbox. Provocative tests include the following:

  Scaphoid lift test: reproduction of pain with dorsal-volar shifting of the scaphoid.

  Watson test: painful dorsal scaphoid displacement as the wrist is moved from ulnar to radial deviation with compression of the tuberosity.
- The diagnosis can usually be made on the basis of anteroposterior and lateral views of the wrist. Oblique views and "scaphoid views," of the scaphoid in radial and ulnar deviation of the wrist, may aid in the diagnosis or may assist in further fracture definition. If the clinical examination suggests fracture but the radiographs are not diagnostic, a trial of immobilization with follow-up radiographs 1 to 2 weeks after

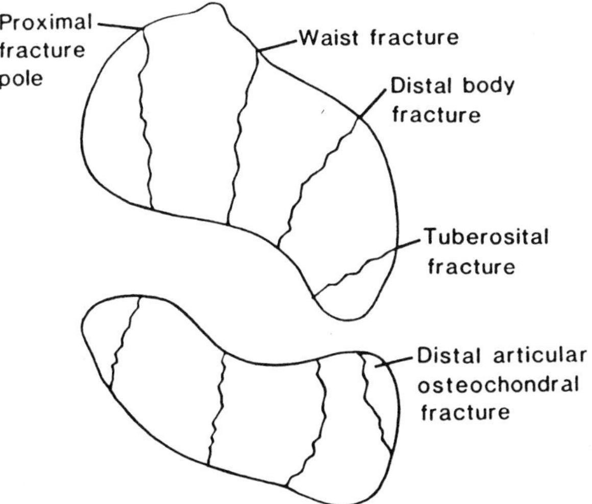

FIG. 21.3. Types of scaphoid fractures. The scaphoid is susceptible to fractures at any level. Approximately 65% occur at the waist, 15% through the proximal pole, 10% through the distal body, 8% through the tuberosity, and 2% in the distal articular surface. (From Rockwood CA Jr, Green DP, Bucholz RW, Heckman JD, eds. *Rockwood and Green's fractures in adults,* 4th ed. Vol. 1. Philadelphia: Lippincott-Raven, 1996:826, with permission.)

the fracture may demonstrate the fracture. Technetium bone scan, magnetic resonance imaging, computed tomography, and ultrasound evaluation may be used to diagnose occult scaphoid fractures.

CLASSIFICATION

- Fracture pattern (Russe)
  - Horizontal oblique
  - Transverse
  - Vertical oblique
- Stability
  - Stable: nondisplaced fractures with no step-off in any plane
  - Unstable: displacement with 1 mm or more step-off with scapholunate angulation >60 degrees or lunatocapitate angulation >15 degrees.
- Location
  - Distal one-third
  - Middle one-third (waist): most common
  - Proximal one-third

Treatment

- Initial treatment in the emergency setting should consist of a thumb spica splint or cast immobilization if swelling is not pronounced. Whether a long-arm cast is necessary remains controversial, although studies demonstrate decreased time to union and lower incidences of nonunion and delayed union with the use of a long arm cast.
- For stable nondisplaced fractures, a long-arm thumb spica cast should be placed with the wrist in neutral deviation and flexion/extension and should be maintained for 6 to 8 weeks. The patient may then be changed to a short-arm thumb spica cast for up to an additional 6 weeks or until radiographic evidence of healing is found.

- Healing rates with nonoperative treatment depend on fracture location as follows:
  - Tuberosity and distal third, 100%;
  - Waist, 80% to 90%;
  - Proximal pole, 60% to 70%.
- Displaced fractures generally require open reduction and internal fixation.
  - The volar approach between the flexor carpi radialis and the radial artery provides good exposure for open reduction and internal fixation and for repair of the radioscapholunate ligament. The volar approach is the least damaging to the vascular supply of the vulnerable proximal pole.
  - Operative fixation may be achieved via the use of Kirschner wires or Herbert compression screws (preferred) with or without the use of a bone graft.
  - Postoperative immobilization consists of a long-arm thumb spica cast for 6 weeks.

Complications

- Delayed union, nonunion, and malunion: reported to occur with greater frequency when a short-arm cast is used as compared with long-arm cast immobilization, as well as with proximal scaphoid fractures. May necessitate operative fixation with bone grafting to achieve union.
- Osteonecrosis: occurs especially with fractures of the proximal pole, due to the tenuous vascular supply. Incidence may be minimized by immobilization in a long-arm thumb spica cast or through early treatment of displaced fractures with open reduction and internal fixation.

Lunate

- Fractures of the lunate are often unrecognized until they progress to osteonecrosis, at which time they are diagnosed as Kienböck disease.
- Lunate fractures are among the most commonly fractured carpal bones, second only to the scaphoid.
- The lunate has been referred to as the "carpal keystone," because it rests in the well-protected concavity of the lunate fossa of the distal radius, anchored by interosseous ligaments to the scaphoid and triquetrum and distally congruent with the convex head of the capitate.
- The vascular supply is derived from the proximal carpal arcade dorsally and volarly with three variable intralunate anastomoses.
- Mechanism of injury is typically a fall onto an outstretched hand with the wrist in hyperextension or a strenuous push with the wrist in extension.
- Clinical evaluation reveals tenderness to palpation on the volar wrist overlying the distal radius and lunate with painful range of motion.

Radiographic Evaluation

- Using anteroposterior and lateral views of the wrist is often inadequate for establishing the diagnosis of lunate fracture because osseous details are frequently obscured by overlapping densities.
- Oblique views may be helpful, but computed tomography, polytomography, or technetium bone scanning best demonstrate a fracture.
- Magnetic resonance imaging has been used with increasing frequency to appreciate the vascular changes associated with injury and healing and is the imaging test of choice for evaluation of Kienböck disease.

STAHL AND LICHTMAN CLASSIFICATION (FIG. 21.4)

Stage I: normal appearance or linear or compression fracture on tomogram
Stage II: sclerosis, slight collapse of radial border
Stage III: fragmentation, collapse, and cystic degeneration; loss of carpal height; proximal migration of capitate; scaphoid rotation (scapholunate dissociation)
Stage IV: advanced collapse; scaphoid rotation; sclerosis; radiocarpal osteophytes

Treatment

- Nondisplaced fractures should be treated in a short-arm cast or splint with follow-up at close intervals to evaluate progression of healing.

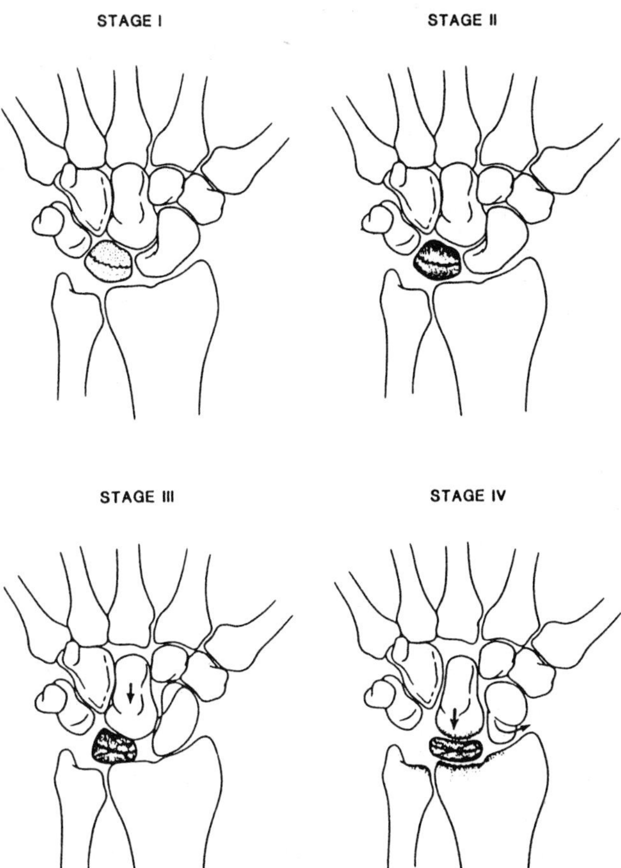

FIG. 21.4. Staging of Kienböck disease (after Lichtman). *Stage I:* Routine x-rays (posteroanterior [PA], lateral) are normal, but tomography may show a linear fracture; usually transverse through the body of the lunate. Magnetic resonance imaging will confirm avascular changes. *Stage II:* Bone density increase (sclerosis) and a fracture line are usually evident on the PA x-ray. PA and lateral tomograms demonstrate sclerosis, cystic changes, and often a clear fracture. No collapse deformity is seen. *Stage III:* Advanced bone density changes are present with fragmentation, cystic resorption, and collapse. The diagnosis is evident from the PA x-ray. Tomograms (PA, lateral) demonstrate the degree of lunate infraction and amount of fracture displacement. Proximal migration of the capitate is present, and mild to moderate rotary alignment of the scaphoid is found. *Stage IV:* Perilunate arthritic changes are present with complete collapse and fragmentation of the lunate. Carpal instability is evident with scaphoid malalignment and capitate displacement into the lunate space. (From Heckman JD, Bucholz RW, eds. *Rockwood, Green, and Wilkins' fractures in adults,* 5th ed. Vol. 1. Philadelphia: Lippincott Williams & Wilkins, 2001:843, with permission.)

- Displaced or angulated fractures must be treated surgically to allow adequate apposition for formation of vascular anastomoses. This may be achieved with open reduction and internal fixation or with distraction with external fixation to allow the fragments to coapt.

Complications

Osteonecrosis. Established Kienböck disease represents the most devastating complication of lunate fractures, with advanced collapse and radiocarpal degeneration. This may require further operative intervention for relief, including radial shortening, radial wedge osteotomy, ulnar lengthening, or salvage procedures, such as proximal row carpectomy, wrist denervation, or arthrodesis.

Triquetrum

- The mechanism of fracture is typically direct trauma to the ulnar wrist or avulsion with associated ligamentous damage.
- Most commonly, the injury occurs with the wrist in extension and ulnar deviation, resulting in an impingement-shear fracture by the ulnar styloid against the dorsal triquetrum.
- Clinical evaluation reveals tenderness to palpation on the dorsoulnar aspect of the wrist and painful range of wrist motion.
- Transverse fractures of the body can generally be identified on anteroposterior views.
- Dorsal triquetral fractures are not easily appreciated on anteroposterior and lateral views of the wrist due to superimposition of the lunate. An oblique pronated lateral view may help to visualize the dorsal triquetrum.

Treatment

- Nondisplaced fractures of the body or dorsal chip fractures may be treated in a short-arm cast or ulnar gutter splint for 6 weeks.
- Displaced fractures may be amenable to open reduction and internal fixation.

Pisiform

- The mechanism of injury is either a direct blow to the volar wrist or a fall onto an outstretched dorsiflexed hand.
- Clinical evaluation demonstrates tenderness on the volar aspect of the ulnar wrist with painful passive extension of the wrist as the flexor carpi ulnaris is placed under tension.
- In the radiographic evaluation, pisiform fractures are not well visualized on standard views of the wrist; special views including a lateral view of the wrist with forearm supination of 20 to 45 degrees or a carpal tunnel view (20-degree supination oblique view demonstrating an oblique projection of the wrist in radial deviation and semisupination) are often necessary.
- Treatment of nondisplaced or minimally displaced fractures consists of an ulnar gutter splint or short-arm cast for 6 weeks. Displaced fractures may require excision, either early, in the case of a severely displaced fragment, or late, in the case of a pisiform fracture that has resulted in painful nonunion.

Trapezium

- The mechanism of injury is axial loading of the adducted thumb, driving the base of the first metacarpal onto the articular surface of the trapezium.
- Avulsion fractures may occur with forceful deviation, traction, or rotation of the thumb.
- Direct trauma to the palmar arch may result in avulsion of the trapezial ridge by the transverse carpal ligament.
- Clinical evaluation reveals tenderness to palpation in the radial wrist, accompanied by painful range of motion at the first carpometacarpal joint.

Radiographic Evaluation

- Fractures are usually identifiable on standard anteroposterior and lateral views.

- Superimposition of the first metacarpal base may be eliminated by obtaining a Robert view or a true anteroposterior view of the first carpometacarpal joint and trapezium, taken with the hand in maximum pronation.
- A carpal tunnel view (see above) may be necessary for adequate visualization of dorsal ridge fractures.

Treatment
- Nondisplaced fractures are generally amenable to thumb-spica splinting or casting to immobilize the first carpometacarpal joint for 6 weeks.
- Indications for open reduction and internal fixation include articular involvement of the carpometacarpal articulation, comminuted fractures, and displaced fractures. These require open reduction and internal fixation to restore articular congruity and to maintain carpometacarpal joint integrity.
- Comminuted fractures may require supplemental bone grafting.

Complications
Posttraumatic osteoarthritis may result in decreased or painful range of motion at the first carpometacarpal joint. Irreparable joint damage may necessitate fusion or excisional arthroplasty.

Trapezoid
- Because of the shape and position of the trapezoid, fractures are rare; axial load transmitted through the second metacarpal may lead to dislocation, more often dorsal, with associated capsular ligament disruption.
- Direct trauma from blast or crush injuries may cause trapezoid fracture, although this often occurs in conjunction with other injuries.
- Clinical evaluation demonstrates tenderness proximal to the base of the second metacarpal; a variable dorsal prominence represents the dislocated trapezoid. Range of motion of the second carpometacarpal joint is painful and limited.

Radiographic Evaluation
- Fractures can be identified on the anteroposterior radiograph based on a loss of the normal relationship between the second metacarpal base and the trapezoid. Comparison with the contralateral uninjured wrist may aid in the diagnosis. The trapezoid or fracture fragments may be superimposed over the trapezium or capitate, and the second metacarpal may be proximally displaced.
- Oblique views, polytomography, or computed tomography may aid in the diagnosis if osseous details are obscured by overlap.

Treatment
- Nondisplaced fractures may be treated with a splint or short-arm cast for 6 weeks.
- Displaced fractures, especially those involving the carpometacarpal articulation, indicate the need for open reduction and internal fixation. These may be addressed with open reduction and internal fixation with Kirschner wires with attention to restoration of articular congruity.

Complications
Posttraumatic osteoarthritis may result at the second carpometacarpal articulation if joint congruity is not restored.

Capitate
- Fracture is uncommon as an isolated injury due to its relatively protected position.
- A fracture of the capitate is more commonly associated with a greater arc injury pattern (transscaphoid, transcapitate perilunate fracture-dislocation). A variation of this is the "naviculocapitate syndrome," in which the capitate and scaphoid are fractured without associated dislocation.
- The mechanism of injury is typically direct trauma or a crushing force that results in associated carpal or metacarpal fractures.

- Clinical evaluation reveals point tenderness and variable painful dorsiflexion of the wrist as the capitate impinges on the dorsal rim of the radius.
- In the radiographic evaluation, the fracture can usually be identified on the anteroposterior radiograph, with evaluation of the head of the capitate on lateral views to determine rotation or displacement.

Treatment

Capitate fractures require reduction to diminish the risk of osteonecrosis. If closed reduction is unattainable, open reduction and internal fixation is indicated, usually with Kirschner wires or compression screws, to restore normal anatomy.

Complications

- Midcarpal arthritis: due to capitate collapse as a result of displacement of the proximal pole.
- Osteonecrosis: rare, but results in functional impairment; emphasizes the need for accurate diagnosis and stable reduction.

Hamate

- The hamate may be fractured through its distal articular surface, through other articular surfaces, or through its hamulus, or hook.
- A distal articular fracture accompanied by fifth metacarpal subluxation may occur when axial force is transmitted down the shaft of the metacarpal, such as with a fist-strike or a fall.
- Fractures of the body of the hamate generally occur with direct trauma or crush injuries to the hand.
- Fractures of the hook of the hamate are a frequent athletic injury sustained when the palm of the hand is struck by an object (e.g., baseball bat, golf club, hockey stick); they generally occur at the base, although avulsion fractures of the tip may occur.
- Patients typically present with pain and tenderness over the hamate. Ulnar and median neuropathy can also be seen, as can rare injuries to the ulnar artery.
- The diagnosis of hamate fracture can usually be made on the basis of the anteroposterior view of the wrist. Fracture of the hamulus is best visualized on the carpal tunnel or 20-degree supination oblique view (oblique projection of the wrist in radial deviation and semisupination). Computed tomography, tomogram, and bone scan are sometimes necessary to visualize the fracture. A hamulus fracture should not be confused with an os hamulus proprium, which represents an ossification center that has failed to fuse.
- Classification of hamate fractures is descriptive.

Treatment

- Nondisplaced hamate fractures may be treated with immobilization in a short-arm splint or a cast for 6 weeks.
- Displaced fractures of the body may be amenable to Kirschner wire or screw fixation. Fractures of the hook of the hamate may be treated with excision of the fragment for displaced fragments or in cases of symptomatic nonunion.

Complications

- Symptomatic nonunion: may be treated with excision of the nonunited fragment.
- Ulnar or median neuropathy: related to the proximity of the hamate to these nerves. May require surgical exploration and release.
- Ruptures of the flexor tendons to the small finger: due to attritional wear at the fracture site.

Perilunate Dislocations and Fracture-Dislocations

- The lunate, which is normally securely attached to the distal radius by ligamentous attachments, is commonly referred to as the carpal keystone, because perilunate and lunate dislocations involve the greatest expenditure of force during wrist injuries.

- A greater arc injury passes through the scaphoid, capitate, and triquetrum and often results in transscaphoid or transscaphoid transcapitate perilunate fracture-dislocations.
- A lesser arc injury follows a curved path through the radial styloid, midcarpal joint, and lunatotriquetral space and results in perilunate and lunate dislocations.
- The most common injury is transscaphoid perilunate dislocation (de Quervain injury).
- Clinical evaluation reveals that scapholunate or perilunate injuries typically cause tenderness just distal to the Lister tubercle. Swelling is generalized about the wrist with variable dorsal prominence of the entire carpus in cases of frank perilunate dislocation.

Radiographic Evaluation

Diagnosis can be made without accompanying radiographs, but anteroposterior and lateral views should be obtained to confirm the diagnosis and rule out associated injuries. Finger-trap traction with 5 to 10 pounds aids in the diagnosis; computed tomography, magnetic resonance imaging, and arthrography are generally unnecessary but may be useful in further defining the injury pattern.

- Anteroposterior view: dislocated lunate appears to be wedge shaped, with an elongated volar lip.
- Lateral view: "spilled teacup sign" with volar tilt of the lunate.
- Clenched-fist anteroposterior view: obtained after closed reduction of the midcarpal joint is useful for checking residual scapholunate or lunotriquetral dissociation and for fractures.

CLASSIFICATION

A sequence of progressive perilunate instability is seen as the injury spreads from the scapholunate joint (radioscapholunate ligament [RSLL]) → midcarpal joint (radioscaphocapitate ligament [RSCL]) → lunotriquetral joint (distal limb of radiolunotriquetral ligament [RLTL]) → dorsal radiolunotriquetral ligament → volar dislocation of the lunate.

Stage I: Disruption of the scapholunate joint—the radioscapholunate and interosseous scapholunate ligaments are disrupted.

Stage II: Disruption of the midcarpal (capitolunate) joint—the radioscaphocapitate ligament is disrupted.

Stage III: Disruption of the lunotriquetral joint—the distal limb of the radiolunotriquetral ligament is disrupted.

Stage IV: Disruption of the radiolunate joint—the dorsal radiolunotriquetral ligament is disrupted, ultimately causing volar dislocation of the lunate.

Treatment

- Closed reduction and casting may be attempted initially for acute injuries, although many authors have noted when performing open reduction for failed closed treatment that the injury was often much greater than was initially appreciated.
- Irreducible or unstable injuries require open reduction, repair, and internal fixation using Kirschner wire fixation, followed by postoperative casting for 3 to 4 weeks.

Complications

- Median neuropathy: may result from carpal tunnel compression, necessitating surgical release.
- Posttraumatic osteoarthritis: may occur as a result of the initial injury or secondary to small retained osseous fragments.
- Chronic perilunate injury: may result from untreated or inadequately treated dislocation or fracture-dislocation and may cause chronic pain, instability, and wrist deformity, often associated with tendon rupture or increasing nerve symptoms. Repair may be possible, but a salvage procedure, such as proximal row carpectomy or radiocarpal fusion, may be necessary.

Carpal Dislocations

- Carpal dislocations represent a continuum of perilunate dislocations, with frank lunate dislocation representing the final stage. All such injuries reflect significant ligamentous injury.
- Associated fractures are common and may represent avulsion injuries (e.g., volar or dorsal intercalated segmental instability with associated radial rim fracture).
- The mechanism of injury is a fall onto an outstretched hand (most common cause), although direct force can cause traumatic carpal dislocations as well.
- Clinical evaluation reveals a patient with painful limited wrist range of motion. Median neuropathy may be present. Specific tests for carpal instability include the following:
  - Midcarpal stress test: dorsal-palmar stressing of the midcarpal joint results in a pathologic clunk representing subluxation of the lunate.
  - Dynamic test for midcarpal instability: wrist extension with radioulnar deviation produces a "catch-up" clunk as the proximal row snaps from flexion to extension.

Radiographic Evaluation

- Most dislocations may be diagnosed on anteroposterior and lateral views of the wrist. Finger-trap traction of 5 to 10 pounds may aid in the diagnosis.
- Polytomography, computed tomography, and magnetic resonance imaging may aid in further injury definition.

Treatment

- Correction of carpal dislocations consists of closed reduction of the midcarpal joint, which is often accomplished with traction combined with direct manual pressure over the capitate and lunate.
- Irreducible dislocations or unstable injuries should be addressed with open reduction and internal fixation using a combined dorsal and volar approach. Dorsally, the osseous anatomy is restored with Kirschner wire fixation. Volarly, the soft tissues are repaired.

Complications

- Posttraumatic osteoarthritis: a consequence of unrecognized associated fractures or malreduction, resulting in functional limitation and pain.
- Recurrent instability: may result from inadequate repair of ligamentous structures on the volar aspect or from insufficient fixation dorsally.

Scapholunate Dissociation

- This injury is a ligamentous analogue of a scaphoid fracture; it represents the most common and most significant ligamentous disruption of the wrist.
- The underlying pathology is a disruption of the radioscapholunate and the interosseous scapholunate ligaments.
- The mechanism of injury is stress loading of the extended carpus in ulnar deviation.
- Clinical findings include ecchymosis and tenderness on the volar wrist. The proximal pole of the scaphoid is prominent dorsally. Signs of scapholunate dissociation include pain induced by a vigorous grasp, decreasing repetitive grip strength, a positive Watson test (*see "Scaphoid Fractures" above*), and painful flexion-extension or ulnar-radial deviation of the wrist.

Radiographic Evaluation

Views should include the tangential posteroanterior, clenched fist anteroposterior, and radial and ulnar deviation. Classic signs of scapholunate dissociation on the anteroposterior view include the following:

- "Terry Thomas sign": widening of the scapholunate space.
- "Cortical ring sign": caused by the abnormally rotated scaphoid overlapping the trapezoid.
- Scapholunate angle >70 degrees visualized on lateral views.

Treatment

- The scaphoid can often be reduced with an audible and palpable click, which is followed by immobilization for 8 weeks. Good results are seen with anatomic reduction.
- Arthroscopically assisted reduction with percutaneous pin fixation has been described with good results.
- An inability to obtain or maintain reduction is an indication for open reduction and internal fixation. This may be accomplished by a combined dorsal and volar approach with reduction and fixation of the scapholunate joint dorsally and repair of the ligaments volarly with a combination of Kirschner wire and suture fixation.

Complications

Recurrent instability: failed closed or open reduction and internal fixation with ligament repair may necessitate ligament augmentation, intercarpal fusion, proximal row carpectomy, or wrist fusion.

Lunotriquetral Dissociation

- These injuries involve disruption of the distal limb of the volar radiolunotriquetral ligament either as a stage III lesser arc injury of perilunate instability or as a result of a force causing excessive radial deviation and intercarpal pronation. The lunotriquetral interosseous and dorsal radiolunotriquetral ligaments are also injured.
- Clinical findings include swelling over the peritriquetral area and tenderness dorsally, typically one finger breadth distal to the ulnar head.
  - Ballottement test (shear or shuck test): dorsal-volar displacement of the triquetrum on the lunate results in increased excursion when compared with the normal contralateral side, as well as painful crepitus.

Radiographic Evaluation

Posteroanterior radiographs of the hand rarely reveal frank gapping of the lunotriquetral space, but a break in the normal smooth contour of the proximal carpal row can be appreciated.

- Radial deviation view: may demonstrate the triquetrum to be dorsiflexed with the intact scapholunate complex palmar-flexed.
- A lateral projection may reveal a volar intercalated segmental instability pattern.

Treatment

- Acute lunotriquetral dissociation with minimal deformity may be treated with a short-arm cast or custom splinting for 6 to 8 weeks.
- Closed reduction with pinning of the lunate to the triquetrum may be necessary to maintain fixation.
- Angular deformity or unacceptable reduction from nonoperative treatment may necessitate open reduction and internal fixation using a combined dorsal and volar approach with pinning of the triquetrum to the lunate and ligamentous repair.

Complications

Recurrent instability: may necessitate ligament reconstruction with capsular augmentation. If recurrent instability persists, lunotriquetral fusion may be necessary, with possible concomitant ulnar shortening to increase the tension of the volar ulnocarpal ligaments.

Ulnocarpal Dissociation

- Avulsion or rupture of the TFCC from the ulnar styloid results in a loss of "sling" support for the ulnar wrist.
- The lunate and triquetrum "fall away" relative to the distal ulna and assume a semisupinated and palmar-flexed attitude with the distal ulna subluxed dorsally.
- Clinical evaluation reveals dorsal prominence of the distal ulna and volar displacement of the ulnar carpus.

Radiographic Evaluation

- Posteroanterior views may reveal avulsion of the ulnar styloid. Dorsal displacement of the distal ulna on true lateral views suggests disruption of the TFCC in the absence of an ulnar styloid avulsion fracture.
- Magnetic resonance imaging may demonstrate a tear of the TFCC and may additionally provide evidence of chondral lesions and effusion.

Treatment

- Operative repair of the TFCC may be achieved via a dorsal approach between the fifth and sixth extensor compartments.
- Open reduction and internal fixation of large displaced ulnar styloid fragments are necessary.

Complications

- Recurrent instability: may occur with or without previous operative intervention and may result in pain and functional debilitation that may be progressive.
- Ulnar neuropathy: transient sensory symptoms may result from irritation of the ulnar nerve in the Guyon canal or at its dorsal sensory branch. Permanent damage is rare, but persistence of symptoms beyond 12 weeks may necessitate exploration.

22. HAND

- Treatment goals for the hand include maintenance of joint motion and function with protection of underlying structures.
- Factors to be considered in appropriate treatment include patient age, hand dominance, occupation, associated soft-tissue injury, patient motivation and reliability, and comorbid conditions.
- Principles of treatment include fracture reduction, elevation of the entire extremity to limit edema, immobilization in the intrinsic positive or safe position, and early mobilization of the injured finger.
- The proximal interphalangeal joint has been referred to as the most important and unforgiving joint in the hand.

EPIDEMIOLOGY

- Metacarpal and phalangeal fractures are common, comprising 10% of all fractures; more than 50% of these are work-related.
- Border digits are most commonly involved, with approximate incidence as follows:
  - Distal phalanx, 45%;
  - Metacarpal, 30%;
  - Proximal phalanx, 15%;
  - Middle phalanx, 10%.
- Twenty-seven percent of finger fractures are treated inappropriately in the emergency department; inaccurate reduction and unsatisfactory splinting are the most common errors (Davis and Stothard).

MECHANISM OF INJURY

The mechanism of hand injuries varies considerably; in general, fracture patterns emerge based on the nature of the traumatic force, as follows:

- Nonepiphyseal: torque, angular force, compressive load, and direct trauma.
- Epiphyseal: avulsion, shear, splitting.

CLINICAL EVALUATION

- A careful history is essential because it may influence treatment. This should include the following:
  - Patient's age;
  - Dominant versus nondominant hand;
  - Patient's occupation;
  - Systemic illnesses;
  - Exact nature of the injury: crush, direct trauma, twist, tear, laceration, etc.;
  - Exact time of injury (for open fractures);
  - Exposure to contamination: barnyard, brackish water, animal/human bite, etc.;
  - Treatment provided: cleansing, antiseptic, bandage, or tourniquet;
  - Financial issues: worker's compensation.
- Physical examination should include the following:
  - Digital viability (capillary refill <2 seconds);
  - Neurologic status (documented by two-point discrimination and individual muscle testing);
  - Rotational and angulatory deformity;
  - Range of motion (documented by goniometer).

RADIOGRAPHIC EVALUATION

- Anteroposterior, lateral, and oblique radiographs of the affected digit or hand should be obtained. Injured digits should be viewed individually, where possible, to minimize overlap of other digits over the area of interest.
- Tomograms may be useful for the evaluation of intraarticular fractures.

DESCRIPTIVE CLASSIFICATION

- Open versus closed injury (see below)
- Bone involved
- Location within bone
- Fracture pattern: comminuted, transverse, spiral, or vertical split
- Presence or absence of displacement
- Presence or absence of deformity (rotation and/or angulation)
- Extra- versus intraarticular fracture
- Stable versus unstable

SWANSON, SZABO, AND ANDERSON CLASSIFICATION OF OPEN HAND FRACTURES

Type I: Clean wound without significant contamination or delay in treatment and no systemic illness.

Type II: One or more of the following is present:

- Contamination with gross dirt/debris, human or animal bite, warm lake/river injury, barnyard injury;
- Delay in treatment >24 hours;
- Significant systemic illness (e.g., diabetes, hypertension, rheumatoid arthritis, hepatitis, asthma).

Rate of infection:

- Type I injuries, 1.4%
- Type II injuries, 14%

Neither primary internal fixation nor immediate wound closure was associated with increased risk of infection in type I injuries. Primary internal fixation was not associated with increased risk of infection in type II injuries.

Primary wound closure is appropriate for type I injuries, with delayed closure appropriate for type II injuries.

ORTHOPAEDIC TRAUMA ASSOCIATION (OTA) CLASSIFICATION OF METACARPAL FRACTURES

Type A: extraarticular
- A1: metacarpal head
  - A1.1: simple
  - A1.2: metaphyseal wedge
  - A1.3: metaphyseal complex
- A2: no classification
- A3: metacarpal base
  - A3.1: simple
  - A3.2: metaphyseal multifragmentary

Type B: articular
- B1: metacarpal head
  - B1.1: oblique/spiral
  - B1.2: sagittal
  - B1.3: coronal
- B2: metacarpal diaphyseal
  - B2.1: spiral/oblique
  - B2.2: transverse
  - B2.3: simple wedge
- B3: metacarpal base
  - B3.1: avulsion
  - B3.2: depression
  - B3.3: split/depression

Type C: articular/extraarticular
- C1: metacarpal head
  - C1.1: articular simple/metaphyseal simple
  - C1.2: articular simple/metaphyseal multifragmentary
  - C1.3: multifragmentary articular and metaphyseal

C2: no classification
C3: metacarpal base
C3.1: articular simple/metaphyseal simple
C3.2: articular simple/metaphyseal multifragmentary
C3.3: articular multifragmentary/metaphyseal simple
C3.4: multifragmentary articular and metaphyseal

OTA CLASSIFICATION OF PHALANGEAL FRACTURES

Type A: extraarticular
A1: proximal aspect
A1.1: simple
A1.2: multifragmentary
A2: diaphyseal
A2.1: spiral/oblique
A2.2: transverse
A2.3: simple wedge
A2.4: multifragmentary
A3: distal aspect
A3.1: spiral
A3.2: multifragmentary
Type B: articular and diaphyseal
B1: proximal partial articular
B1.1: unicondylar
B1.2: bicondylar
B2: no classification
B3: distal partial articular
B3.1: unicondylar
B3.2: bicondylar
Type C: complete articular
C1: proximal complete articular
C1.1: articular simple/metaphyseal simple
C1.2: articular simple/metaphyseal multifragmentary
C1.3: multifragmentary articular and metaphyseal
C2: no classification
C3: distal complete articular
C3.1: simple
C3.2: complex

TREATMENT

General Principles

- *"Fight-bite" injuries.* Any short curved laceration overlying a joint in the hand, particularly the metacarpal-phalangeal joint, must be suspected of having been caused by a tooth. These injuries must be assumed to be contaminated with oral flora and should be addressed with broad-spectrum antibiotics.
- *Stable fractures.* These should be treated as follows:
  - Buddy taping or splinting with repeat radiographs in 1 week.
  - Initially unstable fractures that are reduced and then converted to a stable position should be treated by external immobilization (cast, cast with outrigger splint, gutter splint, or anterior-posterior splints) or percutaneous pinning to prevent displacement and to permit earlier mobilization.
- *Unstable fractures.* Unstable fractures that are irreducible or that exhibit continued instability despite closed treatment or percutaneous pinning should be treated by open reduction and internal fixation, including Kirschner wire fixation, interosseous wiring, tension band technique, interfragmentary screws alone, or plates and screws.

- *Fractures with segmental bone loss.* These continue to be problematic. The primary treatment should be directed to the soft tissues, maintaining length with Kirschner wires or external fixation.

Management of Specific Fracture Patterns

Metacarpal Head

- These fractures include the following:
  - Epiphyseal fractures;
  - Collateral ligament avulsion fractures;
  - Oblique, vertical, and horizontal head fractures;
  - Comminuted fractures;
  - Boxer fractures with joint extension;
  - Fractures associated with bone loss.
- Most fractures require anatomic reduction (if possible) to reestablish joint congruity and thus to minimize posttraumatic arthrosis.
  - Stable reductions of fractures may be splinted in the "protected position," consisting of metacarpal-phalangeal flexion >70 degrees to minimize joint stiffness.
  - Percutaneous pinning may be necessary to obtain stable reduction; severe comminution may necessitate the use of minicondylar plate fixation or external fixation with distraction.
- Early range of motion is essential (Fig. 22.1).

Metacarpal Neck

- Fractures result from direct trauma with volar comminution and dorsal angulation. Most of these fractures can often be reduced closed, but maintenance of reduction may be difficult.
- The degree of acceptable deformity varies according to which metacarpal is injured:
  - Greater than 15-degree angulation for the second and third metacarpals is unacceptable.
  - Greater than 40- to 45-degrees angulation for the fourth and fifth metacarpals is unacceptable.

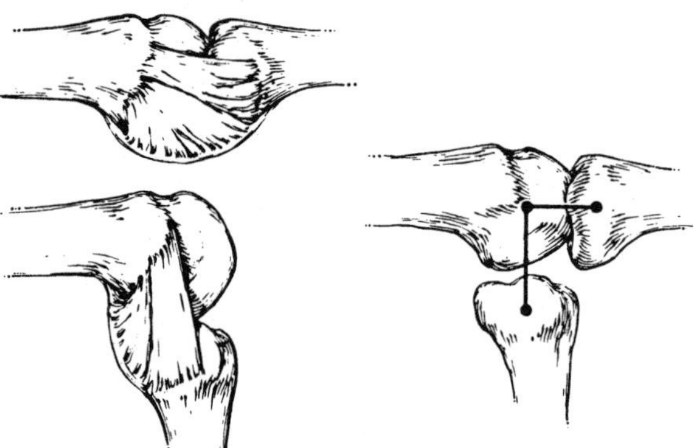

FIG. 22.1. Left: The collateral ligaments of the metacarpophalangeal joints are relaxed in extension, permitting lateral motion, but become taut when the joint is fully flexed. This occurs because of the unique shape of the metacarpal head, which acts as a cam. **Right:** The distance from the pivot point of the metacarpal to the phalanx in extension is less than the distance in flexion, so that the collateral ligament is tight when the joint is flexed. (From Rockwood CA Jr, Green DP, Bucholz RW, Heckman JD, eds. *Rockwood and Green's fractures in adults,* 4th ed. Vol. 1. Philadelphia: Lippincott-Raven, 1996:659, with permission.)

- Unstable fractures require operative intervention with either percutaneous pins (may be intramedullary or transverse into the adjacent metacarpal) or plate fixation.

Metacarpal Shaft

- Nondisplaced or minimally displaced fractures may be reduced and splinted in the protected position.
- Operative indications include rotational deformity and dorsal angulation >10 degrees for the second and third metacarpals or >20 degrees for the fourth and fifth metacarpals.
- Operative fixation may be achieved with either closed reduction and percutaneous pinning (intramedullary or transverse into the adjacent metacarpal) or open reduction and plate fixation.

Metacarpal Base

Fingers are treated as follows:

- Fractures of the base of the second, third, and fourth fingers are generally minimally displaced and are associated with ligament avulsion. Treatment is by splinting and early motion in the majority of cases.
- The reverse Bennett fracture is a fracture-dislocation of the base of the fifth metacarpal/hamate.
  - The metacarpal is displaced proximally by the pull of the extensor carpi ulnaris. The degree of displacement is best ascertained via radiograph with the hand pronated 30 degrees from a fully supinated (anteroposterior) position.
  - This fracture often requires surgical intervention with open reduction and internal fixation.

The thumb is treated as follows:

- *Extraarticular fractures* (Fig. 22.2). These are usually transverse or oblique. Most can be held by closed reduction and casting, but some unstable fractures require closed reduction and percutaneous pinning. The basal joint of the thumb is quite forgiving, and an anatomic reduction of an angulated shaft fracture is not essential.
- *Intraarticular fractures* (Fig. 22.3). Treatment for these fractures differs according to type as follows:
  - Type I: Bennett fracture—fracture line separates major part of metacarpal from volar lip fragment, producing a disruption of the first carpometacarpal joint; first metacarpal is pulled proximally by the abductor pollicis longus.
  - Type II: Rolando fracture—requires greater force than a Bennett fracture; presently used to describe either a comminuted Bennett fracture, a "Y" or "T" fracture, or a fracture with dorsal and palmar fragments.

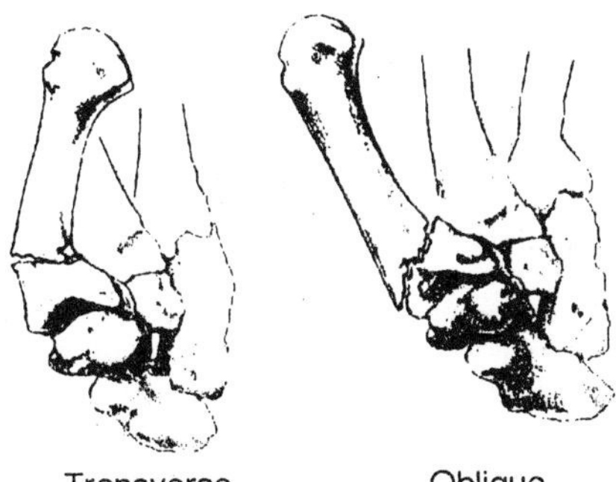

FIG. 22.2. Extraarticular fractures of the base of the thumb. (From Green DP, O'Brien ET. Fractures of the thumb metacarpal. *South Med J* 1972;65:807, with permission.)

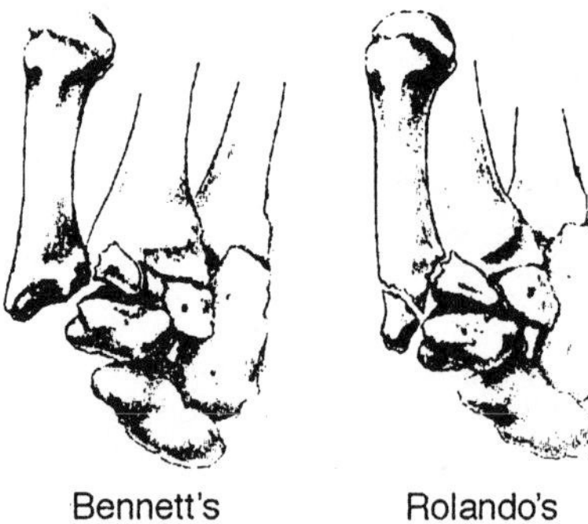

FIG. 22.3. Intraarticular fractures of the base of the thumb. (From Green DP, O'Brien ET. Fractures of the thumb metacarpal. *South Med J* 1972;65:807, with permission.)

Treatment: Both type I and II fractures of the base of the first metacarpal may be treated with either closed reduction and percutaneous pins or open reduction and internal fixation.

Proximal and Middle Phalanges

1. Intraarticular fractures
   - Condylar fractures
     - Single, bicondylar, osteochondral.
     - This type of fracture requires anatomic reduction; open reduction and internal fixation should be performed for >l mm displacement.
   - Comminuted intraarticular phalangeal fractures should be addressed with reconstruction of the articular surface, if possible. Severely comminuted fractures that are deemed non-reconstructible may be treated closed with early protected mobilization.
2. Fracture-dislocations
   - *Volar lip fracture of the middle phalangeal base (dorsal fracture-dislocation)*
     - Treatment: controversial; depends on percentage of articular surface fractured.
     - Hyperextension injuries without a history of dislocation with <30% to 35% articular involvement: buddy tape to adjacent digit.
     - With >30% to 35% articular involvement: some recommend open reduction and internal fixation with reconstruction of the articular surface or a volar plate arthroplasty if the fracture is comminuted; others recommend nonoperative treatment with a dorsal extension block splint if the joint is not subluxed.
   - *Dorsal lip fracture of the middle phalangeal base (volar fracture-dislocation)*
     - Usually the result of central slip avulsion.
     - If less than 1 mm of displacement: may be treated closed with splinting, as in boutonniere injuries.
     - If greater than l mm of displacement or volar subluxation of the proximal interphalangeal joint: indicates need for operative stabilization of the fracture.
3. Extraarticular fractures
   - Fractures at the base of the middle phalanx tend to angulate apex dorsal, whereas fractures at the neck angulate apex volar due to the pull of the sublimis tendon (Fig. 22.4).
   - Closed reduction should be attempted with finger-trap traction initially, followed by splinting.
   - Fractures in which stable closed reduction cannot be achieved or maintained should be addressed with either closed reduction and percutaneous pinning or open reduction and internal fixation with minifragment implants.

Distal Phalanx

1. Intraarticular fractures
   - Dorsal lip

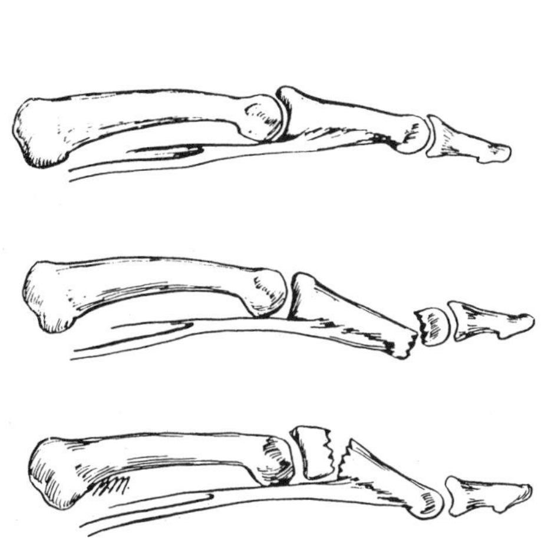

FIG. 22.4. Top: A lateral view, showing the prolonged insertion of the superficialis tendon into the middle phalanx. **Center:** A fracture through the neck of the middle phalanx is likely to have a volar angulation because the proximal fragment is flexed by the strong pull of the superficialis. **Bottom:** A fracture through the base of the middle phalanx is more likely to have a dorsal angulation because of the extension force of the central slip on the proximal fragment and a flexion force on the distal fragment by the superficialis. (From Rockwood CA Jr, Green DP, Bucholz RW, Heckman JD, eds. *Rockwood and Green's fractures in adults,* 4th ed. Vol. 1. Philadelphia: Lippincott-Raven, 1996:627, with permission.)

A mallet finger may result from a fracture of the dorsal lip with disruption of the extensor tendon. Alternatively, a mallet finger may result from a purely tendinous disruption and may therefore not be radiographically apparent.

Treatment remains somewhat controversial.

Some recommend nonoperative treatment for all mallet fingers with full-time extension splinting for 6 to 8 weeks, including those with a significant articular fracture and joint subluxation.

Others believe that joint subluxation is an indication for surgery, even though operative intervention is technically demanding and significant complications associated with surgery have been reported.

- Volar lip

  Associated with flexor digitorum profundus rupture ("jersey finger;" seen in football and rugby players; most commonly involves the ring finger).

  Treatment: primary repair, especially with large displaced bony fragments.

2. Extraarticular fractures
   - Transverse, longitudinal, and comminuted (nail matrix injury very common)
   - Treatment: closed reduction and splinting
3. Nailbed injuries
   - Frequently overlooked or neglected in the face of an obvious fracture, but failure to address such injuries may result in growth disturbances of the nail.
   - Subungual hematomas should be evacuated with cautery or a hot paper clip.
   - If the nail-plate has been avulsed at its base, it should be removed, cleansed with povidone-iodine, and retained for use as a biologic dressing.
   - Nailbed disruptions should be carefully sutured with 7-0 chromic catgut under magnification.
   - Polypropylene artificial nail dressings may be used if the original nail-plate is not usable as a biologic dressing.

COMPLICATIONS

- *Malunion.* Angulation can disturb intrinsic balance and can also result in prominence of metacarpal heads in the palm with pain on gripping. Rotational or angulatory deformities, especially of the second and third metacarpals, may result in functional and cosmetic disturbances, emphasizing the need to maintain as near anatomic relationships as possible.

- *Nonunion.* This is uncommon but may occur, especially with extensive soft-tissue injury and bone loss and with open fractures with gross contamination and infection. This complication may necessitate debridement, bone grafting, or flap coverage.
- *Infection.* Grossly contaminated wounds require meticulous management and appropriate antibiotics depending on the injury setting (e.g., barnyard contamination, brackish water, bite wounds), local wound care with debridement as necessary, and possible delayed closure.
- *Metacarpal-phalangeal joint extension contracture.* This may result if splinting is not in the protected position (i.e., metacarpal phalangeal joints at >70 degrees) due to soft-tissue contracture.
- *Loss of motion.* This is secondary to tendon adherence, especially at the level of the proximal interphalangeal joint.
- *Posttraumatic osteoarthritis.* This may result from a failure to restore articular congruity.

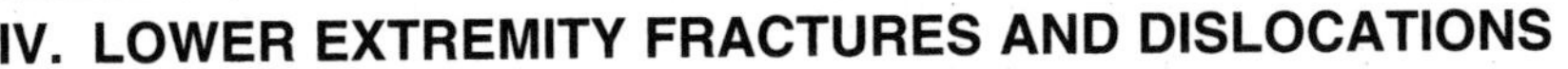

IV. LOWER EXTREMITY FRACTURES AND DISLOCATIONS

23. HIP DISLOCATIONS

EPIDEMIOLOGY

- Incidence is directly related to the incidence of motor vehicle accidents, because these comprise the most common mechanism of injury.
- Up to 50% of patients sustain concomitant fractures elsewhere at the time of dislocation.
- Anterior dislocations constitute 10% to 15% of traumatic dislocations of the hip; posterior dislocations account for the remainder.
- Sciatic nerve injury is present in 10% to 20% of posterior dislocations.

ANATOMY

- The hip articulation has a ball-and-socket configuration with stability conferred by bony and ligamentous restraints, as well as by the congruity of the femoral head with the acetabulum.
- The acetabulum is formed from the confluence of the ischium, ilium, and pubis at the triradiate cartilage.
- Forty percent of the femoral head is covered by the bony acetabulum at any position of hip motion.
- The effect of the labrum is to deepen the acetabulum and to increase the stability of the joint.
- The hip joint capsule is formed by thick longitudinal fibers supplemented by much stronger ligamentous condensations (iliofemoral, pubofemoral, and ischiofemoral ligaments) that run in a spiral fashion, preventing excessive hip extension.
- The main vascular supply to the femoral head originates from the medial and lateral femoral circumflex arteries, branches of the profunda femoral artery. An extracapsular vascular ring is formed at the base of the femoral neck with ascending cervical branches that pierce the hip joint at the level of the capsular insertion. These branches ascend along the femoral neck and enter the bone just inferior to the cartilage of the femoral head. The artery of the ligamentum teres, a branch of the obturator artery, may contribute blood supply to the epiphyseal region of the femoral head.
- The sciatic nerve exits the pelvis at the greater sciatic notch. A certain degree of variability exists in the relationship of the nerve with the piriformis muscle and short external rotators of the hip. Most frequently, the sciatic nerve exits the pelvis deep into the muscle belly of the piriformis.

MECHANISM OF INJURY

- Hip dislocations are almost always due to high energy trauma, such as a motor vehicle accident, a fall from a height, or an industrial injury. Force transmission to the hip joint occurs with application to one of three common sources as follows:
  - The anterior surface of the flexed knee striking an object;
  - The sole of the foot, with the ipsilateral knee extended;
  - The greater trochanter.
- Less frequently, the dislocating force may be applied to the posterior pelvis with the ipsilateral foot or knee acting as the counterforce.
- The direction of dislocation—anterior versus posterior—is determined by the direction of the pathologic force and the position of the lower extremity at the time of injury.

Anterior Dislocations

- These comprise 10% to 15% of traumatic dislocations of the hip.
- The hip is externally rotated and abducted.
- The degree of hip flexion determines whether a superior or inferior type of anterior hip dislocation results:
  - Inferior (obturator) dislocation is the result of simultaneous abduction, external rotation, and hip flexion.

Superior (iliac or pubic) dislocation is the result of simultaneous abduction, external rotation, and hip extension.

Posterior Dislocations

- These are much more frequent than are anterior hip dislocations.
- They result from trauma to the flexed knee (e.g., dashboard injury) with the hip in varying degrees of flexion, as follows:
  - If the hip is in the neutral or slightly adducted position at the time of impact, a dislocation without acetabular fracture is likely to occur.
  - If the hip is in slight abduction, an associated fracture of the posterior-superior rim of the acetabulum typically occurs.

CLINICAL EVALUATION

- A full trauma survey is essential due to the high energy nature of these injuries. Many patients are obtunded or unconscious when they arrive in the emergency room as a result of associated injuries. Concomitant intraabdominal, chest, and other musculoskeletal injuries, such as acetabular, pelvic, or spine fractures, are common.
- Patients presenting with dislocations of the hip typically are unable to move the lower extremity and are in severe discomfort.
- The classic appearance of an individual with a posterior hip dislocation is a patient in severe pain with the hip in a position of flexion, internal rotation, and adduction. Patients with an anterior dislocation hold the hip in marked external rotation with mild flexion and abduction. The appearance and alignment of the extremity, however, can be dramatically altered by ipsilateral extremity injuries.
- A careful neurovascular examination is essential, because injury to the sciatic nerve or femoral neurovascular structures may occur at the time of dislocation. Sciatic nerve injury may occur with stretching of the nerve over the posteriorly dislocated femoral head (Fig. 23.1).
- Posterior wall fragments from the acetabulum may also pierce or partially lacerate the nerve.
- Usually the peroneal portion of the nerve is affected, with little, if any, dysfunction of the tibial nerve. Rarely, injury to the femoral artery, vein, or nerve may occur as

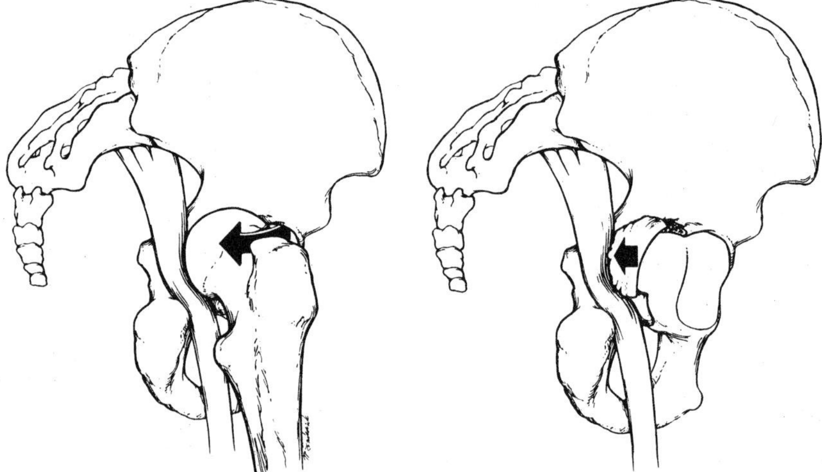

FIG. 23.1. Left: Sciatic nerve impingement by the posteriorly dislocated femoral head. **Right:** Sciatic nerve impingement by a posterior acetabular fracture fragment in a posterior fracture-dislocation of the hip. (From Rockwood CA Jr, Green DP, Bucholz RW, Heckman JD, eds. *Rockwood and Green's fractures in adults,* 4th ed. Vol. 2. Philadelphia: Lippincott-Raven, 1996:1756, with permission.)

a result of an anterior dislocation. Ipsilateral knee, patella, and femur fractures are common. Pelvic fractures and spine injuries may also be seen.

RADIOGRAPHIC EVALUATION

- An anteroposterior radiograph of the pelvis, as well as a cross-table lateral of the affected hip, is essential.
- On the anteroposterior view of the pelvis, the following items should be noted:
  - Femoral heads should appear similar in size, and the joint spaces should be symmetric throughout. In posterior dislocations, the affected femoral head will appear smaller than the normal femoral head. In anterior dislocation, the femoral head will appear slightly larger than the normal hip.
  - The Shenton line should be smooth and continuous.
  - The relative appearance of the greater and lesser trochanters may indicate pathologic internal or external rotation of the hip. The adducted or abducted position of the femoral shaft should also be noted.
  - Evaluation of the femoral neck must rule out the presence of a femoral neck fracture before any manipulative reduction.
- A cross-table lateral view of the affected hip may help distinguish a posterior from an anterior dislocation.
- Forty-five–degree internal and external oblique (Judet) views may help to ascertain the presence of osteochondral fragments, the integrity of the acetabulum, and the congruence of the joint spaces.
- Femoral head depressions and fractures may also be seen.
- Computed tomography is usually obtained after successful closed reduction of a dislocated hip. If closed reduction is not possible and an open reduction is planned, a computed tomography should be obtained to assess the femoral head, the presence of possible intraarticular fragments, and the congruence of the femoral head and acetabulum and to rule out associated femoral head and acetabular fractures.
- The role of magnetic resonance imaging in the evaluation of hip dislocations has not been established; it may prove useful in the evaluation of the integrity of the labrum and the vascularity of the femoral head.

GENERAL CLASSIFICATION

Hip dislocations are classified based on the relationship of the femoral head to the acetabulum and on whether associated fractures are present.

THOMPSON AND EPSTEIN CLASSIFICATION OF POSTERIOR HIP DISLOCATIONS (FIG. 23.2)

Type I: simple dislocation with or without an insignificant posterior wall fragment
Type II: dislocation associated with a single large posterior wall fragment
Type III: dislocation with a comminuted posterior wall fragment
Type IV: dislocation with fracture of the acetabular floor
Type V: dislocation with fracture of the femoral head

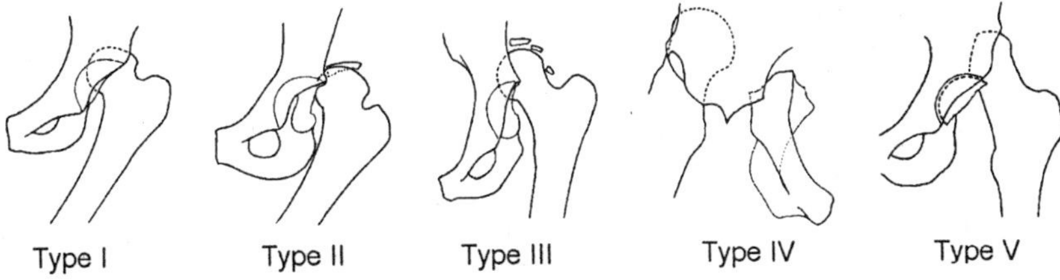

FIG. 23.2. Thompson and Epstein classification of posterior hip dislocations.

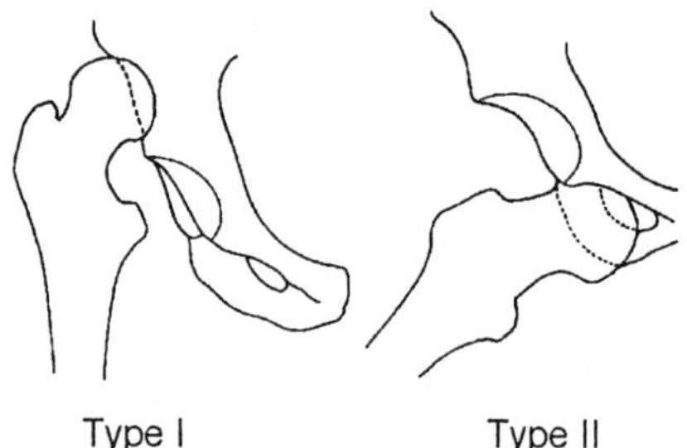

FIG. 23.3. Epstein classifications of anterior hip dislocations. (From Rockwood CA, Green DP, eds. *Fractures in adults*, 3rd ed. Philadelphia: Lippincott, 1991: 1576–1579, with permission.)

EPSTEIN CLASSIFICATION OF ANTERIOR HIP DISLOCATIONS (FIG. 23.3)

Type I: superior dislocations, including pubic and subspinous
- IA: no associated fractures
- IB: associated fracture or impaction of the femoral head
- IC: associated fracture of the acetabulum

Type II: inferior dislocations, including obturator and perineal
- IIA: no associated fractures
- IIB: associated fracture or impaction of the femoral head
- IIC: associated fracture of the acetabulum

COMPREHENSIVE CLASSIFICATION OF HIP DISLOCATIONS

This classification combines both anterior and posterior dislocations and incorporates physical findings both before and after reduction.

Type I: no significant associated fractures; no clinical instability after concentric reduction

Type II: irreducible dislocation without significant femoral head or acetabular fracture (reduction must be attempted under general anesthesia)

Type III: unstable hip after reduction or with incarcerated fragments of cartilage, labrum, or bone

Type IV: associated acetabular fracture requiring reconstruction to restore hip stability or joint congruity

Type V: associated femoral head or femoral neck injury

ORTHOPAEDIC TRAUMA ASSOCIATION (OTA) CLASSIFICATION OF HIP DISLOCATIONS (FIG. 23.4)

30-D10: anterior
30-D11: posterior
30-D30: obturator

TREATMENT

- Reduction should be expedient to decrease the risk of osteonecrosis of the femoral head; whether this should be accomplished by closed or open methods remains controversial. Most recommend an immediate attempt at a closed reduction, although some believe that all fracture-dislocations of the hip should have immediate open surgery to remove fragments from the joint and to reconstruct fractures.
- Long-term prognosis worsens significantly if reduction (closed or open) is delayed more than 12 hours. Associated acetabular or femoral head fractures can be treated in the subacute phase.

Closed Reduction

Regardless of the direction of the dislocation, the reduction can be attempted using inline traction with the patient lying supine. The preferred method is to perform a closed reduction under general anesthesia; if this is not feasible, reduction under intravenous sedation is possible. Three popular methods for achieving closed reduction of the hip follow.

Allis Method
Traction is applied in line with the deformity. The patient is placed supine with the surgeon standing above the patient on the stretcher. Initially, the surgeon applies in-line traction while the assistant applies countertraction by stabilizing the patient's pelvis. While increasing the traction force, the surgeon should slowly increase the degree of flexion to approximately 70 degrees. Gentle rotational motions of the hip and slight adduction will often help the femoral head clear the lip of the acetabulum. A lateral force to the proximal thigh may assist in reduction. An audible "clunk" is a sign of a successful closed reduction.

Stimson Gravity Technique
The patient is placed prone on the stretcher with the affected leg hanging off the side of the stretcher. This brings the extremity into a position of both hip and knee flexion of 90 degrees each. In this position the assistant immobilizes the pelvis and the surgeon applies an anteriorly directed force on the proximal calf. Gentle rotation of the limb may assist in reduction.

Bigelow and Reverse Bigelow Maneuvers
These have been associated with iatrogenic femoral neck fractures and are not as frequently used as reduction techniques. In the Bigelow maneuver, the patient is supine and the surgeon applies longitudinal traction on the limb. The adducted and internally rotated thigh is then flexed at least 90 degrees. The femoral head is levered into the acetabulum by abduction, external rotation, and extension of the hip. In the reverse Bigelow maneuver, used for anterior dislocations, traction is again applied in the line of the deformity. The hip is then adducted, sharply internally rotated, and extended.

Following Closed Reduction
After closed reduction of the hip, postreduction radiographs should be obtained to confirm adequate reduction. The hip should be examined for stability while the patient is still sedated or under anesthesia. If an obvious large, displaced acetabular fracture is found, the stability examination need not be performed.

- Stability is checked by flexing the hip to 90 degrees in neutral position. A strong posteriorly directed force is then applied. If any sensation of subluxation is detected, the patient will require additional diagnostic studies and possibly surgical exploration or traction.
- After successful closed reduction and completion of the stability examination, the patient should undergo computed tomographic evaluation. If the hip is unstable, then skeletal traction with a tibial pin is used.

Open Reduction
- Indications for open reduction of a dislocated hip include the following:
  - Dislocation irreducible by closed means;
  - Nonconcentric reduction;
  - Fracture of the acetabulum or femoral head that requires either excision or open reduction and internal fixation;
  - Ipsilateral femoral neck fracture.
- A standard posterior approach (Kocher-Langenbeck) will allow exploration of the sciatic nerve, removal of posteriorly incarcerated fragments, treatment of major posterior labral disruptions or instability, and repair of posterior acetabular fractures.
- An anterior (Smith-Peterson) approach is recommended for isolated femoral head fractures. A concern when using an anterior approach for a posterior dislocation is the possibility that complete vascular disruption will occur. By avoiding removal of the capsule from the femoral neck and trochanters (i.e., taking down the capsule from the acetabular side), injury to the lateral circumflex artery or its branches should not occur.
- An anterolateral (Watson-Jones) approach is useful for most anterior dislocations and for combined fracture of both the femoral head and neck.
- A direct lateral (Hardinge) approach will allow exposure anteriorly and posteriorly through the same incision.

(*text continues on page 170*)

Joint: Hip (30-D)

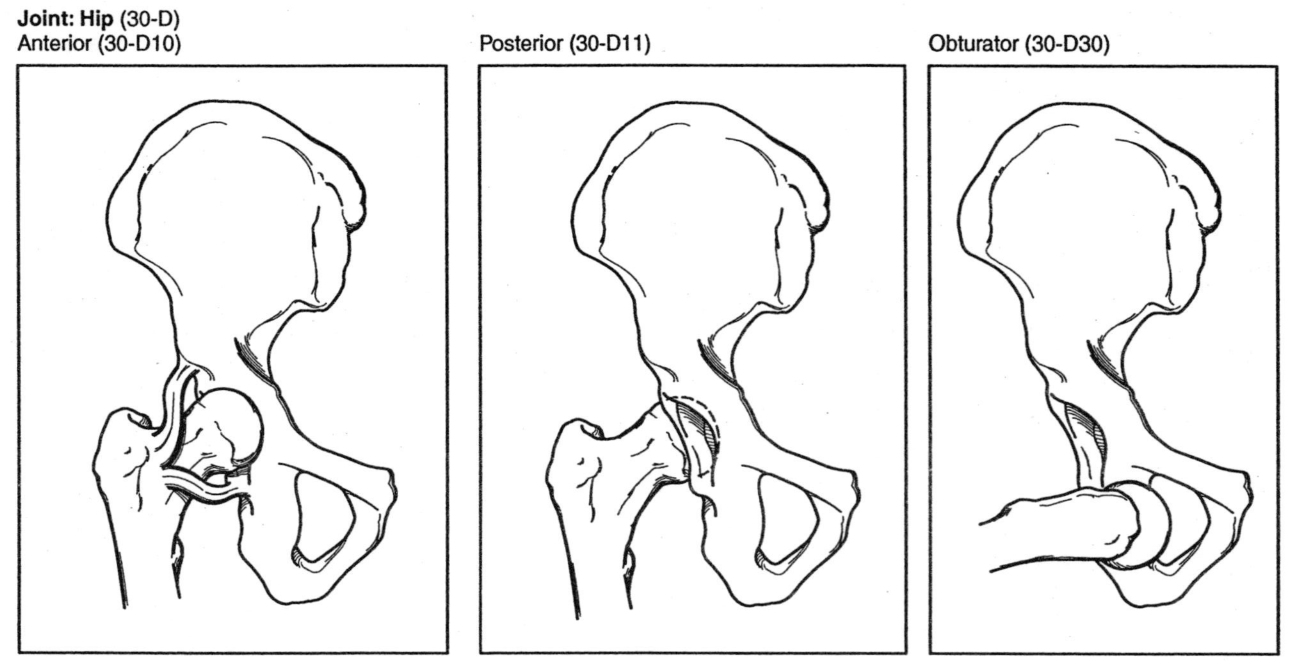

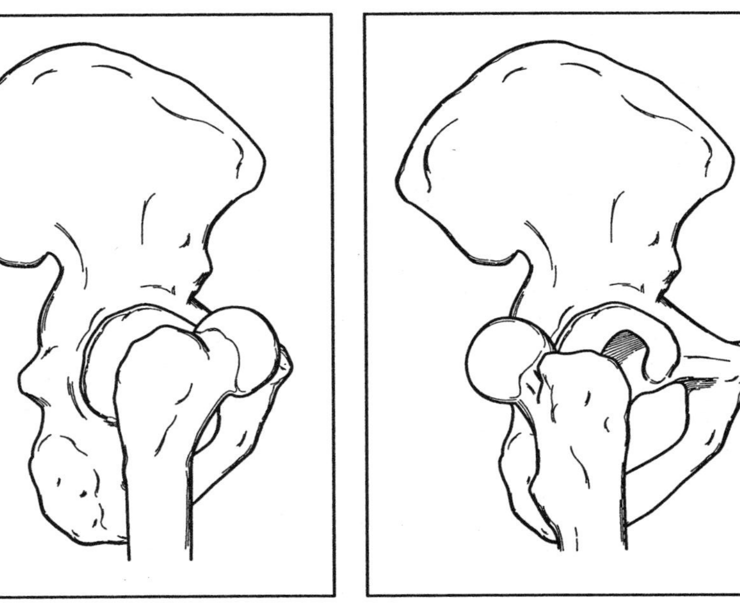

FIG. 23.4. The Orthopaedic Trauma Association classification of hip dislocations. (From Heckman JD, Bucholz RW, eds. *Rockwood, Green, and Wilkin's fractures in adults*, 5th ed. Philadelphia: Lippincott Williams & Wilkins, 2001, with permission.)

- In the case of an ipsilateral displaced or nondisplaced femoral neck fracture, closed reduction of the hip should not be attempted. The hip fracture should be provisionally fixed through a lateral approach on a fracture table. A gentle reduction is then performed, and definitive fixation of the femoral neck fracture can subsequently be performed.
- Management after open reduction ranges from short periods of simple bedrest to various durations of skeletal traction to hip spica immobilization. No correlation exists between early weight bearing and osteonecrosis. Therefore, partial weight bearing is advised. Other advice includes the following:
  - If reduction is concentric and stable: a short period of bedrest should followed by protected weight bearing for 4 to 6 weeks.
  - If reduction is concentric but unstable: skeletal traction should be used for 6 to 8 weeks to allow time for acetabular fractures to heal; this is followed by subsequent progressive protective weight bearing.

Prognosis

- The functional outcome after hip dislocation ranges from an essentially normal hip to a severely painful and degenerated joint.
- A 70% to 80% good or excellent outcome is reported in simple posterior dislocations. When posterior dislocations are associated with femoral head fractures or acetabular fractures, however, the associated fractures generally compromise the outcome.
- Anterior dislocations of the hip are noted to have a high incidence of associated femoral head injuries (transchondral or indentation types). The only patients with excellent results in these series are those without associated femoral head injuries.

COMPLICATIONS

- Osteonecrosis: observed in 5% to 40% of injuries, with increased risk associated with increased duration of dislocation (>6 to 24 hours), although some suggest that osteonecrosis may result from the initial injury and not from prolonged dislocation. Osteonecrosis may become clinically apparent up to 5 years after injury. Repeated reduction attempts may also increase its incidence.
- Posttraumatic osteoarthritis: most frequent long-term complication of hip dislocations; incidence is dramatically higher when dislocations are associated with acetabular fractures or transchondral fractures of the femoral head.
- Recurrent dislocation: rare (<2%), although patients with decreased femoral anteversion may suffer a recurrent posterior dislocation, whereas those with increased femoral anteversion may be prone to recurrent anterior dislocations.
- Neurovascular injury: sciatic nerve injuries found in 10% to 20% of hip dislocations. They are usually caused by a stretching of the nerve from a posteriorly dislocated head or from a displaced fracture fragment. Prognosis is unpredictable, but most report 40% to 50% full recovery.
- Electromyographic and nerve conduction velocity studies are indicated at 3 to 4 weeks for baseline information and prognostic guidance. If no clinical or electrical improvement is seen by 1 year, surgical intervention may be considered. If a sciatic nerve injury occurs only after a closed reduction is performed, then entrapment of the nerve is likely and surgical exploration is indicated.
- Injury to the femoral nerve and femoral vascular structures have been reported with anterior dislocations.
- Femoral head fractures: occur in 10% of posterior dislocations (shear fractures) and in 25% to 75% of anterior dislocations (indentation fractures).
- Heterotopic ossification: occurs in 2% of patients; is related to the initial muscular damage and hematoma formation. Surgery increases its incidence. Treatment of choice is indomethacin prophylaxis for 6 weeks. Some recommend 1,000 cGy of radiation in single or divided doses immediately following operation.
- Thromboembolism: may occur after hip dislocation due to traction-induced intimal injury to the vasculature. Patients should be given adequate prophylaxis consisting of compression stockings, sequential compression devices, and chemoprophylaxis (e.g., low molecular weight heparin preparations), especially if placed in traction.

24. FEMORAL HEAD

EPIDEMIOLOGY

- Almost all femoral head fractures are associated with hip dislocations.
- Fracture complicates 10% of posterior hip dislocations.
- Most fractures are of the shear or cleavage type, although recently, more indentation- or crush-type fractures have been recognized with the increased use of computed tomography.
- Indentation fractures are more commonly associated with anterior hip dislocations (25% to 75%).

ANATOMY

- The femoral head receives its blood supply from three sources (Fig. 24.1), as follows:
  - Medial femoral circumflex artery: supplies the majority of the superior weight-bearing portion;
  - Lateral femoral circumflex artery and the artery of the ligamentum teres: supply the remainder.
- Seventy percent of the femoral head articular surface is involved in load transfer; therefore, damage to this surface may lead to the development of posttraumatic arthritis.

Mechanism of Injury

- Most femoral head fractures are secondary to motor vehicle accidents, with axial load transmission proximally through the femur.
- If the thigh is neutral or adducted, a posterior hip dislocation with or without a femoral head fracture may result. These fractures may be the result of avulsion by the ligamentum teres or of cleavage over the posterior acetabular edge.
- In anterior dislocations, impacted femoral head fractures may occur because of a direct blow from the acetabular margin.

CLINICAL EVALUATION

- A formal trauma evaluation is frequently necessary because most femoral head fractures are a result of high energy trauma; injury to other body systems frequently occurs.
- In addition to hip dislocation, femoral head fractures are also associated with acetabular fractures, knee ligament injuries, patella fractures, and femoral shaft fractures.
- A careful neurovascular examination is essential because posterior hip dislocations may result in neurovascular compromise.

RADIOGRAPHIC EVALUATION

- Anteroposterior and Judet (45-degree oblique) views of the pelvis should be obtained.
- Hip dislocation is almost always present.
- The anteroposterior radiograph of the pelvis may demonstrate femoral head fragments in the acetabular fossa.
- If closed reduction of the joint is successful, computed tomography may be necessary to evaluate the reduction status of the femoral head fracture and to rule out the presence of intraarticular fragments that may hinder adequate reduction.
- Tomography or sagittal computed tomographic reconstruction may also be helpful in delineating the femoral head fracture.

PIPKIN CLASSIFICATION (FIG. 24.2)

Type I: hip dislocation with fracture of the femoral head caudad to the fovea capitis femoris

Type II: hip dislocation with fracture of the femoral head cephalad to the fovea capitis femoris

Type III: type I or II injury associated with fracture of the femoral neck

Type IV: type I or II injury associated with fracture of the acetabular rim

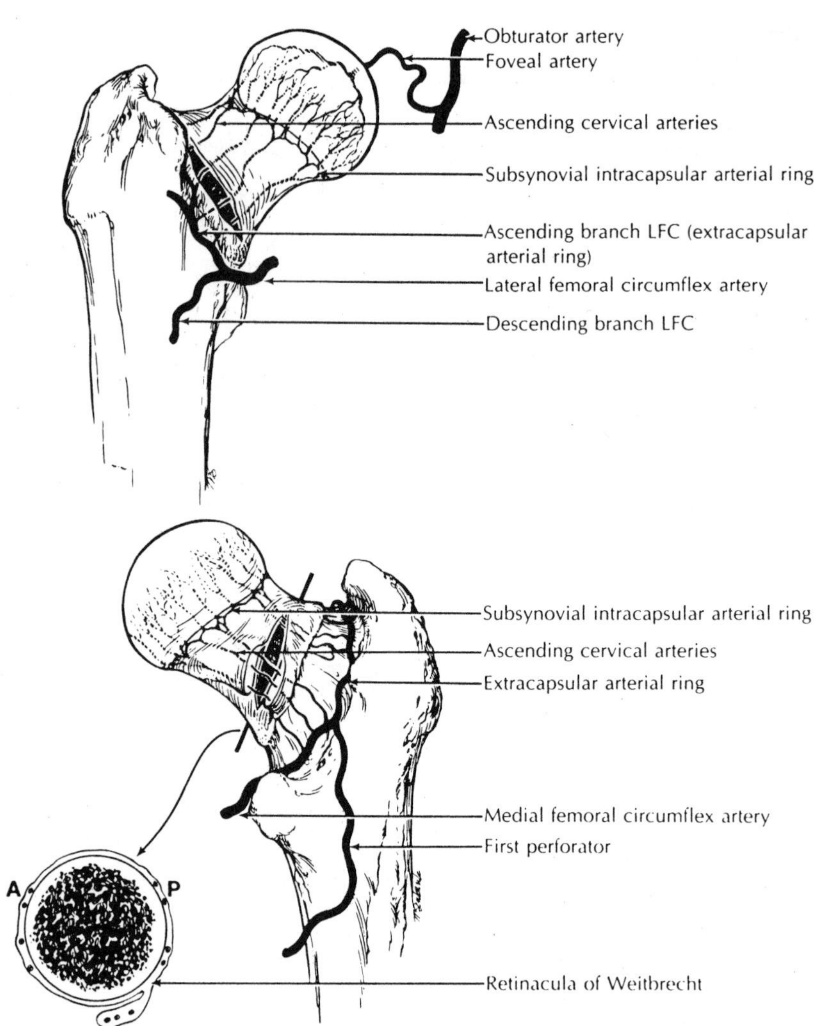

FIG. 24.1. Vascular anatomy of the femoral head and neck. **Top:** Anterior aspect. **Bottom:** Posterior aspect. Abbreviation: *LFC*, lateral femoral circumflex artery. (From Rockwood CA Jr, Green DP, Bucholz RW, Heckman JD, eds. *Rockwood and Green's fractures in adults*, 4th ed. Vol. 2. Philadelphia: Lippincott-Raven, 1996:1662, with permission.)

BRUMBACK ET AL. CLASSIFICATION

Type 1A: posterior hip dislocation with femoral head fracture involving the inferomedial (non–weight-bearing) portion of the head and minimal or no fracture of the acetabular rim with stable hip joint after reduction

Type 1B: type 1A with significant acetabular fracture and hip instability

Type 2A: posterior hip dislocation with femoral head fracture involving the superomedial (weight-bearing) portion of the head and minimal or no fracture of the acetabular rim with stable hip joint after reduction

Type 2B: type 2A with significant acetabular fracture and hip instability

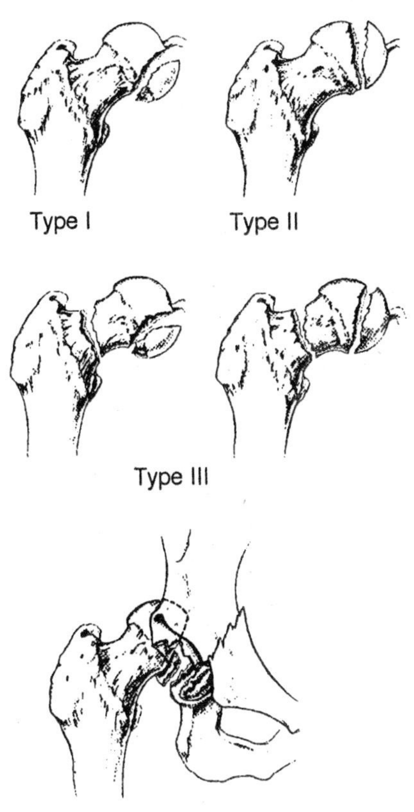

FIG. 24.2. Pipkin classification of femoral head fractures. (From Hansen S, Swiontkowski M. *Orthopedic trauma protocols*. New York: Raven Press, 1993:238, with permission.)

Type 3A: any hip dislocation with femoral neck fracture
Type 3B: any hip dislocation with femoral neck and head fracture
Type 4A: anterior dislocation of the hip with indentation of the superolateral weight-bearing surface of the femoral head
Type 4B: anterior dislocation of the hip with transchondral shear fracture of the weight-bearing surface of the femoral head
Type 5: central fracture-dislocations of the hip with fracture of the femoral head

ORTHOPAEDIC TRAUMA ASSOCIATION (OTA) CLASSIFICATION OF FEMORAL HEAD FRACTURES (FIG. 24.3)

Type C1: femoral head split fracture
- C1.1: avulsion of the ligamentum teres
- C1.2: with rupture of the ligamentum teres
- C1.3: large fragment

Type C2: femoral head depression fracture
- C2.1: posterior and superior
- C2.2: anterior and superior
- C2.3: split depression

Type C3: femoral head fracture with femoral neck fracture
- C3.1: split and transcervical neck fracture
- C3.2: split and subcapital neck fracture
- C3.3: depression and neck fracture

1. Avulsion of ligamentum teres (31-C1.1)

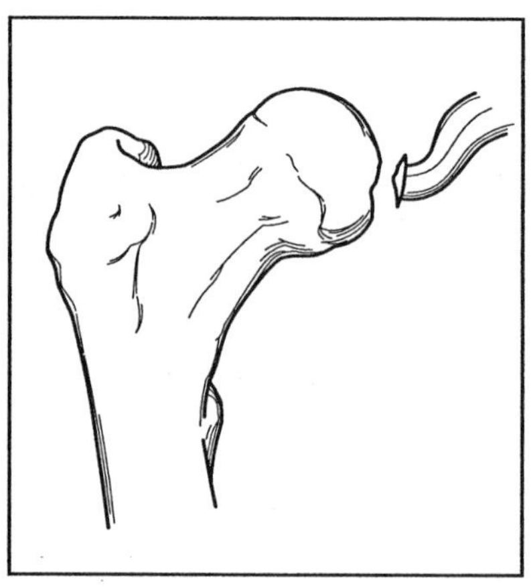

3. Large fragment (31-C1.3)

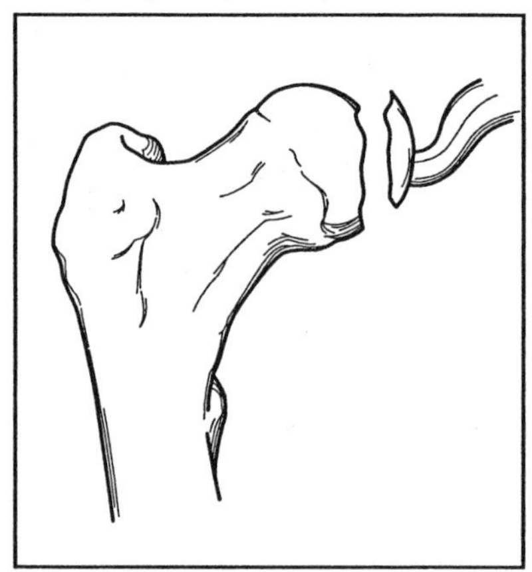

2. With rupture of ligamentum teres (31-C1.2)

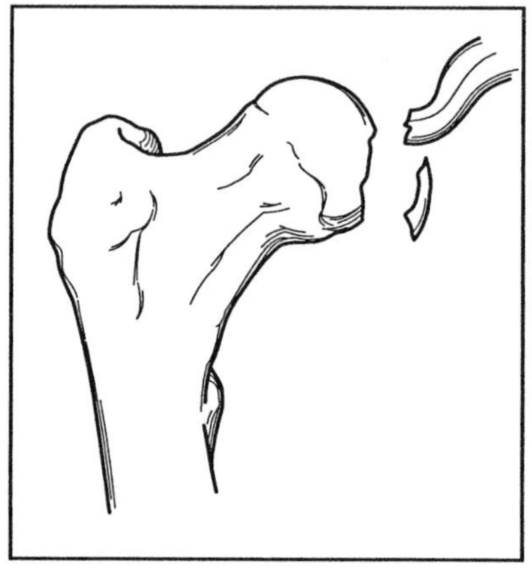

FIG. 24.3. The Orthopaedic Trauma Association classification of femoral head fractures. (From Heckman JD, Bucholz RW, eds. *Rockwood, Green, and Wilkin's fractures in adults*, 5th ed. Philadelphia: Lippincott Williams & Wilkins, 2001, with permission.)

TREATMENT

Pipkin Type I

- If reduction is adequate (<1 mm step-off), closed treatment is recommended.
- If the reduction is not adequate, open reduction and internal fixation with small cancellous screws or Herbert screws using an anterior approach are recommended.
- In cases of multiple trauma, open reduction and internal fixation may also be indicated to allow mobilization of a young patient.
- Very small fragments may be excised if they do not sacrifice stability.

Pipkin Type II

- The same recommendations apply for the nonoperative treatment of type II fractures as for type I fractures, except that only an anatomic reduction as seen on computed tomography and repeat radiographs can be accepted for nonoperative care.
- Open reduction with internal fixation is generally the treatment of choice.

Pipkin Type III

- The prognosis for this fracture is poor and depends on the degree of displacement of the femoral neck fracture.
- In young patients, an emergent open reduction with internal fixation of the femoral neck is performed, followed by internal fixation of the femoral head. This can be done using an anterolateral (Watson-Jones) approach.
- In older patients with a badly displaced femoral neck fracture, prosthetic replacement is indicated.

Pipkin Type IV

- This fracture must be treated in tandem with its associated acetabular fracture.
- The acetabular fracture should dictate the surgical approach, and the femoral head fracture, even if nondisplaced, should be internally fixed to allow early motion of the hip joint.

Femoral Head Fractures Associated with Anterior Dislocations

- These fractures are difficult to manage.
- Indentation fractures, typically located on the superior aspect of the femoral head, require no specific treatment; but the fracture size and location have prognostic implications.
- Displaced transchondral fractures that result in a nonconcentric reduction require open reduction and either excision or internal fixation, depending on fragment size and location.

COMPLICATIONS

- *Osteonecrosis*

  Posterior hip dislocations with an associated femoral head fracture are at high risk for developing osteonecrosis and posttraumatic degenerative arthritis. The prognosis for these injuries varies. Pipkin types I and II are reported to have the same prognosis as a simple dislocation. Pipkin type IV injuries seem to have roughly the same prognosis as acetabular fractures without a femoral head fracture. Pipkin type III injuries have a poor prognosis with a 50% rate of posttraumatic osteonecrosis.

  Ten percent of anterior dislocations develop osteonecrosis. Risk factors include a time delay in reduction and repeated reduction attempts.
- *Posttraumatic osteoarthritis.* Risk factors include transchondral fracture, indentation fracture greater than 4 mm in depth, and osteonecrosis.

25. FEMORAL NECK FRACTURES

EPIDEMIOLOGY

- More than 250,000 hip fractures occur in the United States each year; this number is projected to double by the year 2050.
- The average age of occurrence is 77 years for women and 72 years for men.
- Eighty percent of these fractures occur in women; the incidence doubles for each decade of life after the fifth decade.
- The incidence in younger patients is very low and is mainly associated with high energy trauma.

ANATOMY

- The upper femoral epiphysis closes by the age of 16 years.
- The neck-shaft angle is 130 ± 7 degrees.
- Femoral anteversion is 10 ± 6 degrees.
- Minimal periosteum exists about the femoral neck; thus, any callus that forms must do so by endosteal proliferation.
- Calcar femorale is a vertically oriented plate of dense cancellous bone from the posteromedial portion of the femoral shaft radiating superiorly toward the greater trochanter.
- The capsule is attached anteriorly to the intertrochanteric line and posteriorly, 1 to 1.5 cm proximal to the intertrochanteric line.
- The three ligaments that attach in this region are as follows:
  - Iliofemoral—Y-ligament of Bigelow (anterior);
  - Pubofemoral—anterior;
  - Ischiofemoral—posterior.
- Vascular supply is as follows:
  - At the base of the femoral neck, an extracapsular ring is formed anteriorly by the ascending branch of the lateral femoral circumflex artery and posteriorly by the medial femoral circumflex artery.
  - The ascending cervical branches from this ring pierce the hip capsule near its distal insertion, becoming the retinacular arteries coursing along the femoral neck. Most arteries supplying the femoral head are posterosuperior in location.
  - A subsynovial intracapsular arterial ring is formed by these retinacular arteries at the base of the femoral head. As they enter the femoral head, they become the epiphyseal branches.
  - The lateral epiphyseal arteries that arise from the posterosuperior ascending cervical branches supply most of the femoral head.
  - The artery of the ligamentum teres, usually a branch of the obturator, offers a small supplemental contribution to the femoral head and is limited to the area around the fovea capitis.
- Forces acting across the hip joint are as follows:
  - Straight leg raise: 1.5 times body weight.
  - One-legged stance: 2.5 times body weight.
  - Two-legged stance: 0.5 times body weight.
  - Running: 5.0 times body weight.
- The internal anatomy of the femoral neck indicates that the direction of the trabeculae parallels the direction of weight bearing. Primary and secondary compressive and tensile groups exist. The bony trabeculae are laid down along the lines of maximal internal stress, crossing each other at right angles. They are perpendicular to the surface of the bone or articular cartilage (Fig. 25.1).
- The association between osteoporosis and these fractures is clear. Eighty-four percent of patients with femoral neck fractures have mild to severe osteoporosis. Patients with femoral neck fractures are more osteoporotic than age- and sex-matched control subjects, although no causal relationship between osteoporosis and femoral neck fractures has been demonstrated.

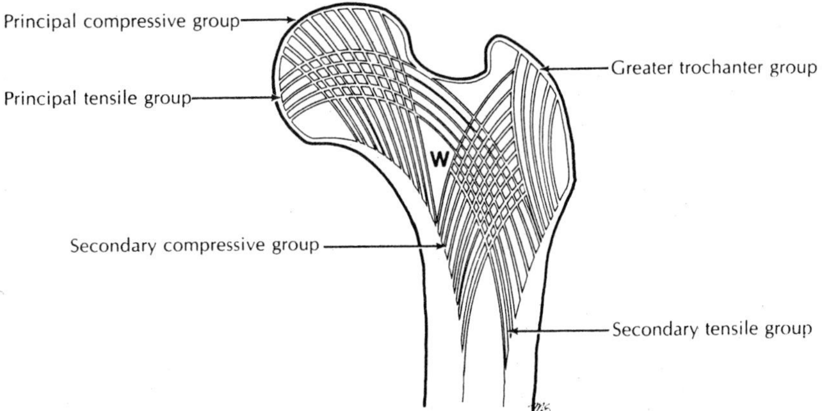

FIG. 25.1. Anatomy of the bony trabeculae in the proximal end of the femur. In a non-osteoporotic femur, all five groups of bony trabeculae are readily evident on x-ray. The Ward triangle (*W*) is a small area in the neck of the femur that contains thin and loosely arranged trabeculae only. (From Rockwood CA Jr, Green DP, Bucholz RW, Heckman JD, eds. *Rockwood and Green's fractures in adults*, 4th ed. Vol. 2. Philadelphia: Lippincott-Raven, 1996:1667, with permission.)

MECHANISM OF INJURY

- Low energy trauma is most common in older patients:
  - Direct: fall onto the greater trochanter or forced external rotation of the lower extremity impinging an osteoporotic neck onto the posterior lip of the acetabulum (i.e., fall causes the fracture)
  - Indirect: muscle contraction overcomes the strength of the bone (i.e., fracture causes the fall)
- High energy trauma (e.g., motor vehicle accident, a fall from a significant height) accounts for femoral neck fractures in both younger and older patients.
- Cyclical loading-stress fractures are seen in athletes, military recruits, and ballet dancers; patients with osteoporosis and osteopenia are at particular risk.

CLINICAL EVALUATION

- Patients with acute hip fractures typically are unable to ambulate, with obvious shortening and external rotation of the lower extremity. Patients with impacted or stress fractures may demonstrate more subtle findings, such as anterior capsular tenderness, pain with axial compression, and lack of deformity, and may be able to bear weight.
- Pain is evident on range of motion, with possible pain on axial compression and tenderness to palpation of the groin.
- An accurate history is more important in the low energy fracture that usually occurs in older individuals. Obtaining a history of loss of consciousness, prior syncopal episodes, chest pain, prior hip pain (pathologic fracture), and preinjury ambulatory status, as well as a medical history, is essential. In younger patients involved in high energy events, physical and radiographic examinations are usually of more value.

RADIOGRAPHIC EVALUATION

- An anteroposterior view with the hip in internal rotation and a cross-table lateral should be obtained.
- Posterior comminution and angulation may be evaluated on the cross-table lateral view.
- Magnetic resonance imaging may be undertaken in the first 24 hours if plain radiographs are negative with a high index of suspicion.

- Technetium bone scans may be performed to rule out occult fracture; these are best done 48 hours after injury.

CLASSIFICATION BY ANATOMIC LOCATION

- Subcapital
- Transcervical
- Basicervical

PAUWELS CLASSIFICATION (FIG. 25.2)

Based on angle of fracture from horizontal.

Type I: 30 degrees
Type II: 50 degrees
Type III: 70 degrees

Increasing shear forces with increasing angle lead to more instability.

GARDEN CLASSIFICATION (FIG. 25.3)

Based on degree of valgus displacement.

Type I: incomplete/impacted
Type II: complete nondisplaced on anteroposterior and lateral views
Type III: complete with partial displacement; trabecular pattern of the femoral head does not line up with that of the acetabulum
Type IV: completely displaced; trabecular pattern of the head assumes a parallel orientation with that of the acetabulum

ORTHOPAEDIC TRAUMA ASSOCIATION CLASSIFICATION OF FEMORAL NECK FRACTURES (FIG. 25.4)

Type B1: subcapital with slight displacement
  B1.1: impacted in valgus ≥15 degrees
  B1.2: impacted in valgus <15 degrees
  B1.3: nonimpacted
Type B2: transcervical
  B2.1: basicervical
  B2.2: midcervical adduction
  B2.3: midcervical shear

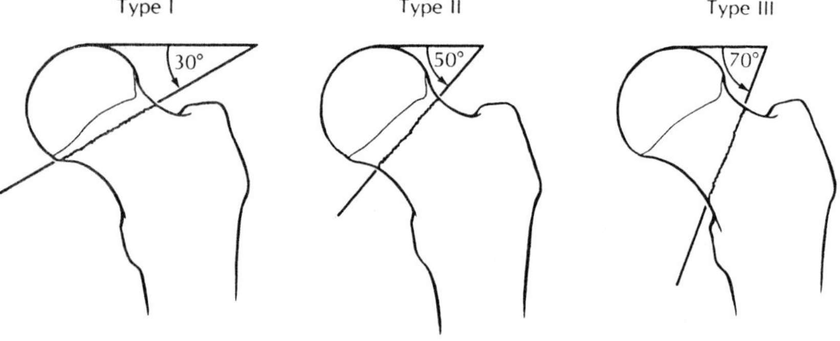

FIG. 25.2. The Pauwels classification of femoral neck fractures is based on the angle the fracture forms with the horizontal plane. As a fracture progresses from type I to type III, the obliquity of the fracture line increases and, theoretically, the shear forces at the fracture site also increase. (From Rockwood CA Jr, Green DP, Bucholz RW, Heckman JD, eds. *Rockwood and Green's fractures in adults*, 4th ed. Vol. 2. Philadelphia: Lippincott-Raven, 1996:1670, with permission.)

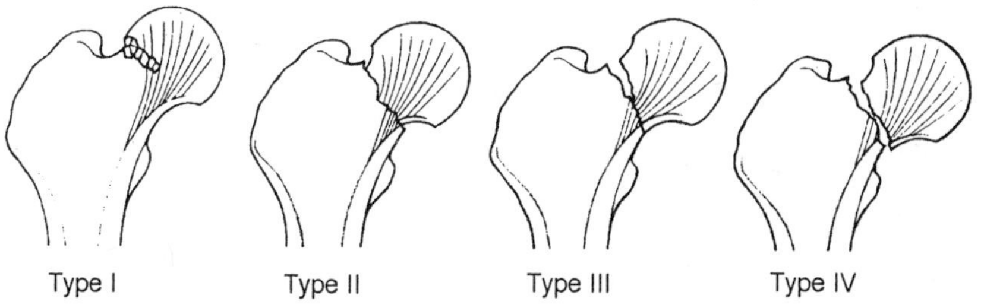

FIG. 25.3. Garden classification of femoral neck fractures. (From Hansen S, Swiontkowski M. *Orthopaedic trauma protocols*. New York: Raven Press, 1993:238, with permission.)

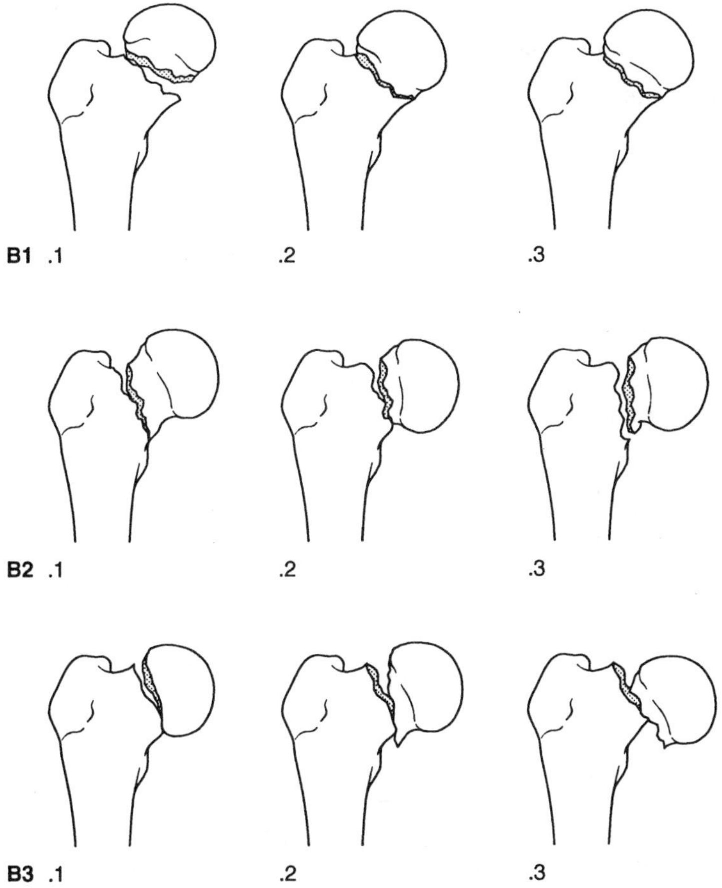

B1 .1 .2 .3

B2 .1 .2 .3

B3 .1 .2 .3

FIG. 25.4. The Orthopaedic Trauma Association classification for femoral neck fractures. The B1 group fracture is a non- to minimally displaced subcapital fracture. The B2 group includes transcervical fractures through the middle or base of the neck, and the B3 group includes all displaced nonimpacted subcapital fractures. Subgroups further specify fracture geometry. The diagrams represent common examples of the defined fracture pattern. To use this system effectively, the text of the classification must be read and applied. (Adapted from Müller ME, Nazarian S, Koch P, et al. *The comprehensive classification of fractures of long bones*. New York: Springer-Verlag, 1990:118, with permission.)

Type B3: subcapital, nonimpacted displaced
- B3.1: moderate displacement in varus and external rotation
- B3.2: moderate displacement with vertical translation and external rotation
- B3.3: marked displacement

CURRENT CLASSIFICATION

- Nondisplaced and impacted valgus femoral neck fractures: much better prognostic situation
- Displaced: any detectable displacement

TREATMENT

The goals of treatment are to protect from additional damage, to minimize discomfort, to restore hip function, and to allow rapid mobilization by obtaining early anatomic reduction and stable internal fixation or by prosthetic replacement.

Fatigue/Stress Fractures

- Tension (seen at the superior lateral neck on an internally rotated anteroposterior view): significant risk for displacement; *in situ* screw fixation recommended.
- Compression (seen as a haze of callus at the inferior neck): lower risk for displacement without additional trauma; protective crutch ambulation recommended until asymptomatic.

Impacted/Nondisplaced Fractures

- Approximately 8% to 20% of "impacted" fractures will displace without treatment—impossible to identify which will displace in advance.
- Less than 10% of fractures develop osteonecrosis secondary to kinking of the lateral epiphyseal vessels and tethering of the medial vessels in a valgus position.
- *In situ* fixation with three cancellous screws is indicated; exceptions are pathologic fractures, severe osteoarthritis/rheumatoid arthritis, Paget disease, and other metabolic conditions, all of which require prosthetic replacement.

Displaced Fractures

- Young patient with high energy injury and normal bone: urgent closed/open reduction with internal fixation and capsulotomy.
- Elderly patients are treated using the following criteria:
  - High functional demands and good bone density: timely medical evaluation followed by prompt closed/open reduction and internal fixation.
  - Normal to intermediate longevity but poor bone density, chronic illness, and lower functional demands: modular unipolar or bipolar hemiarthroplasty.
  - Low demand and poor bone quality: hemiarthroplasty using a one-piece unipolar prosthesis.
  - Severely ill, demented, and bedridden: consider nonoperative treatment, excisional arthroplasty, or prosthetic replacement for intolerable pain.

Operative Treatment

- Reduction
  - Reduction should be achieved as soon as possible to avoid osteonecrosis. Risk of osteonecrosis may increase with increasing time to reduction.
  - Reduction maneuver—flexion with gentle traction and external rotation to disengage the fragments and then slow extension and internal rotation to achieve reduction. Reduction must be confirmed on the anteroposterior and lateral images.
  - Guidelines for acceptable reduction:
    - Garden alignment index: on the anteroposterior view, valgus is more mechanically acceptable; on the lateral, maintain anteversion while avoiding any posterior translation of the fracture surfaces.
    - Posterior comminution must be assessed.
- Internal fixation
  - Multiple screw fixation is the most accepted method of fixation. Threads should cross the fracture site to allow for compression.

Three parallel screws are the optimal number for fixation. Additional screws add little additional stability and increase the chances of penetrating the joint.

Sliding-screw sideplate devices—not recommended, even though used by some. If used, a second pin or screw should be inserted superiorly to control rotation during screw insertion.

- Prosthetic replacement
  1. The advantages of hemiarthroplasty over open reduction and internal fixation include the following:
     - May allow faster full weight bearing;
     - Eliminates nonunion, osteonecrosis, and failure of fixation risks;
     - Second operations required in 18% of cases with open reduction and internal fixation after a displaced femoral neck fracture.
  2. The disadvantages of hemiarthroplasty include the following:
     - More extensive procedure, greater blood loss, and more perioperative complications;
     - Not useful in younger patients.
  3. Indications for prosthetic replacement include the following:
     - Displaced femoral neck fracture in the elderly;
     - Pathologic fracture;
     - Severe medical condition;
     - Nonambulatory status before fracture;
     - Neurologic condition (dementia, ataxia, hemiplegia, parkinsonism).
  4. Contraindications include the following:
     - Active sepsis;
     - Active young person;
     - Preexisting acetabular disease (e.g., rheumatoid arthritis).
  5. Bipolar versus unipolar replacement is as follows:
     - Bipolar theoretically reduces acetabular erosion; therefore, it is useful in relatively young active patients.
     - Unipolar is more economical in the elderly less active patient.
  6. Primary total hip replacement is useful in the following situations:
     - Preexisting ipsilateral degenerative disease;
     - Contralateral hip disease;
     - Preexisting ipsilateral acetabular metastatic disease.

COMPLICATIONS

- Nonunion: usually apparent by 12 months as groin or buttock pain, pain on hip extension, or pain with weight bearing. May complicate up to 5% of nondisplaced fractures and up to 25% of displaced fractures. Elderly patients presenting with nonunion may be adequately treated with arthroplasty, whereas younger patients may benefit from cancellous bone grafting, proximal femoral osteotomy, or muscle pedicle graft.
- Osteonecrosis: may present as groin, buttock, or proximal thigh pain, complicating up to 10% of nondisplaced fractures and up to 27% of displaced fractures. Not all cases develop evidence of radiographic collapse. Treatment should be guided by symptomatology.
  - Early without x-ray changes: physical therapy, non-weight bearing, possible core decompression.
  - Late with x-ray changes: elderly patients treated with arthroplasty, whereas younger patients treated with osteotomy, possible arthrodesis, or arthroplasty.
- Fixation failure: usually related to failure of osteoporotic bone around implants or technical problems (malreduction, short implants, threads crossing the fracture). This may be treated with attempted repeat open reduction and internal fixation or prosthetic arthroplasty.
- Thromboembolic phenomenon: present in 30% to 50% of patients but only symptomatic in 7% to 12%. Patients awaiting surgery should have thromboembolic prophylaxis.

26. INTERTROCHANTERIC FRACTURES

EPIDEMIOLOGY

- Intertrochanteric fractures account for nearly 50% of all fractures of the proximal femur.
- The average age of incidence is 66 to 76 years.
- The ratio of occurrence in women to men ranges from 2:1 to 8:1, likely due to postmenopausal metabolic changes in bone.

ANATOMY

- These fractures occur in the region between the greater and lesser trochanters of the proximal femur, occasionally extending into the subtrochanteric region.
- These are extracapsular fractures that occur in cancellous bone with an abundant blood supply. As a result, nonunion and osteonecrosis are not major problems, as in femoral neck fractures.
- Deforming muscle forces will usually produce shortening, external rotation, and a varus position at the fracture site.
- Abductors tend to displace the greater trochanter laterally and proximally.
- The iliopsoas displaces the lesser trochanter medially and proximally.
- The hip flexors, extensors, and adductors pull the distal fragment proximally.
- Fracture stability is determined by the presence of posteromedial bony contact, which acts as a buttress against fracture collapse.

MECHANISM OF INJURY

- Direct: trauma to the greater trochanter. The overwhelming majority result from a fall.
- Indirect: muscle forces transmitted to the intertrochanteric area.

CLINICAL EVALUATION

- Patients typically present as nonambulatory with the injured lower extremity markedly foreshortened in external rotation.
- Range of motion is typically painful with variable crepitus, and the hip presents with variable swelling and ecchymosis.
- Common associated injuries include fractures of the distal radius, proximal humerus, ribs, and spine (compression fractures). Careful assessment of the patient is necessary to ensure that these diagnoses are not overlooked.
- Patients may have experienced delays of up to days before being discovered, usually on the floor and without oral intake. The examiner must therefore be cognizant of potential dehydration, nutritional and pressure ulceration issues, and hemodynamic instability because intertrochanteric fractures may be associated with as much as a full unit of hemorrhage into the fracture site.

RADIOGRAPHIC EVALUATION

- Anteroposterior views of the pelvis and hip (internal rotation) and a cross-table lateral view should be obtained.
- Technetium bone scan or magnetic resonance imaging may be of clinical utility in delineating nondisplaced or occult fractures that are not readily apparent on plain radiographs.

BOYD AND GRIFFIN CLASSIFICATION (FIG. 26.1)

Type I: a single fracture along the intertrochanteric line, stable and easily reducible

Type II: major fracture line along the intertrochanteric line with comminution in the coronal plane

Type III: fracture at the level of the lesser trochanter with variable comminution and extension into the subtrochanteric region (reverse obliquity)

Type IV: fracture extending into the proximal femoral shaft in at least two planes

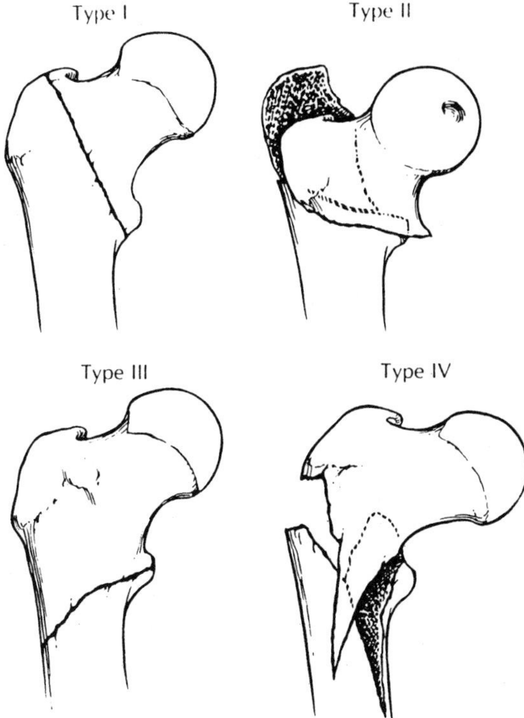

FIG. 26.1. The Boyd and Griffin classification of trochanteric fractures. (From Boyd HB, Griffin LL. Classification and treatment of trochanteric fractures. *Arch Surg* 1949;58: 853–866, with permission.)

EVANS CLASSIFICATION (FIG. 26.2)

Based on pre- and postreduction stability—that is, the convertibility of an unstable fracture configuration to a stable reduction.

Type I: Primary fracture line extending from lesser trochanter proximally and laterally; subdivided based on initial stability and stability after reduction.
Type II: Reverse obliquity fractures; inherently unstable despite an adequate reduction due to the pull of the abductors on the proximal fragment and to the pull of the adductors on the distal fragment.

KYLE CLASSFICATION

Type I: nondisplaced, stable
Type II: displaced into varus with a small lesser trochanteric fragment; stable
Type III: displaced into varus with posteromedial comminution, greater trochanteric fracture; unstable
Type IV: type III with subtrochanteric extension

ORTHOPAEDIC TRAUMA ASSOCIATION CLASSIFICATION OF INTERTROCHANTERIC FRACTURES (FIG. 26.3)

Type A1: pertrochanteric simple (the typical oblique fracture line extending from the greater trochanter to the medial cortex; the lateral cortex of the greater trochanter remains intact—two fragments)

(*text continues on page 186*)

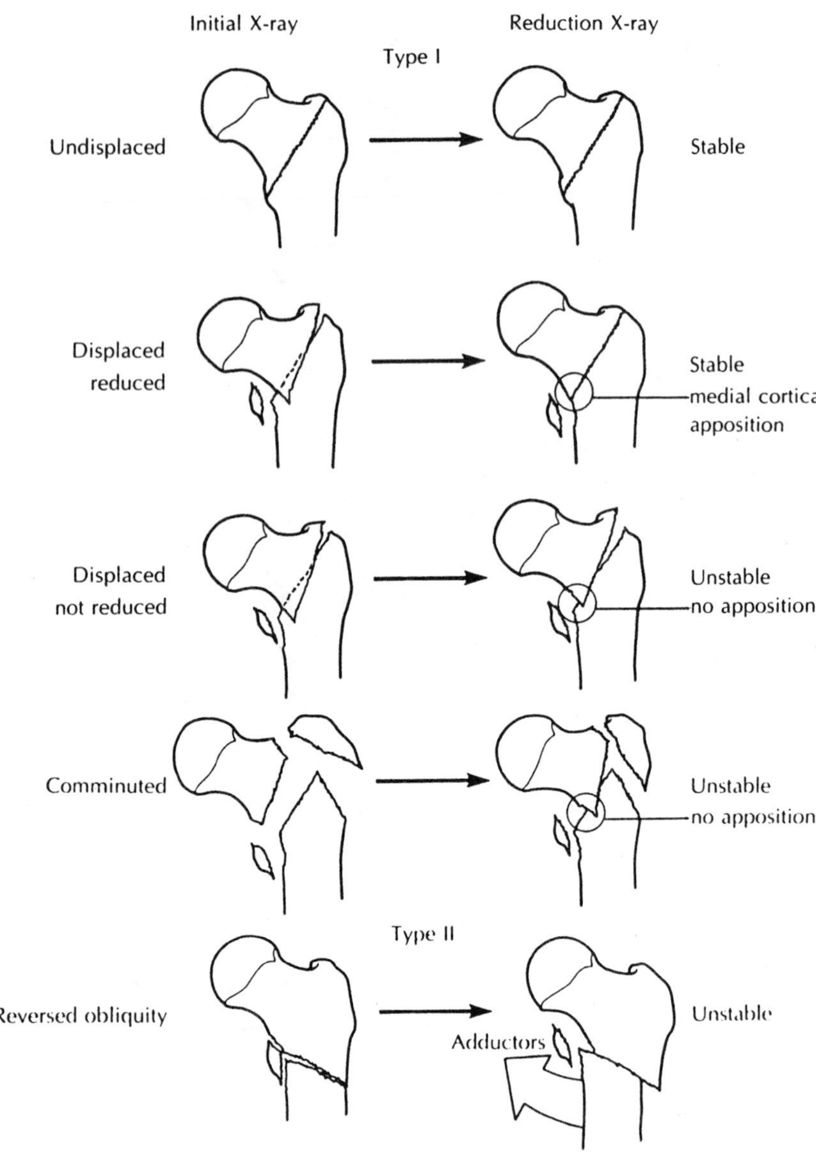

FIG. 26.2. The Evans classification of intertrochanteric fractures is divided into two main types depending on the direction of the fracture. In type I, the fracture line extends upward and outward from the lesser trochanter. In type II, the fracture line is one of reversed obliquity. Stability in type I fractures is obtained by anatomic medical cortical reduction. Type II fractures have a tendency toward medial displacement of the femoral shaft and hence retain a degree of instability. (From Rockwood CA Jr, Green DP, Bucholz RW, Heckman JD, eds. *Rockwood and Green's fractures in adults*, 4th ed. Vol. 2. Philadelphia: Lippincott-Raven, 1996:1721, with permission.)

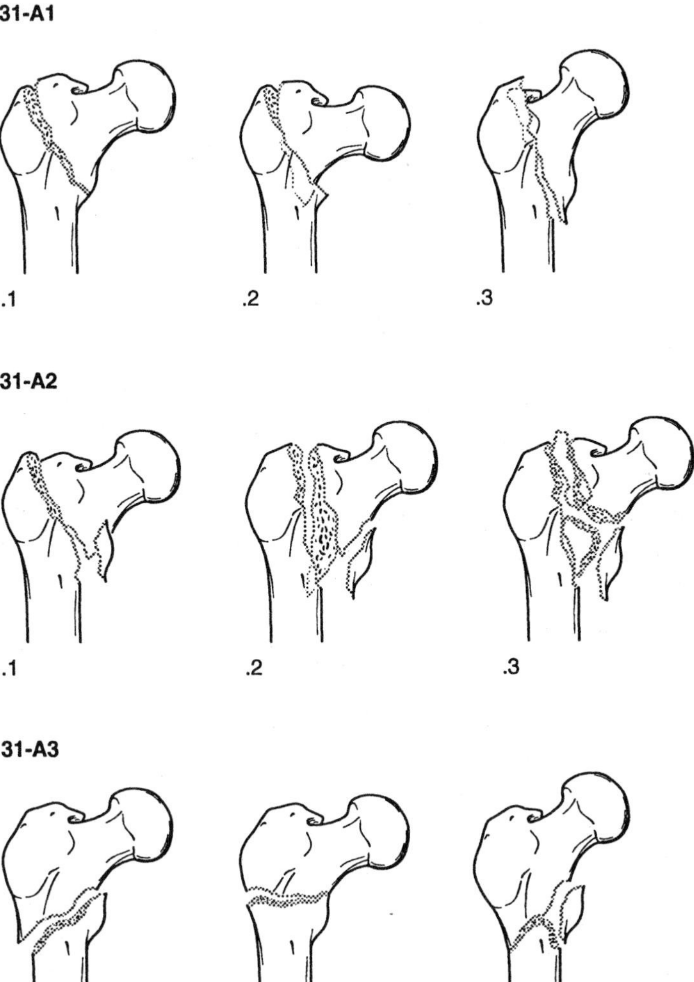

FIG. 26.3. In the Orthopaedic Trauma Association (OTA) alphanumeric fracture classification, intertrochanteric hip fractures are type 31A. These fractures are divided into three groups, and each group is further divided into subgroups based on obliquity of the fracture line and degree of comminution. Group 1 fractures are simple (two-part) fractures, with the typical oblique fracture line extending from the greater trochanter to the medial cortex; the lateral cortex of the greater trochanter is intact. Group 2 fractures are comminuted with a posteromedial fragment; the lateral cortex of the greater trochanter, however, remains intact. Fractures in this group are generally unstable, depending on the size of the medial fragment. Group 3 fractures are those in which the fracture line extends across both the medial and lateral cortices; this group includes the reverse obliquity pattern. (Adapted from OTA. Fracture and dislocation compendium. *J Orthop Trauma* 1996;10:31–35, with permission.)

A1.1: along the intertrochanteric line
A1.2: through the greater trochanter
A1.3: below the lesser trochanter

Type A2: pertrochanteric multifragmentary (the typical oblique fracture line extending from the greater trochanter to the medial cortex; the lateral cortex of the greater trochanter remains intact—separate posteromedial fragment)

A2.1: with one intermediate fragment
A2.2: with several intermediate fragments
A2.3: extending more than 1 cm below the lesser trochanter

Type A3: intertrochanteric (fracture line extends across both the medial and lateral cortices)

A3.1: simple oblique (reverse obliquity pattern)
A3.2: simple transverse
A3.3: multifragmentary

TREATMENT

Nonoperative Treatment

- Indicated only for patients who are at extreme medical risk for surgery; may also be considered for demented nonambulators.
- Early bed-to-chair mobilization is critical to avoid increased risks and complications of prolonged recumbency, including potential poor pulmonary toilet, atelectasis, venous stasis, and pressure ulceration.
- Resultant hip deformity is both expected and accepted.
- This treatment is associated with a higher mortality rate than operative treatment.

Operative Treatment

- The goal is stable internal fixation to allow early mobilization and full weight-bearing ambulation. Stability of fracture fixation depends on the following:
  - Bone quality;
  - Fracture pattern;
  - Fracture reduction;
  - Implant design;
  - Implant placement.
- The sliding hip screw is the most commonly used device for both stable and unstable fracture patterns. It is available in plate angles from 130 to 150 degrees.
  - Provides optimal strain distribution with compressive forces across the medial calcar and low tensile strain at the lateral cortex.
  - Most important technical aspect of screw insertion is placement within 1 cm of subchondral bone; provides secure fixation and central position in the femoral head.
  - Four percent to 12% incidence of loss of fixation reported, most commonly with unstable fracture patterns.
  - Most failures of fixation attributable to technical problems of screw placement and/or to inadequate impaction of the fracture fragments at the time of screw insertion.
- Intramedullary hip screw—the features of a sliding hip screw and an intramedullary nail.
  - Advantages are both technical and mechanical: theoretically they can be inserted in a closed manner with limited fracture exposure, decreased blood loss and less tissue damage than a sliding hip screw. In addition, these devices are subjected to a lower bending moment than the sliding hip screw due to their intramedullary location.
  - Studies have demonstrated no clinical advantage of the intramedullary hip screw when compared with the sliding hip screw.
  - Use of intramedullary hip screws has been associated with an increased risk of femur fracture at the nail tip or distal locking screw insertion point.
- Prosthetic replacement successfully used for patients who have had failed open reduction and internal fixation and who are unsuitable for repeat internal fixation.
  - A calcar replacement hemiarthroplasty or bipolar endoprosthesis is the implant of choice due to the level of the fracture.

Primary prosthetic replacement for comminuted unstable intertrochanteric fractures has yielded up to 94% good functional results.

Disadvantages include morbidity associated with a more extensive operative procedure and the risk of postoperative prosthetic dislocation.

- Biomechanical studies clearly demonstrate the improved stress distributions of anatomic reduction over displacement osteotomies.

Special Considerations

- Large posteromedial fragments in younger individuals should receive fixation with cerclage wires or a lag screw to restore the posteromedial buttress.
- Greater trochanteric displacement should be fixed using tension band techniques.
- Reverse obliquity fractures are best treated as subtrochanteric fractures.
- Ipsilateral fractures of the femoral shaft, though more common in association with femoral neck fractures, should be ruled out when the injury is due to high energy trauma.

COMPLICATIONS

- Loss of fixation: most commonly due to varus collapse of the proximal fragment with cut-out of the lag screw from the femoral head with incidence of fixation failure reported to be as high as 20% in unstable fracture patterns. Lag screw cut-out from the femoral head generally occurs within three months of surgery and is usually due to one the following:

  Eccentric placement of the lag screw within the femoral head.

  Improper reaming that creates a second channel.

  Inability to obtain a stable reduction.

  Excessive fracture collapse such that the sliding capacity of the device is exceeded.

  Inadequate screw-barrel engagement, which prevents sliding.

  Severe osteopenia, which precludes secure fixation.

  Management choices include acceptance of the deformity; revision open reduction and internal fixation, which may require methylmethacrylate; and conversion to prosthetic replacement. Acceptance of the deformity should be considered in marginal ambulators who are a poor surgical risk. Revision open reduction and internal fixation is indicated in younger patients, whereas conversion to prosthetic replacement (unipolar, bipolar, or total hip replacement) is preferred in the elderly patient with osteopenic bone.
- Nonunion: rare; occurring in less than 2% of patients; often found in patients with unstable fracture patterns. The diagnosis should be suspected in a patient with persistent hip pain and radiographs revealing a persistent radiolucency at the fracture site 4 to 7 months after fracture fixation. With adequate bone stock, repeat internal fixation combined with a valgus osteotomy and bone grafting may be considered. In most elderly individuals, conversion to a calcar replacement prosthesis is preferred.
- Malrotation deformity: results from internal rotation of the distal fragment at the time of internal fixation. When so severe that it interferes with ambulation, revision surgery with plate removal and rotational osteotomy of the femoral shaft should be considered.
- Osteonecrosis of the femoral head: rare after intertrochanteric fracture.
- Lag screw-sideplate separation.
- Lag screw migration into the pelvis.
- Laceration of the superficial femoral artery by a displaced lesser trochanter fragment.

27. TROCHANTERIC FRACTURES

GREATER TROCHANTER

Epidemiology

- Isolated greater trochanteric fractures are rare.
- They occur in a bimodal distribution:
  - Pediatric: ages 7 to 17 years; occur as a result of avulsion of the entire greater trochanteric apophysis.
  - Adult: elderly; occur as a result of trauma, typically associated with later trochanteric fractures of the proximal femur.

Anatomy

- The pull of the abductors typically results in characteristic displacement of the trochanteric fragment in a proximally and laterally displaced abducted position.
- The attachment of the short external rotators may account for rotational displacement.
- Displacement is typically limited by the remaining intact fibers of the gluteus medius that attach distal to the fracture line.

Mechanism of Injury

- Direct: low energy (falls in the elderly) or high energy (motor vehicle accidents or falls from heights in younger adults) trauma.
- Indirect: sudden, eccentric muscle contraction in a skeletally immature individual.

Clinical Evaluation

- Patients typically complain of pain about the lateral aspect of the hip and buttock, which may increase with range of hip motion and weight bearing.
- Swelling, tenderness, and variable ecchymosis may be present, with potential hip flexion due to muscle spasm.

Radiographic Evaluation

- Anteroposterior view of the pelvis (for comparison with the opposite hip) and anteroposterior and cross-table lateral views of the involved hip.
- The greater trochanter is typically displaced as was previously discussed.

DESCRIPTIVE CLASSIFICATION

- Associated fractures
- Displacement
- Angulation
- Rotation
- Comminution

Treatment

Nonoperative Treatment

- Treatment is usually nonoperative and involves the use of nonnarcotic analgesics and assisted weight bearing. Full weight bearing usually is achieved by 4 to 6 weeks following injury.
- Because only a portion of the greater trochanter is usually involved, abductor muscle function is largely preserved; even fractures displaced >1 cm can be expected to heal by osseous or fibrous union with restoration of abductor function.

Operative Treatment

- Operative management should be considered in younger active patients who have a widely displaced greater trochanter (>1 cm).
- Through a lateral incision, operative fixation may be achieved via the use of screws, wires, or heavy suture. Tension band wiring of the displaced fragment and the attached abductor muscles is the preferred technique.

- Postoperatively, the patient is allowed to bear weight gradually with the use of crutches for 3 to 4 weeks.

Complications

- *Malunion.* Fractures that are widely displaced and are treated nonoperatively may heal in proximal or abducted positioning, resulting in residual abductor weakness due to loss of mechanical advantage. Although this is rarely clinically significant, patients with severe weakness and gait alterations may be treated with osteotomy and internal fixation.
- *Nonunion.* This is extremely rare; it is related to wide displacement (>1 cm) without reduction and fixation.

LESSER TROCHANTERIC FRACTURES

Epidemiology

- Isolated fractures of the lesser trochanter are seen most often in children and in young adults.
- Peak incidence is between 12 and 16 years of age, with 85% of cases occurring before the age of 20 years.
- These fractures are uncommon in the elderly population and are directly related to the degree of osteoporosis or the presence of pathologic lesions of the proximal femur.

Anatomy

- In cases of severe osteoporosis, rarefaction of the trabecular structure of the lesser trochanter may occur, resulting in diminished mechanical strength and a predisposition to failure by avulsion mechanisms.
- The lesser trochanter is the site of insertion of the iliopsoas, the primary function of which is hip flexion.

Mechanism of Injury

- Young adults and adolescents: occurs secondary to forceful iliopsoas contracture, resulting in avulsion of the lesser trochanteric apophysis.
- Elderly: associated with pathologic lesions of the proximal femur, including tumor or severe osteoporosis, that diminish mechanical strength such that the fracture may occur with normal loading.

Clinical Evaluation

- Patients typically present as ambulatory but with tenderness and vague swelling in the femoral triangle.
- The Ludloff test of iliopsoas insufficiency is used; the patient who is sitting on the edge of the examining table is unable to flex the hip off the table against gravity resistance. Some active flexion of the hip may be retained in the face of complete fracture as the distal-most fibers of the iliacus may insert 2 cm distal and anterior to the lesser trochanter.

Radiographic Evaluation

- Anteroposterior and lateral views of the affected hip should be obtained.
- In cases of complete fracture, the lesser trochanteric fragment may be displaced proximally and medially.
- The radiographs should be scrutinized for evidence of pathologic lesion or generalized osteopenia.

DESCRIPTIVE CLASSIFICATION

- Displacement
- Angulation
- Rotation

Treatment

- If a pathologic process is identified, treatment will be based on the nature of the lesion and extent of involvement.
- If no evidence of a pathologic lesion is found, treatment should be symptomatic and should be directed at regaining range of hip motion and ambulatory function.
- Most authors agree that bedrest (without immobilization) and increasing weight bearing as tolerated will result in full, painless, active hip flexion at 3 weeks following injury.
- Open reduction and internal fixation has been advocated by some authors for severe displacement, although most agree that this is unnecessary.

Complications

Nonunion: extremely rare; no specific treatment is indicated as sufficient hip flexion is typically present for daily activities.

28. SUBTROCHANTERIC FRACTURES

EPIDEMIOLOGY

- Subtrochanteric fractures associated with high energy injuries have a high affinity with multisystem injuries and other skeletal injuries to the pelvis, spine, or long bones.
- Ten percent of high energy subtrochanteric fractures are due to gunshot injuries.

ANATOMY

- A subtrochanteric femur fracture is a fracture between the lesser trochanter and a point 5 cm distal to the lesser trochanter.
- The subtrochanteric segment of the femur is the site of very high biomechanical stresses. The medial and posteromedial cortices are the sites of high compressive forces, whereas the lateral cortex experiences high tensile forces. Strain-gauge studies have shown that the compressive stresses in the medial cortex are significantly higher than are the tensile stresses in the lateral cortex. Therefore, in treating these fractures, restoration of the medial cortex in subtrochanteric fractures is important.
- The subtrochanteric area of the femur is composed mainly of cortical bone. Therefore, less vascularity is found in this region, and the potential for healing is diminished when compared with intertrochanteric fractures.
- The deforming muscle forces on the proximal fragment include abduction by the gluteus, external rotation by the short external rotators, and flexion by the iliopsoas. The distal fragment is pulled proximally and into varus by the adductors.

MECHANISM OF INJURY

- Low energy mechanisms: elderly patients suffering a minor fall in which the fracture occurs through weakened bone.
- High energy mechanisms: younger patients with normal bone incurring injuries from motor vehicle accidents, gunshot wounds, or falls from a height.
- Pathologic fracture: accounts for 17% to 35% of all subtrochanteric fractures.

CLINICAL EVALUATION

- Patients involved in high energy trauma should receive full trauma evaluation.
- Patients typically present nonambulatory with varying degrees of gross deformity of the lower extremity.
- Range of motion is extremely painful, with tenderness to palpation and swelling of the proximal thigh.
- Because substantial forces are required to produce this fracture pattern in younger patients, associated injuries should be expected and should be carefully evaluated, especially those of the hip and knee.
- Field dressings or splints should be completely removed, and the injury site should be examined for evidence of soft-tissue compromise or open injury.
- The thigh represents a capacious compartment into which volume loss due to hemorrhage may be significant; thus, monitoring for hypovolemic shock should be undertaken, with invasive monitoring as necessary.
- Provisional splinting until definitive fixation should be performed to limit further soft-tissue damage and hemorrhage.
- A careful neurovascular examination is important to rule out associated injuries, although neurovascular compromise related to the subtrochanteric fracture is uncommon.

RADIOGRAPHIC EVALUATION

- An anteroposterior view of the pelvis and anteroposterior and lateral views of the hip should be obtained.
- Associated injuries should be evaluated; and if any are suspected, appropriate radiographic evaluation should ensue.

FIELDING CLASSIFICATION (FIG. 28.1)

Based on the location of the primary fracture line in relation to the lesser trochanter.

Type I: at level of the lesser trochanter
Type II: <2.5 cm below the lesser trochanter
Type III: 2.5 to 5 cm below the lesser trochanter

SEINSHEIMER CLASSIFICATION (FIG. 28.2)

Based on the number of major bone fragments and the location and shape of the fracture lines.

Type I: nondisplaced fracture or any fracture with <2 mm of displacement of the fracture fragments
Type II: two-part fractures
- IIA: two-part transverse femoral fracture
- IIB: two-part spiral fracture with the lesser trochanter attached to the proximal fragment
- IIC: two-part spiral fracture with the lesser trochanter attached to the distal fragment

Type III: three-part fractures
- IIIA: three-part spiral fracture in which the lesser trochanter is part of the third fragment, which has an inferior spike of cortex of varying length
- IIIB: three-part spiral fracture of the proximal third of the femur, where the third part is a butterfly fragment

Type IV: comminuted fracture with four or more fragments
Type V: subtrochanteric-intertrochanteric fracture, including any subtrochanteric fracture with extension through the greater trochanter

RUSSELL-TAYLOR CLASSIFICATION

Created in response to the development of first- and second-generation interlocked nails.

Type I: fractures with an intact piriformis fossa in which the following are found:
- IA: lesser trochanter is attached to the proximal fragment.
- IB: lesser trochanter is detached from the proximal fragment.

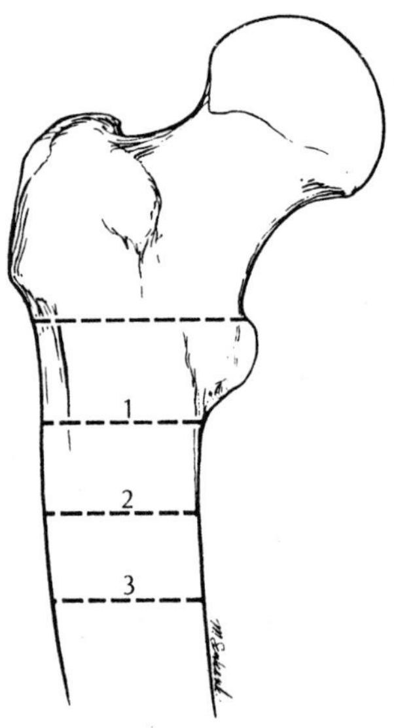

FIG. 28.1. Fielding classification of subtrochanteric fractures. (From Rockwood CA Jr, Green DP, Bucholz RW, Heckman JD, eds. *Rockwood and Green's fractures in adults*, 4th ed. Vol. 2. Philadelphia: Lippincott-Raven, 1996:1742, with permission.)

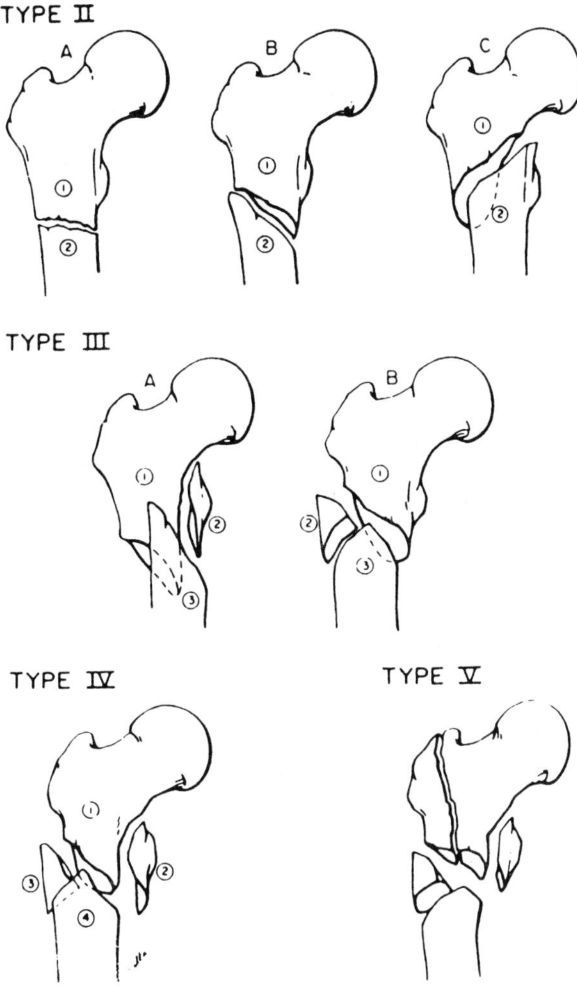

FIG. 28.2. Seinsheimer classification of subtrochanteric fractures. (From Heckman JD, Bucholz RW, eds. *Rockwood, Green, and Wilkins' fractures in adults*, 5th ed. Philadelphia: Lippincott Williams & Wilkins, 2001, with permission.)

Type II: fractures that extend into the piriformis fossa as follows:
- IIA: a stable medial construct (posteromedial cortex) found.
- IIB: comminution of the piriformis fossa and lesser trochanter, associated with varying degrees of femoral shaft comminution.

ORTHOPAEDIC TRAUMA ASSOCIATION CLASSIFICATION OF SUBTROCHANTERIC FRACTURES

Based on fracture pattern and degree of comminution; it does not take into account the degree of fracture displacement.

Type A: two-part fractures
- A1: spiral

A2: oblique
A3: transverse
Type B: fractures with a butterfly fragment
B1: spiral wedge
B2: bending wedge
B3: comminuted wedge
Type C: complex comminuted fractures
C1: comminuted spiral
C2: segmental
C3: irregular pattern

TREATMENT

Nonoperative Treatment

- Skeletal traction in the 90-degree/90-degree position is followed by spica casting or cast bracing.
- Nonoperative treatment is reserved only for elderly patients who are very poor operative candidates.
- Nonoperative treatment generally results in increased morbidity and mortality and in nonunion, delayed union, and malunion with varus angulation, rotational deformity, and shortening.

Operative Treatment

Interlocking Nails

- First generation (centromedullary) nail is indicated for subtrochanteric fractures with both trochanters intact.
- Second generation (cephalomedullary) nail (i.e., reconstruction nail) is indicated for fractures with loss of the posteromedial cortex.
- Second-generation nails can also be used for fractures extending into the piriformis fossa, but they are technically more difficult to insert.

Ninety-five–degree Fixed Angle Plates

- Russell-Taylor type II fractures are difficult to stabilize with an intramedullary device and are perhaps better treated with a sliding hip screw or a 95-degree fixed-angle device.
- A 95-degree condylar blade plate and dynamic compression screw are best suited for fractures involving both trochanters so that an accessory cancellous screw can be inserted beneath the blade into the calcar to increase proximal fixation.
- These devices function as a tension band when the posteromedial cortex is restored. A dynamic compression screw is technically easier to insert than is the blade plate.

Sliding Hip Screw

- A sliding mechanism allows impaction of fracture surfaces and medial displacement of the femoral shaft relative to the proximal fragment, which serves to reduce the bending moment on the implant and thus to decrease the possibility of varus displacement or device failure.
- However, the sliding mechanism must cross the fracture site and the plate must not be fixed to the proximal fragment for impaction to occur, a situation that can be obtained only in proximal subtrochanteric fractures—specifically, in those with both subtrochanteric and intertrochanteric involvement.
- Reconstructing the posteromedial cortical buttress to minimize the risk of varus displacement and device failure is essential when it is used to reduce more distal fractures or comminuted fractures.

Zickel Nail

- Used less frequently than formerly; superseded by improved devices. Problems include comminution of the greater trochanter and difficulty in controlling rotational stability of the distal fragment.
- A high incidence of refracture occurs during nail extraction, likely due to the geometry of the nail. Used mainly for pathologic fractures, elderly patients, and some nonunions.

Condylocephalic Nails
- Ender nail, a representative type.
- Complications: distal or proximal nail migration; loss of fixation; knee pain.

Bone Grafting
- Closed reduction techniques have decreased the need for bone grafting because fracture fragments are not devascularized to the same extent as in open reduction.
- The bone graft, if needed, should be inserted through the fracture site, usually before plate application.

Open Subtrochanteric Fractures
- These fractures are rare and are almost always associated with either penetrating injury or high energy trauma from a motor vehicle accident or a fall from a height.
- Treatment is immediate surgical debridement and osseous stabilization.
- One should use the minimal amount of fixation necessary to stabilize the subtrochanteric fracture adequately.
- With the advent of smaller diameter cephalomedullary nails, a nonreamed interlocked nail may be used for the treatment of these types of open subtrochanteric fractures.

COMPLICATIONS
- Loss of fixation:
  - Plate and screw devices: implant failure usually occurs secondary to screw cutout from the femoral head and neck in patients with osteopenic bone. Treatment for failure of fixation involves removal of hardware, revision internal fixation with either a plate and screws or an interlocked nail, and bone grafting.
  - Interlocked nails: loss of fixation is commonly related to failure to lock the device statically, comminution of the entry portal, or the use of small-diameter nails.
- Nonunion: may be evident by a patient's inability to resume full weight bearing within 3 to 6 months and his or her symptoms of unremitting pain about the proximal thigh and pain with attempted weight bearing. Nonunion usually occurs in the femoral shaft portion of the fracture.
- Those that develop after intramedullary nailing can be treated by implant removal, followed by repeat reaming and placement of a larger diameter intramedullary nail.
- Malunion: patient complains of limp, leg length discrepancy, or rotational deformity.
  - A valgus osteotomy and revision internal fixation with bone grafting is the treatment of choice for a varus malreduction.
  - Leg length discrepancy is a complex problem that is more likely to occur after a fracture with extensive femoral shaft comminution that has been stabilized with a dynamically locked rather than a statically locked nail construct.
  - Malrotation may occur with the use of a plate and screws or an intramedullary nail if the surgeon is not alert to this potential complication.

29. PELVIS

EPIDEMIOLOGY

Most pelvic fractures arise as a result of high energy trauma as follows:
57%, motor vehicle accidents;
18%, pedestrian injuries;
9%, motorcycle accidents;
9%, falls from a height;
4%, crush mechanisms.

ANATOMY

- The *pelvic ring* is composed of the sacrum and two innominate bones joined anteriorly at the symphysis and posteriorly at the paired sacroiliac joints.
- The *innominate* bone is formed at maturity by the fusion of three ossification centers: the ilium, the ischium, and the pubis through the triradiate cartilage at the dome of the acetabulum.
- The *pelvic brim* is an imaginary division formed by the arcuate lines that join the sacral promontory posteriorly and the superior pubis anteriorly. Below this is the *true* or *lesser* pelvis, in which is contained the pelvic viscera. Above this is the *false* or *greater* pelvis, which represents the inferior aspect of the abdominal cavity.
- Inherent stability of the pelvis is conferred by vital ligamentous structures. These may be divided into four groups according to the ligamentous attachments as follows:
  1. *Sacrum to ilium.* The strongest and most important ligamentous structures are found in the posterior aspect of the pelvis connecting the sacrum to the innominate bones.
     - The *sacroiliac ligamentous complex* is divided into posterior (short and long) and anterior ligaments. Posterior ligaments provide most of the stability.
     - The *sacrotuberous ligament* runs from the posterolateral aspect of the sacrum and the dorsal aspect of the posterior iliac spine to the ischial tuberosity. This ligament, in association with the posterior sacroiliac ligaments, is especially important in helping maintain vertical stability of the pelvis.
     - The *sacrospinous ligament* is triangular, running from the lateral margins of the sacrum and coccyx and inserting on the ischial spine. It is most important for maintaining rotational control of the pelvis if the posterior sacroiliac ligaments are intact.
  2. *Sacrum to ischium.*
  3. *Sacrum to coccyx.*
  4. *Pubis to pubis.* Symphysis pubis.
- Additional stability is conferred by ligamentous attachments between the lumbar spine and pelvic ring:
  1. The *iliolumbar ligaments* originate from the L-4 and L-5 transverse processes and insert on the posterior iliac crest.
  2. The *lumbosacral ligaments* originate from the transverse process of L-5 to the ala of the sacrum.
- The transversely placed ligaments resist rotational forces and include the short posterior sacroiliac, anterior sacroiliac, iliolumbar, and sacrospinous ligaments.
- The vertically placed ligaments resist vertical shear and include the long posterior sacroiliac, sacrotuberous, and lateral lumbosacral ligaments.

PELVIC STABILITY

- A stable injury is defined as one that can withstand normal physiologic forces without abnormal deformation.
- Penetrating trauma infrequently results in pelvic ring destabilization.
- An unstable injury may be characterized by the type of displacement, as follows:
  - Rotationally unstable (open and externally rotated or compressed and internally rotated);
  - Vertically unstable.

Mcbroom and Tile Research Results

The results from sectioning ligaments of the pelvis to determine relative contributions to pelvic stability (these include bony equivalents to ligamentous disruptions) were as follows:

- Symphysis: pubic diastasis <2.5 cm;
- Symphysis and sacrospinous ligaments: >2.5 cm of pubic diastasis (note that these are rotational movements and not vertical or posterior displacements);
- Symphysis, sacrospinous, sacrotuberous, and posterior sacroiliac: unstable vertically, posteriorly, and rotationally.

MECHANISM OF INJURY

- Injuries may be divided into low energy injuries, which typically result in fractures of individual bones, and high energy fractures, which may lead to pelvic ring disruption.
  - Low energy injuries may result from sudden muscular contractions in young athletes, resulting in domestic falls and in avulsion injuries and straddle-type injuries.
  - High energy injuries typically result from motor vehicle accidents, struck pedestrian mechanisms, motorcycle accidents, falls from heights, and crush mechanisms.
- Impact injuries result when a moving victim strikes a stationary object or vice versa. Direction, magnitude, and nature of the force all contribute to the type of fracture.
- Crush injuries occur when a victim is trapped between the injurious force and an unyielding environment, such as the ground or pavement. In addition to those factors mentioned previously, the position of the victim, the duration of the crush, and whether the force was direct or a "roll-over" (resulting in a changing force vector) are important for understanding the fracture pattern.
- Specific injury patterns vary as follows by the direction of force application:
  1. Anteroposterior force can cause the following:
     - External rotation of the hemipelvis.
     - Pelvis springs open, hinging on the intact posterior ligaments.
  2. Lateral compression force is the most common and results in impaction of cancellous bone through the sacroiliac joint and sacrum. The injury pattern depends on the location of force application as follows:
     - Posterior half of the ilium: classic lateral compression with minimal soft-tissue disruption. This is a stable configuration.
     - Anterior half of the iliac wing: rotation of the hemipelvis inward; may disrupt the posterior sacroiliac ligamentous complex. If this force continues to push the hemipelvis across to the contralateral side, it will push the contralateral hemipelvis out into external rotation, producing lateral compression on the ipsilateral side and an external rotation injury on the contralateral side.
     - Greater trochanteric region: may be associated with a transverse acetabular fracture.
  3. An external rotation abduction force commonly occurs in motorcycle accidents and is applied as follows:
     - Force application through the femoral shafts and head when the leg is caught and externally rotated and abducted.
     - Tends to tear the hemipelvis from the sacrum.
  4. A shear force acts as follows:
     - Leads to a completely unstable fracture with triplanar instability secondary to disruption of the sacrospinous and sacrotuberous ligaments.
     - Bone strength is less than ligamentous strength in the elderly individual; fails first.
     - Bone strength is greater in a young individual; thus, ligamentous disruptions usually occur.

CLINICAL EVALUATION

1. Assess the patient: **A**irway, **B**reathing, **C**irculation, **D**isability. This should include a full trauma evaluation as necessary.

2. Initiate resuscitation: address life-threatening injuries.
3. Evaluate injuries to head, chest, abdomen, and spine.
4. Identify all injuries to extremities and pelvis with careful assessment of distal neurovascular status.
   - Pelvic instability may result in a leg-length discrepancy involving shortening on the involved side or a markedly internally or externally rotated pelvis. Ipsilateral lower extremity fractures must be ruled out.
   - The anteroposterior-lateral compression test for pelvic instability should be performed only once.
     "The first clot is the best clot." Once disrupted, subsequent thrombus formation of a retroperitoneal hemorrhage is difficult due to hemodilution by administered intravenous fluid and exhaustion of the body's coagulation factors by the original thrombus.
   - Massive flank or buttock contusions and swelling with hemorrhage are indicative of significant bleeding.
   - Palpation of the posterior aspect of the pelvis may reveal a large hematoma, a defect representing the fracture, or a dislocation of the sacroiliac joint. Palpation of the symphysis may also reveal a defect.
   - The perineum must be carefully inspected for the presence of a lesion representing an open fracture.
5. Monitor hemodynamic status. Retroperitoneal hemorrhage may be associated with massive intravascular volume loss. The usual etiology of retroperitoneal hemorrhage secondary to pelvic fracture is a disruption of the venous plexus in the posterior pelvis. It may also be caused by a large-vessel injury, such as external or internal iliac disruption. Large-vessel injury causes rapid massive hemorrhage with frequent loss of the distal pulse and marked hemodynamic instability. This often necessitates immediate surgical exploration to gain proximal control of the vessel before repair. The superior gluteal artery is occasionally injured and can be managed with rapid fluid resuscitation, appropriate stabilization of the pelvic ring, or embolization. Options for immediate control include the following:
   Application of military antishock trousers (MAST). This is typically performed in the field.
   Application of an anterior external fixator.
   Wrapping a sheet circumferentially around the pelvis.
   Application of a pelvic C-clamp.
   Open reduction and internal fixation. These may be undertaken if patient will be undergoing emergent laparotomy for other indications; they are frequently contraindicated by themselves as loss of a tamponade effect may encourage hemorrhage.
   Distal femoral traction, if necessary.
   Angiography/embolization. These measures should be considered if hemorrhage continues despite closing of the pelvic volume.
6. Assess neurologic injury: lumbosacral plexus and nerve root injuries may be present but may not be apparent in an unconscious patient.
7. Assess for genitourinary and gastrointestinal injury as follows:
   - Bladder injury: 20% incidence with pelvic trauma.
   - Urethral injury: 10% incidence with pelvic fractures; males much more frequent than females. To do so, check the following:
     Examine for blood at the urethral meatus or for expression of blood on catheterization.
     Examine for a high-riding or "floating" prostate on rectal examination.
     Clinical suspicion should be followed by a retrograde urethrogram.
   - Bowel injury: perforations in the rectum or anus due to osseous fragments are technically open injuries and should be treated as such. Infrequently, entrapment of the bowel in the fracture site with gastrointestinal obstruction may occur.

RADIOGRAPHIC EVALUATION

Standard trauma radiographs include an anteroposterior view of the chest, a lateral view of the cervical spine, an anteroposterior view of the abdomen, and an anteroposterior view of the pelvis.

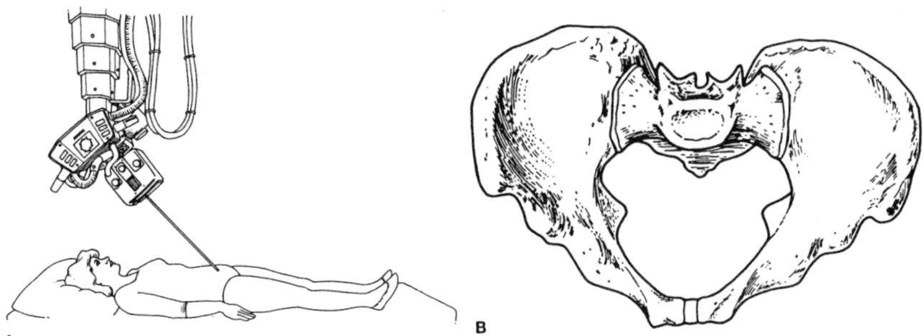

FIG. 29.1. Inlet view of the pelvis. **A.** Technique (after Tile). **B.** Artist's sketch. (From Rockwood CA Jr, Green DP, Bucholz RW, Heckman JD, eds. *Rockwood and Green's fractures in adults*, 4th ed. Vol. 2. Philadelphia: Lippincott-Raven, 1996:1599, with permission.)

- Anteroposterior radiograph of the pelvis. Note the following:
  - Anterior lesions: pubic rami fractures and symphysis displacement;
  - Sacroiliac joint and sacral fractures;
  - Iliac fractures;
  - L-5 transverse process fractures.
- Special views of the pelvis include the following:
  - Obturator and iliac oblique views: may be used on cases of suspected acetabular fractures (see Chapter 30).
  - Inlet radiograph (Fig. 29.1):
    - Taken in the supine position with the tube directed 60 degrees caudally, perpendicular to the pelvic brim.
    - Useful for determining anterior or posterior displacement of the sacroiliac joint, sacrum, or iliac wing.
    - May determine internal rotation deformities of the ilium and sacral impaction injuries.
  - Outlet radiograph (Fig. 29.2):
    - Taken in the supine position with the tube directed 45 degrees cephalad.
    - Useful for determination of vertical displacement of the hemipelvis.
    - May allow for visualization of subtle signs of pelvic disruption, such as a slightly widened sacroiliac joint, discontinuity of the sacral borders, nondisplaced sacral fractures, or disruption of the sacral foramina.

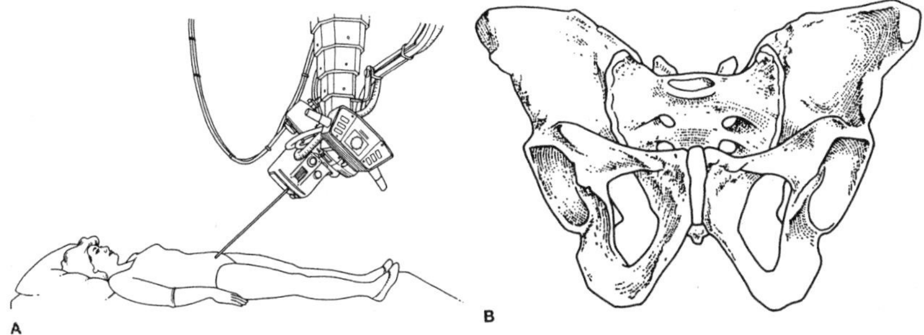

FIG. 29.2. Outlet view of the pelvis. **A.** Technique (after Tile). **B.** Artist's sketch. (From Rockwood CA Jr, Green DP, Bucholz RW, Heckman JD, eds. *Rockwood and Green's fractures in adults*, 4th ed. Vol. 2. Philadelphia: Lippincott-Raven, 1996:1599, with permission.)

- Computed tomography: revolutionized the assessment of the posterior structures of the pelvis by allowing superior visualization and resolution with the possibility of three-dimensional reconstruction.
- Magnetic resonance imaging: limited clinical utility due to limited access to a critically injured patient, prolonged duration of imaging, and equipment constraints. However, may provide superior imaging of genitourinary and pelvic vascular structures.
- Stress views: push-pull radiographs performed under general anesthesia to assess vertical stability.
    - Tile defined instability as ≥0.5 cm of motion.
    - Bucholz, Kellam, and Browner consider ≥1 cm of vertical displacement to be unstable.

YOUNG AND BURGESS CLASSIFICATION (FIG. 29.3)

Based on the mechanism of injury:

1. Lateral compression (LC): implosion of pelvis secondary to laterally applied force that shortens the anterior sacroiliac, sacrospinous, and sacrotuberous ligaments. May see transverse fractures of the pubic rami ipsilateral or contralateral to posterior injury.
    - Type I: Sacral impaction on the side of impact; transverse fractures of pubic rami; stable.
    - Type II: Posterior iliac wing fracture (crescent) on the side of impact with variable disruption of the posterior ligamentous structures resulting in variable mobility of the anterior fragment to internal rotation stress; maintains vertical and external rotational stability; may be associated with an anterior sacral crush injury.

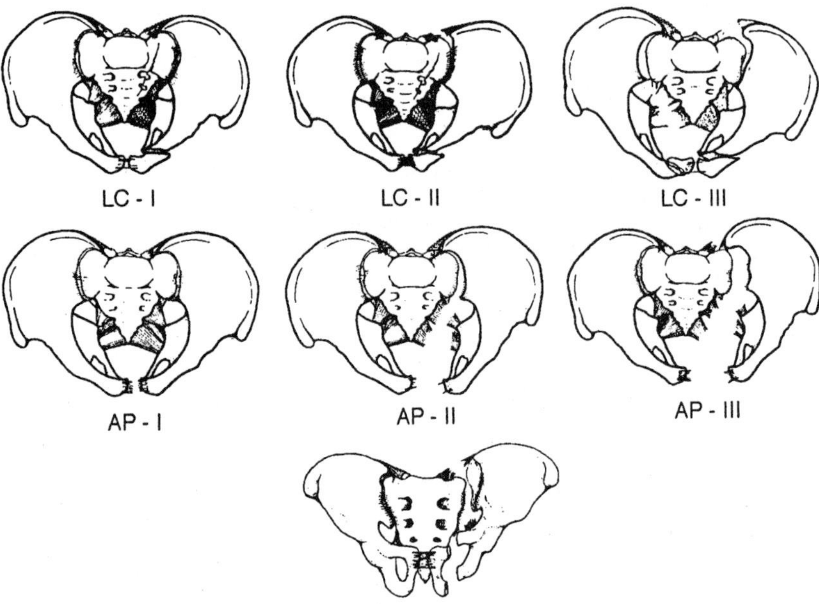

FIG. 29.3. Young and Burgess classification of pelvic ring fractures. (From Young JWR, Burgess AR. *Radiologic management of pelvic ring fractures*. Baltimore: Urban & Schwarzenberg, 1987, with permission.)

Type III: LC-I or LC-II injury on the side of impact; force continued to contralateral hemipelvis to produce an external rotation injury ("windswept pelvis") due to sacroiliac, sacrotuberous, and sacrospinous ligamentous disruption. Instability may result in hemorrhage and neurologic injury secondary to traction injury on the side of sacroiliac injury.

2. Anteroposterior compression: anteriorly applied force from direct impact or indirectly transferred via the lower extremities or ischial tuberosities resulting in external rotation injuries, symphyseal diastasis, or longitudinal rami fractures.
   Type I: <2.5 cm of symphyseal diastasis; vertical fractures of one or both pubic rami; intact posterior ligaments.
   Type II: >2.5 cm of symphyseal diastasis; widening of sacroiliac joints due to anterior sacroiliac ligament disruption; disruption of the sacrotuberous, sacrospinous, and symphyseal ligaments with intact posterior sacroiliac ligaments results in "open book" injury with internal and external rotational instability; vertical stability is maintained.
   Type III: Complete disruption of the symphysis, sacrotuberous, sacrospinous, and sacroiliac ligaments resulting in extreme rotational instability and lateral displacement; no cephaloposterior displacement; completely unstable with the highest rate of associated neurovascular injuries and blood loss.
3. Vertical shear: vertically or longitudinally applied forces due to falls onto an extended lower extremity, impacts from above, or motor vehicle accidents with an extended lower extremity against the floorboard or dashboard. These injuries are typically associated with complete disruption of the symphysis, sacrotuberous, sacrospinous, and sacroiliac ligaments resulting in extreme instability, most commonly in a cephaloposterior direction due to inclination of the pelvis; high associated incidence of neurovascular injury and hemorrhage.
4. Combined mechanical: combination of injuries often due to crush mechanisms; most common is vertical shear and lateral compression.

TILE CLASSIFICATION

Type A: stable.
- A1: fractures of the pelvis not involving the ring; avulsion injuries.
- A2: stable, minimal displacement of the ring.

Type B: rotationally unstable, vertically stable.
- B1: external rotation instability; open-book injury.
- B2: lateral compression injury; internal rotation instability; ipsilateral only.
- B3: lateral compression injury; bilateral rotational instability (bucket handle).

Type C: rotationally and vertically unstable.
- C1: unilateral injury.
- C2: bilateral injury; one side rotationally unstable, with contralateral side vertically unstable.
- C3: bilateral injury; both sides rotationally and vertically unstable with associated acetabular fracture.

ORTHOPAEDIC TRAUMA ASSOCIATION CLASSIFICATION OF PELVIC FRACTURES

Type A: fracture of pelvic ring, stable.
- A1: fracture of innominate bone, avulsion.
- A2: fracture of innominate bone, direct impact.
- A3: transverse fracture of sacrum and coccyx.

Type B: fracture of the pelvic ring, partially stable.
- B1: unilateral, partial disruption of posterior arch, external rotation (open book injury).
- B2: unilateral, partial disruption of posterior arch, internal rotation (lateral compression injury).
- B3: bilateral, partial lesion of posterior arch.

Type C: Fracture of the pelvic ring, unstable disruption of posterior arch.
- C1: unilateral, complete disruption of posterior arch.
- C2: bilateral, ipsilateral complete, contralateral incomplete disruption of posterior arch.
- C3: bilateral, complete disruption of posterior arch.

TREATMENT

The recommended management of pelvic fractures varies from institution to institution, highlighting the fact that these are difficult injuries to treat.

Tile: Stabilization Options

1. Stable (A1, A2): stable, minimally displaced fractures with minimal disruption of the bony and ligamentous stability of the pelvic ring may successfully be treated with protected weight bearing and symptomatic treatment.
2. Open book (B1)
   - Symphyseal diastasis <2 cm: protected weight bearing and symptomatic treatment.
   - Symphyseal diastasis >2 cm: external fixation or symphyseal plate (preferred for laparotomy for associated injuries and no open injury).
3. Lateral compression (B2, B3)
   - Ipsilateral only: elastic recoil restores pelvic anatomy. No stabilization necessary.
   - Contralateral (bucket handle): posterior sacral complex commonly compressed.
     - Leg-length discrepancy <1.5 cm: no stabilization necessary.
     - Leg-length discrepancy >1.5 cm: external fixation versus open reduction and internal fixation (ORIF).
4. Rotationally and vertically unstable (C1, C2, C3): external fixation with or without skeletal traction or ORIF.

General Treatment Options

- *External fixation.* A common external frame design is a rectangular construct mounted on two to three 5-mm pins spaced 1 cm apart along the anterior iliac crest. Postoperative plan for immobilization is as follows:
  - ***Lateral compression.*** External fixation for 3 to 6 weeks is advised with mobilization dependent on the patient's comorbid injuries.
  - ***Anteroposterior compression.*** External fixation is for 8 to 12 weeks, depending on the integrity of the posterior sacroiliac ligaments.
  - ***Vertical shear.*** External fixation is for 12 weeks with mobilization guided by radiographic evidence of healing. This may require combination with open reduction and internal fixation for adequate stabilization.
  - ***Complications.*** An external fixator may be removed before completion of the treatment plan secondary to pin tract infection, loosening, or conversion to internal fixation.
- *Internal fixation.* This significantly increases the forces resisted by the pelvic ring when compared with external fixation. Biomechanical studies suggest the following treatments:
  - ***Iliac wing fractures.*** Open reduction and internal fixation using interfragmentary compression screws and neutralization plates.
  - ***Diastasis of the pubic symphysis.*** Plate fixation if undergoing laparotomy and if no open injury or cystostomy tube.
  - ***Sacral fractures.*** Transiliac bar fixation may be inadequate or may cause compressive neurologic injury; in these cases, plate fixation or sacroiliac screw fixation may be indicated.
  - ***Unilateral sacroiliac dislocation.*** Internal fixation with cancellous screws or anterior sacroiliac plate fixation.
  - ***Bilateral posterior unstable disruptions.*** Fixation of the displaced portion of the pelvis to the sacral body may be accomplished by posterior screw fixation.

- *Open fractures.* In addition to fracture stabilization, hemorrhage control, and resuscitation, priority must be given to evaluation of the anus, rectum, vagina, and genitourinary system.
  - Anterior and lateral wounds generally are protected by muscle and are not contaminated by internal sources.
  - Posterior and perineal wounds may be contaminated by rectal and vaginal tears and genitourinary injuries.
  - Colostomy may be necessary for large bowel perforations or injuries to the anorectal region.
- *Postoperative plan.* In general, early mobilization is desired.
  - Aggressive pulmonary toilet should be pursued with incentive spirometry, early mobilization, encouraged deep inspirations and coughing, and suctioning or chest physical therapy as necessary.
  - Prophylaxis against thromboembolic phenomena should be performed with a combination of elastic stockings, sequential compression devices, and low molecular weight heparin or subcutaneous heparin if hemodynamic status allows. Duplex ultrasound examinations may be necessary. Thrombus formation may necessitate anticoagulation and/or vena caval filter placement.
  - Weight-bearing status may be advanced as follows:
    - Full weight bearing on the uninvolved lower extremity within several days.
    - Partial weight bearing on the involved lower extremity for at least 6 weeks.
    - Full weight bearing on the affected extremity without crutches by 12 weeks.
    - Patients with bilateral unstable pelvic fractures should be mobilized from bed to chair with aggressive pulmonary toilet until radiographic evidence of fracture healing is noted.
    - Partial weight bearing on the less injured side is generally tolerated by 12 weeks.

COMPLICATIONS

- *Infection.* Incidence is variable, ranging from 0% to 25%, although the presence of wound infection does not preclude a successful result. Presence of contusion or shear injuries to soft tissues is a risk factor for infection if a posterior approach is used. This risk is minimized by percutaneous posterior ring fixation.
- *Thromboembolism.* Disruption of the pelvic venous vasculature with immobilization constitutes a major risk factor for the development of deep venous thromboses. Sequential compression devices to the lower extremities may decrease this risk, although chemical anticoagulation is often contraindicated due to bleeding issues.
- *Malunion.* Significant disability may result, with complications including chronic pain, limb length inequalities, gait disturbances, sitting difficulties, low back pain, and pelvic outlet obstruction.
- *Nonunion.* This is rare, although it tends to occur more in younger patients (average age of 35 years) with sequelae of pain, gait abnormalities, and nerve root compression or irritation. Stable fixation and bone grafting is usually necessary for union.

30. ACETABULUM

EPIDEMIOLOGY

- Fractures of the acetabulum present a challenge to the orthopedic surgeon.
- Forty percent of posterior dislocations are associated with sciatic nerve injury.

ANATOMY

From the lateral aspect of the pelvis, the innominate osseous structural support of the acetabulum may be conceptualized as a two-columned construct (Judet and Letournel) forming an inverted Y (Fig. 30.1) and described as follows:

- Anterior column (iliopubic component): extends from the iliac crest to the symphysis pubis and includes the anterior wall of the acetabulum.
- Posterior column (ilioischial component): extends from the superior gluteal notch to the ischial tuberosity and includes the posterior wall of the acetabulum.
- Acetabular dome: the superior weight-bearing portion of the acetabulum at the junction of the anterior and posterior columns, including contributions from each.

MECHANISM OF INJURY

- The fracture pattern depends on the position of the femoral head at the time of injury, the magnitude of the force, and the age of the patient.
- Direct impact to the greater trochanter with the hip in neutral position can cause a transverse type of acetabular fracture (an abducted hip causes a low transverse fracture, whereas an adducted hip produces a high transverse fracture). An externally rotated hip causes anterior column injury. An internally rotated hip causes posterior column injury.
- With indirect trauma (e.g., a "dashboard"-type injury to the flexed knee), as the degree of hip flexion increases, the posterior wall is fractured in an increasingly inferior position. Similarly, as the degree of hip flexion decreases, the superior portion of the posterior wall is more likely to be involved.

CLINICAL EVALUATION

- A trauma evaluation may be necessary, with attention to airway, breathing, circulation, and disability, depending on the mechanism of injury.
- Patient factors, such as age, degree of trauma, presence of associated injuries, and general medical condition, are important because they affect treatment decisions and prognosis.
- Careful assessment of neurovascular status is necessary because sciatic nerve injury may be present in up to 40% of posterior column disruptions. Femoral nerve involvement with anterior column injury is rare, although compromise of the femoral artery by a fractured anterior column has been described.
- The presence of associated ipsilateral injuries must be ruled out, paying particular attention to the ipsilateral knee in which posterior instability and patellar fractures are common.
- Soft-tissue injuries (e.g., abrasions, contusions, presence of subcutaneous hemorrhage) may provide insight as to the mechanism of injury.

RADIOGRAPHIC EVALUATION

- Anteroposterior inlet and outlet views may help in ruling out associated pelvic fractures.
- In the anteroposterior view, anatomic landmarks include the iliopectineal line (limit of the anterior column), the ilioischial line (limit of the posterior column), the anterior lip, the posterior lip, and the line that depicts the superior weight-bearing surface of the acetabulum terminating as the medial teardrop.
- The iliac oblique radiograph (45-degree external rotation view) best demonstrates the posterior column (ilioischial line), the iliac wing, and the anterior wall of the acetabulum (Fig. 30.2).

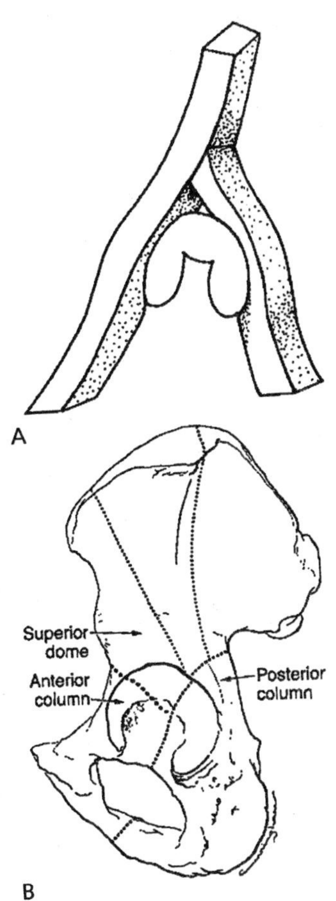

FIG. 30.1. A. Diagram of the two columns as an inverted Y supporting the acetabulum. **B.** Lateral aspect of the hemipelvis and acetabulum. The posterior column is characterized by the dense bone at the greater sciatic notch and follows the *dotted line* distally through the center of the acetabulum, the obturator foramen, and the inferior pubic ramus. The anterior column extends from the iliac crest to the symphysis pubis and includes the entire anterior wall of the acetabulum. Fractures involving the anterior column commonly exit below the anterior-inferior iliac spine as shown by the *heavy dotted line*. (From Heckman JD, Bucholz RW, eds. *Rockwood, Green, and Wilkin's fractures in adults*, 5th ed. Philadelphia: Lippincott Williams & Wilkins, 2001, with permission.)

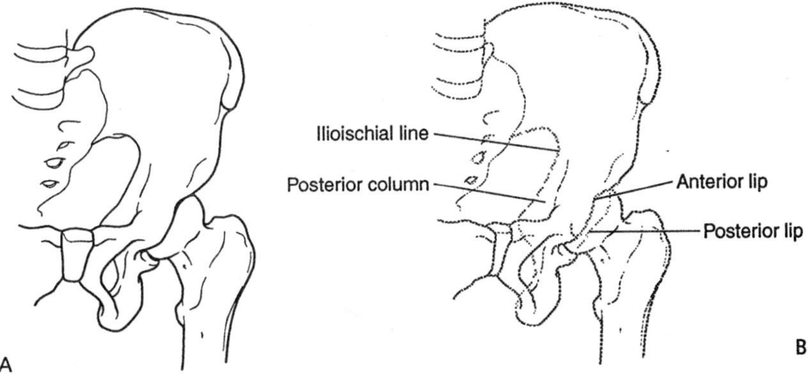

FIG. 30.2. A. Diagram of the anatomic landmarks of the left hemipelvis on the iliac oblique view. **B.** This view best demonstrates the posterior column of the acetabulum, outlined by the ilioischial line, the iliac crest, and the anterior lip of the acetabulum. (From Tile M. *Fractures of the pelvis and acetabulum*. Baltimore: Williams & Wilkins, 1995:455-457, with permission.)

- The obturator oblique view (45-degree internal rotation view with a 15-degree cephalad tilt) is best for evaluating the anterior column and posterior wall of the acetabulum (Fig. 30.3).
- Computed tomography may provide additional information regarding size and position of column fractures, impacted fractures of the acetabular wall, retained bone fragments in the joint, degree of comminution, and sacroiliac joint disruption. Dislocation not readily appreciated by standard radiography may sometimes be seen. Three-dimensional reconstruction allows for digital subtraction of the femoral head, resulting in full delineation of the acetabular surface.

JUDET-LETOURNEL CLASSIFICATION (FIG. 30.4)

Based on degree of columnar damage, 10 fracture patterns occur—5 "elementary" and 5 "associated."
Elementary patterns:

1. Posterior wall
2. Posterior column
3. Anterior wall
4. Anterior column
5. Transverse

Associated patterns:

1. T-shaped
2. Posterior column and posterior wall
3. Transverse and posterior wall
4. Anterior column:
   Posterior
   Hemitransverse
5. Both columns

Elementary Fractures

- Posterior wall fracture
  - This involves primarily the posterior wall inferior to the acetabular dome.
  - "Marginal impaction" is often present in posterior fracture-dislocations (articular cartilage impacted into underlying cancellous bone).
  - In a series by Brumback, marginal impaction was identified in 23% of posterior fracture-dislocations requiring open reduction. This was best appreciated on computed tomography.

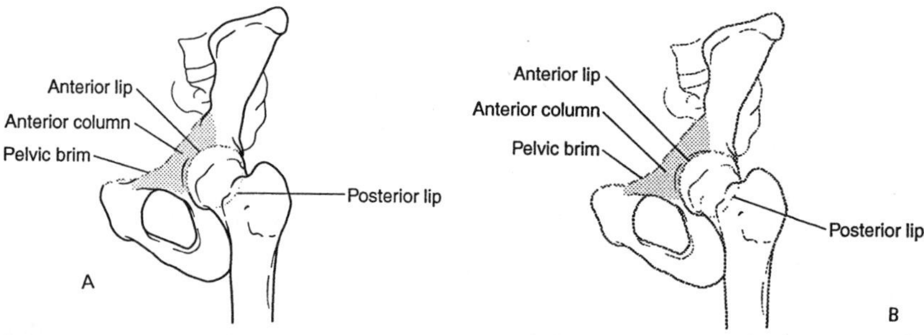

FIG. 30.3. A. Diagram of the anatomy of the pelvis on the obturator oblique view. **B.** In this view, particularly note the pelvic brim indicating the border of the anterior column and the posterior lip of the acetabulum. (From Tile M. *Fractures of the pelvis and acetabulum*. Baltimore: Williams & Wilkins, 1995:455-457, with permission.)

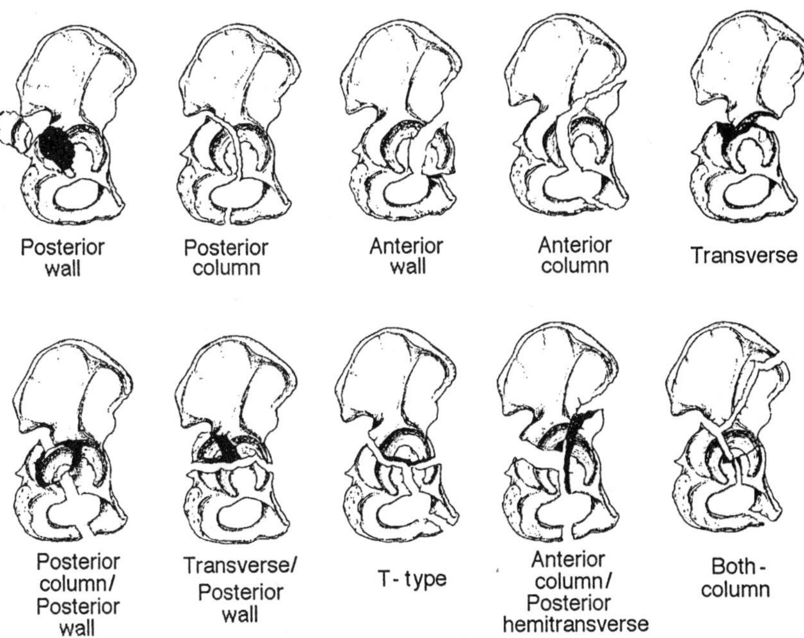

FIG. 30.4. Judet and Letournel classification of acetabular fractures. (From Browner BD, Jupiter JB, Levine AM, et al., eds. *Skeletal trauma*. Philadelphia: W.B. Saunders, 1992:902–903, with permission.)

- Posterior column fracture
  - Typically detaches the entire posterior column in one fragment.
  - May be associated with central femoral head dislocation.
- Anterior wall fracture
  - Associated with disruption of the iliopectineal line.
  - Often associated with anterocentral displacement of the femoral head between the anterior wall and the hinge of the quadrilateral plate.
  - Teardrop often displaced medially with respect to the ilioischial line.
  - Anterior wall fragment best visualized on the obturator oblique view.
- Anterior column fracture
  - This is associated with disruption of the iliopectineal line.
  - This is often associated with anteromedial displacement of the femoral head.
  - Fracture is classified according to the level at which the superior margin of the fracture line divides the innominate bone—low, intermediate, or high pattern.
  - The more superior the fracture line ascends, the greater the involvement of the weight-bearing aspect of the acetabulum.
  - Computed tomography may be helpful in delineating the degree of articular surface involvement.
- Transverse fracture
  - The innominate bone is separated into two fragments that divides the acetabular articular surface in one of three ways:
    1. Transtectal: through the acetabular dome;
    2. Juxtatectal: through the junction of the acetabular dome and fossa acetabuli;
    3. Infratectal: through the fossa acetabuli.
  - The more superior the fracture line, the greater the displacement of the acetabular dome.

The femoral head follows the inferior ischiopubic fragment and may dislocate centrally.
The ilioischial line and teardrop maintain a normal relationship.
Computed tomography typically demonstrates an anteroposterior fracture line.

Associated Fractures

- Associated posterior column and posterior wall fractures
  Two elementary fracture patterns are present. The posterior wall is usually markedly displaced and/or rotated in relation to the posterior column. This injury represents one pattern of posterior hip dislocation that is frequently accompanied by injury to the sciatic nerve.
- T-shaped fracture
  Combines a transverse fracture of any type (transtectal, juxtatectal, or infratectal) with an additional vertical fracture line that divides the ischiopubic fragment into two parts. The vertical component, or stem, may exit anteriorly, inferiorly, or posteriorly depending on the vector of the injurious force. The vertical component is best seen on the obturator oblique view.
- Associated transverse and posterior wall fractures
  The obturator oblique view best demonstrates the position of the transverse component and the posterior wall element. Based on computed tomography, in two-thirds of the cases the femoral head dislocates posteriorly; in one-third of the cases, the head dislocates centrally.
  Marginal impaction may exist; this is best evaluated by computed tomography.
- Associated anterior column and posterior hemitransverse fractures
  Combines an anterior wall or anterior column fracture (of any type) with a fracture line that divides the posterior column exactly as it would a transverse fracture. It is termed a hemitransverse because the "transverse" component involves only one column.
  Of noteworthy importance is the fact that, in this fracture, a piece of acetabular articular surface remains nondisplaced and becomes the key for operative reduction of other fragments.
- Both-column fracture
  This is the most complex type of acetabular fracture, formerly called a "central acetabular fracture."
  Both columns are separated from each other and from the axial skeleton, resulting in a "floating" acetabulum.
  The "spur" sign above the acetabulum on an obturator oblique radiograph is diagnostic.

ORTHOPAEDIC TRAUMA ASSOCIATION CLASSIFICATION OF ACETABULAR FRACTURES

Type A: partial articular, one column
- A1: posterior wall
- A2: posterior column
- A3: anterior

Type B: partial articular, transverse
- B1: transverse
- B2: T-shaped
- B3: anterior column, posterior hemitransverse

Type C: complete articular, both columns
- C1: high
- C2: low
- C3: sacroiliac joint involvement

TREATMENT (FIG. 30.5)

The goal of treatment is anatomic restoration of the articular surface to prevent posttraumatic arthritis.

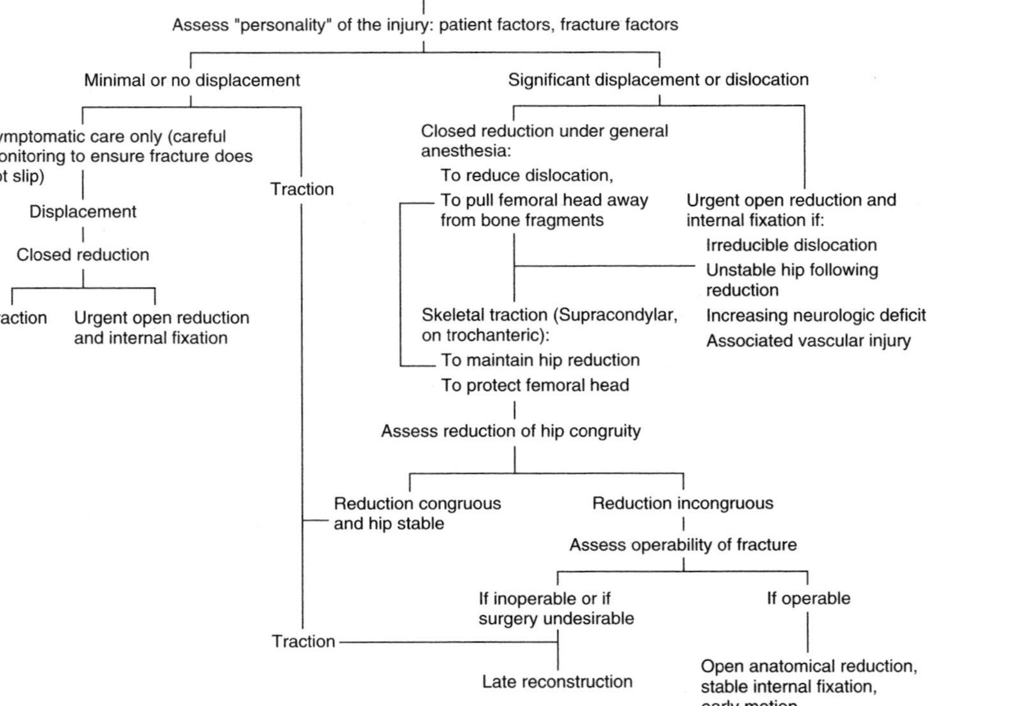

FIG. 30.5. Algorithm of the author's preferred method of treatment of acetabular fracture. (From Rockwood CA Jr, Green DP, Bucholz RW, Heckman JD, eds. *Rockwood and Green's fractures in adults*, 4th ed. Vol. 2. Philadelphia: Lippincott-Raven, 1996:1641, with permission.)

Initial Management

The patient is placed in skeletal traction for 2 to 3 days to allow for initial soft-tissue healing, to permit associated injuries to be addressed, to maintain the length of the limb, and to sustain femoral head reduction within the acetabulum.

Nonoperative Treatment

- A system for roughly quantifying the acetabular dome after fracture can be used by applying three measurements: the medial, anterior, and posterior roof arcs, measured on the anteroposterior, obturator oblique, and the iliac oblique views, respectively.
  - The roof arc is formed by the angle between two lines, one drawn vertically through the geometric center of the acetabulum and the other from the fracture line to the geometric center.
  - Roof arc angles are of limited utility for evaluation of both column fractures and posterior wall fractures.
- Nonoperative treatment may be appropriate in the following situations:
  - Displacement of less than 2 mm to 5 mm in the dome, depending on the location of the fracture and on patient factors, with maintenance of femoral head congruency out of traction and an absence of intraarticular osseous fragments.
  - Distal anterior column or transverse (infratectal) fractures in which femoral head congruency is maintained by the remaining medial buttress.
  - Maintenance of the medial, anterior, and the posterior roof arcs greater than 45 degrees.

Operative Treatment

- Surgical treatment is indicated for the following:
  - Anatomic reduction of a displaced (>3 mm) unstable fracture.
  - Removal of an interposed intraarticular loose fragment.
  - Restoration of a congruous proximal femoral articulation.
  - Reduction of a fracture-dislocation that is irreducible by closed methods.
- Unless coexistent hip dislocation exists, open reduction and internal fixation (ORIF) should be undertaken no sooner than 2 to 3 days postinjury and usually no later than 10 days. Fracture callus usually poses a problem to ORIF about 3 weeks following injury. Preoperative skeletal traction is helpful.
- Approaches to the acetabulum include the Kocher-Langenbach (posterior, posterolateral), ilioinguinal (anterior), and extended iliofemoral. No single approach provides ideal exposure of all fracture types. Proper preoperative classification of the fracture configuration is essential to selecting the best surgical approach.

Stability

- Instability is most common in posterior types but may be present when large fractures of the quadrilateral plate allow central subluxation of the femoral head or in anterior types with major anterior wall fractures.
- Central instability results when a quadrilateral plate fracture is of sufficient size to allow for central subluxation of the femoral head. A medial buttress with a spring plate or cerclage wire is necessary to restore stability.
- Anterior instability results from a large anterior wall fracture or as part of an anterior type with a posterior hemitransverse fracture.

Congruity

- Incongruity of the hip may result in early degenerative changes and posttraumatic osteoarthritis. Evaluation is best made by computed tomography. Acceptance of incongruity is based on the location within the acetabulum.
- Displaced dome fractures rarely reduce with traction; surgery is usually necessary for adequate restoration of the weight-bearing surface.
- High transverse or T-type fractures are shearing injuries that are grossly unstable when involving the superior weight-bearing dome. Nonoperative reduction is virtually impossible, whereas operative reduction can be extremely difficult.
- With displaced both-column fractures (floating acetabulum), surgery is indicated for restoration of congruence if the roof fragment is displaced and if secondary congruence cannot be obtained or if the posterior column is grossly displaced.

- Retained osseous fragments may result in incongruity or in an inability to maintain concentric reduction of the femoral head. Avulsions of the ligamentum teres do not need to be removed unless they are of substantial size.
- Femoral head fractures generally require ORIF to maintain sphericity and congruity.
- Soft-tissue interposition may necessitate operative removal of the interposed tissues.

Postoperative Care

- Indomethacin versus irradiation for heterotopic ossification prophylaxis.
- Low molecular weight heparin, sequential compression devices, and compressive stockings for thromboembolic prophylaxis.
- Mobilization out of bed as associated injuries allow, with pulmonary toilet and incentive spirometry.
- Weight bearing to affected extremity withheld until radiographic signs of union are present, generally by 6 to 8 weeks postoperatively.
- Postoperative traction maintained if the patient has poor bone stock, gross comminution, or questionable fixation. Progressive weight bearing in these cases not usually started until 12 weeks postoperatively, as dictated by radiographic evidence of healing.

COMPLICATIONS

- Surgical wound infection: risk increased secondary to the presence of associated abdominal and pelvic visceral injuries. Local soft-tissue injury from the original impact force may cause closed degloving or local abrasions. Postoperative hematoma formation occurs frequently, further contributing to potential wound infection.
- Nerve injury:
  - Sciatic nerve: the Kocher-Langenbach approach with prolonged or forceful traction can cause a sciatic nerve palsy (most often the peroneal branch; incidence is 16% to 33%). The use of somatosensory evoked potentials may decrease the risk of sciatic injury in posterior approaches.
  - Femoral nerve: the ilioinguinal approach may result in traction injury to the femoral nerve. Rarely, the femoral nerve may be lacerated by an anterior column fracture.
  - Superior gluteal nerve: most vulnerable in the greater sciatic notch. Injury to this nerve during trauma or surgery may result in paralysis of the hip abductors, often causing severe disability.
- Heterotopic ossification: incidence ranges from 3% to 69%, highest with the extended iliofemoral approach and second highest with the Kocher-Langenbach. The highest risk is a young male undergoing a posterolateral extensile approach in which muscle is removed. It is almost nonexistent with the ilioinguinal approach. Both indomethacin and low-dose radiation have been helpful in reducing the incidence of this complication.
- Avascular necrosis: devastating complication occurring in 6.6% of cases, mostly with posterior types associated with high energy injuries.
- Chondrolysis: may occur with nonoperative or operative treatment, resulting in posttraumatic osteoarthritis. Concentric reduction with restoration of articular congruity may minimize this complication.

31. FEMORAL SHAFT

EPIDEMIOLOGY

- Associated injuries are common; they may be present in up to 5% to 15% of cases, with patients presenting with multisystem trauma and spine, pelvis, and ipsilateral lower extremity injuries.
- Ligamentous and meniscal injuries of the ipsilateral knee are present in 50% of patients with closed femoral shaft fractures.

ANATOMY

- The femur is the largest tubular bone in the body; it is surrounded by the largest mass of muscle. An important feature of the femoral shaft is its anterior bow. Additionally, the medial cortex is under compression, whereas the lateral cortex is under tension.
- A femoral shaft fracture is defined as a fracture of the diaphysis occurring between 5 cm distal to the lesser trochanter and 5 cm proximal to the adductor tubercle.
- The femoral shaft is subjected to major muscular forces that deform the thigh after a fracture. Understanding these forces allows one to use appropriate traction in the initial management of femoral shaft fractures (Fig. 31.1) as follows:
  - Abductors (gluteus medius and minimus): insert on the greater trochanter and abduct the proximal femur after subtrochanteric fractures and proximal shaft fractures.
  - Iliopsoas: flexes and externally rotates the proximal fragment in femoral shaft fractures by its attachment to the lesser trochanter.
  - Adductors: span most shaft fractures and exert a strong axial and varus load to the bone by traction on the distal fragment.
  - Gastrocnemius: acts on distal shaft fractures and supracondylar fractures by angulating the distal fragment into flexion.
  - Fascia lata: acts as a tension band by resisting the medial angulating forces of the adductors.
- The thigh musculature is divided into the following three distinct fascial compartments:
  - Anterior compartment: composed of the quadriceps femoris, iliopsoas, sartorius, and pectineus with the femoral artery, vein, and nerve and the lateral femoral cutaneous nerve.
  - Medial compartment: contains the gracilis, adductors longus, brevis, magnus, and obturator externus muscles along with the obturator artery, vein, and nerve and the profunda femoris artery.
  - Posterior compartment: includes the biceps femoris, semitendinosus, and semimembranosus; a portion of the adductor magnus muscle; branches of the profunda femoris artery; the sciatic nerve; and the posterior femoral cutaneous nerve.
- Compartment syndromes are much less common than in the leg due to the high volume of the three fascial compartments of the thigh. Severe bleeding into these compartments is necessary to raise intracompartmental pressures, and profound intravascular volume loss can occur.
- The vascular supply to the femoral shaft is derived mainly from the profunda femoral artery. The nutrient vessel usually enters the bone proximally and posteriorly along the linea aspera. This artery then arborizes proximally and distally to provide the endosteal circulation to the shaft. The periosteal vessels also enter the bone along the linea aspera and supply blood to the outer one-third of the cortex. The endosteal vessels supply the inner two-thirds of the cortex.
- The endosteal blood supply is disrupted after most femoral shaft fractures, and the periosteal vessels proliferate to act as the primary source of blood for healing. The medullary supply is eventually restored late in the healing process.
- Femoral shaft fractures heal readily if the blood supply is not excessively compromised. Therefore, avoiding extreme periosteal stripping, especially posteriorly where

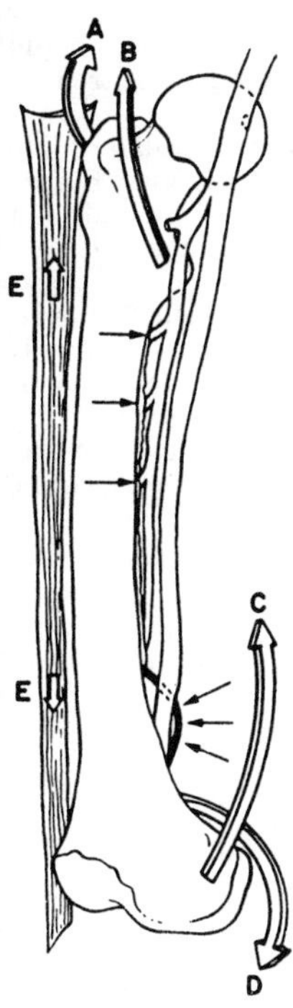

FIG. 31.1. Deforming muscle forces on the femur: abductors. **A.** Iliopsoas. **B.** Adductors. **C.** Gastrocnemius origin. **D.** The medial angulating forces are resisted by the fascia lata. **E.** Potential sites of vascular injury after fracture are at the adductor hiatus and the perforating vessels of the profunda femoris. (From Heckman JD, Bucholz RW, eds. *Rockwood, Green, and Wilkins' fractures in adults*, 5th ed. Philadelphia: Lippincott Williams & Wilkins, 2001, with permission.)

the arteries enter the bone at the linea aspera, is important. The intermuscular septum should not be dissected off the linea aspera unless imperative for surgical exposure.

MECHANISM OF INJURY

- Femoral shaft fractures in adults are almost always the result of high energy trauma. These fractures occur secondary to motor vehicle accidents, gunshot injuries, or falls from a height. Pathologic fractures, especially in the elderly, commonly occur at the relatively weak metaphyseal-diaphyseal junction. Any fracture that occurs and that is inconsistent with the degree of trauma (e.g., a femoral fracture that occurs as a result of stepping off a curb) should arouse suspicion for the possibility of pathologic fracture. Occasionally, femoral shaft fractures may occur in pathologic bone or as a result of persistent microtrauma ("stress fractures").
- Stress fractures due to fatigue failure as the emphasis on physical fitness rises are an increasingly important cause of femoral shaft fracture. Usually located in the proximal femoral or midshaft areas, stress fractures occur mainly in military recruits or runners. Most patients report a recent increase in training intensity just prior to the onset of thigh pain.

CLINICAL EVALUATION

- A full trauma survey may be indicated as these fractures tend to be the result of high energy trauma. A careful physical examination for associated injuries is essential.
- The diagnosis of femoral shaft fracture is usually obvious, with the patient presenting as nonambulatory with pain, variable gross deformity, swelling, and shortening of the affected extremity.

- A careful neurovascular examination is essential, although neurovascular injury is not commonly associated with a femoral shaft fracture. The examiner should be aware that muscular spasm and pain may result in diminished motor strength on examination.
- Ipsilateral limb injuries are common. Thorough examination of the ipsilateral hip and knee should be performed, including systematic inspection and palpation. Range-of-motion or ligamentous testing is often not feasible in the setting of a femoral shaft fracture and may result in displacement if attempted. Knee ligament injuries are common, however, and must be assessed after fracture fixation.
- Major blood loss into the voluminous compartments of the thigh may occur. The average blood loss in one series was greater than 1,200 mL; 40% of patients ultimately required transfusions. Therefore, a careful preoperative assessment of hemodynamic stability is essential, regardless of the presence or absence of associated injuries. Additionally, significant bleeding into the thigh after a femoral shaft fracture may elevate the compartment pressure above the critical level. This may require the measurement of intracompartmental pressures.

RADIOGRAPHIC EVALUATION

Anteroposterior and lateral views of the femur, hip, and knee should be obtained. Cross-table lateral views of the femur and hip should be acquired to minimize displacement, soft-tissue trauma, and hemorrhage.

DESCRIPTIVE CLASSIFICATION

- Open versus closed
- Location: proximal, middle, or distal one-third; supraisthmal or infraisthmal
- Pattern: spiral, oblique, or transverse
- Angulation: varus, valgus, or rotational deformity
- Displacement: shortening or translation
- Comminuted, segmental, or butterfly fragment

WINQUIST AND HANSEN CLASSIFICATION (FIG. 31.2)

Based on comminution; most useful for determining the need for interlocking nails.

Type I: minimal or no comminution
Type II: cortices of both fragments at least 50% intact
Type III: 50% to 100% cortical comminution
Type IV: circumferential comminution with no cortical contact at the fracture site

ORTHOPAEDIC TRAUMA ASSOCIATION CLASSIFICATION OF FEMORAL SHAFT FRACTURES

Type A: simple fracture
  Al: spiral

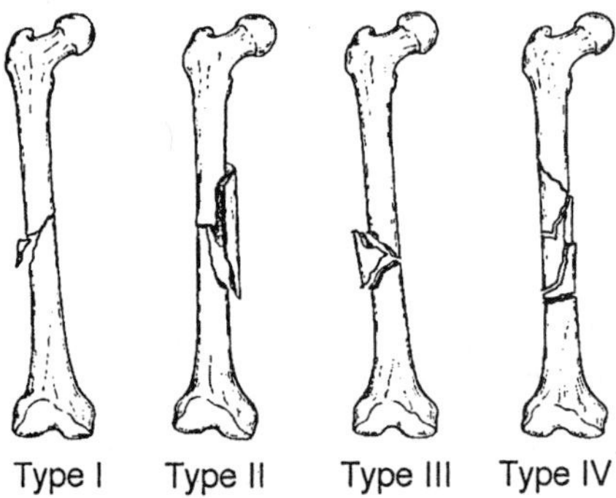

FIG. 31.2. Winquist and Hansen classification of femoral shaft fractures. (From Browner BD, Jupiter JB, Levine AM, et al. *Skeletal trauma*. Philadelphia: W.B. Saunders, 1992:1537, with permission.)

A2: oblique (>30 degrees)
A3: transverse (<30 degrees)
Type B: wedge fracture
B1: spiral
B2: bending
B3: fragmented
Type C: complex fracture
C1: spiral
C2: segmental
C3: irregular

TREATMENT

Nonoperative

Skin Traction

- Historically used, but the major disadvantage is inability to apply sufficient forces to the limb to effect reduction without causing slippage or skin necrosis.
- Currently used in adults only for emergency fracture immobilization in the field for patient comfort and to facilitate patient transport.
- For definitive fracture management, indicated only in young children (Bryant or split Russell traction).

Skeletal Traction

- Skeletal traction, formerly used to treat femoral shaft fractures, is used today for early fracture care before a definitive operative procedure can be performed.
- It may also be used for patients who are too sick for surgery, although these patients are very poor candidates for the prolonged bedrest necessary for the skeletal traction method of treatment.
- The goal of skeletal traction is to restore femoral length and to limit rotational and angular deformities.
- Skeletal traction may be applied through the distal femur or proximal tibia. The distal femur affords more direct longitudinal pull but has been associated with higher rates of knee stiffness after fracture union due to pin-tract scarring through the vastus muscles. Proximal tibial traction through the tibial tubercle is contraindicated with concomitant ligamentous injury to the ipsilateral knee.
- Both methods carry the theoretical risk of pin-tract infection that involves the knee joint.
- Union rates of closed fractures of the femur treated by skeletal traction have been reported to be between 97% and 100% in most studies, although delayed union occurred in up to 30% of cases due to continual distraction across the fracture site.
- Problems with skeletal traction include knee stiffness, limb shortening, prolonged hospitalization, respiratory and skin ailments, and malunion.

Cast Brace

- The cast brace is an external support device that permits progressive weight bearing by partially unloading the fracture through circumferential support of the soft tissues.
- Indications for cast bracing include open fractures, distal third fractures, and comminuted midshaft fractures of the femur. Proximal, simple transverse, or oblique fractures are less amenable to cast bracing due to high stress concentration and a propensity to angulate. The cast brace is best used after an initial period of skeletal traction.
- Consistently high rates of union (>90%), usually by 13 to 14 weeks, have been reported in numerous studies.
- Problems with cast bracing include loss of reduction and subsequent malunion, shortening, and angulation.

Operative

Intramedullary Nailing

- An intramedullary nail acts as a load-sharing device as opposed to a compression plate, which is a load-bearing device. In addition, the central placement of the nail within the femoral canal results in lower tensile and shear stresses on the implant. Benefits of intramedullary nails include less extensive exposure and dissection, lower infection rate, and less quadriceps scarring.
- Other advantages include early functional use of the extremity (mobilization of the patient out of bed within 24 hours), restoration of length and alignment with comminuted fractures, rapid fracture healing, and low refracture rate.
- Flexible (unreamed) devices include Enders nails and Rush rods, which are based on three-point fixation. Their use is limited by the success of the locked reamed nail.
- Reamed locked nails are the best treatment for most shaft fractures. Most studies show union rates of 98%, with infection rates of <1%. Interlocking nails with both proximal and distal transfixation screws allow optimal control of rotation and shortening in comminuted fractures.
- Controversy exists surrounding the use of reaming in a patient with concomitant pulmonary injury because reaming theoretically may produce fat embolization.
- Unreamed locked nails can be used in grade I, II, and IIIA open femoral fractures. The interlocking screws are not strong enough for full weight bearing; therefore, full weight bearing is delayed until fracture callus formation involving three cortices is seen.
- The use of a fracture table allows convenient application of traction and fracture manipulation; in addition, supine positioning of the patient often allows adequate access for concomitant surgical procedures and anesthesia concerns. However, access to the hip for antegrade intramedullary fixation is more restricted, especially in obese individuals.
- The use of a flat table allows lateral positioning of the patient, with increased access to the hip and piriformis fossa for antegrade intramedullary fixation, especially in obese individuals. However, access for concomitant procedures and anesthesia is more restricted, thus limiting its utility in multisystem trauma. Lateral positioning is relatively contraindicated in cases of pulmonary injury, pelvic or spine fractures, and contralateral femur fractures.
- Retrograde intramedullary fixation obviates many of the difficulties encountered with access to the hip. In addition, it allows for hardware in the proximal femur (e.g., fixation for ipsilateral femoral neck fracture). Fractures of the distal femur are not amenable to retrograde nailing. Potential problems with this technique include knee pain and stiffness.

External Fixation

- External fixation provides excellent bony fixation and wound access, as well as early mobilization. Therefore, external fixation is the method of choice for grade IIIB and IIIC open femur fractures.
- Proper application of the external fixator includes placing the pins as close to the fracture site as possible, prestressing the pins, and placing the fixation bar as close to the bone as possible. Based on the fracture pattern, the external fixator may be placed laterally (stiffest in medial to lateral plane) or anteriorly (stiffest in sagittal plane).
- Complications include distraction of the fracture, pin-tract infection (up to 50%), pin loosening, and loss of knee motion, possibly due to the tethering of the quadriceps muscle to the femoral shaft.
- The increased rate of complications may be secondary to the increased severity of injuries treated with external fixation.

Compression Plating

- Compression plating was widely used to treat femur fractures in the 1960s and 1970s because of dissatisfaction with the nonoperative modes of treatment. Advantages of this technique include early mobilization, rigid fixation of the fracture, and improvement in knee motion.

- Complications of compression plating include failure of fixation, infection, nonunion, devitalization of fracture fragments with excessive periosteal stripping, and stress shielding with possible refracture.
- The best indication for compression plating is a fracture involving the distal metaphyseal-diaphyseal junction of the femur. With the advent of intramedullary nailing, compression plating is now rarely used to treat femoral shaft fractures.

Ipsilateral Fractures of the Proximal or Distal Femur

- Ipsilateral fractures of the femoral neck have been reported in 2.5% to 5% of cases of femoral shaft fracture. Options for operative fixation include antegrade intramedullary nailing with multiple screw fixation of the femoral neck (miss-a-nail technique), antegrade cephalomedullary nailing, retrograde nailing with multiple screw fixation of the femoral neck, or compression plating with screw fixation of the femoral neck. A sliding hip screw may be used with intertrochanteric fractures with "stacking" or overlapping of the plates. Most authors recommend at least provisional fixation of the neck fracture with one screw or Kirschner wires to prevent displacement while the shaft fracture is being addressed.
- Ipsilateral fractures of the distal femur are uncommon in the setting of femoral shaft fracture; they may exist as a distal extension of the shaft fracture or as a distinct fracture. Options for fixation include fixation of both fractures with a single plate, fixation of the shaft and distal femoral fractures with separate plates (or with a blade plate for the distal femoral fracture), intramedullary nailing of the shaft fracture with open reduction and internal fixation of the distal femoral fracture, or interlocked intramedullary nailing spanning both fractures (high supracondylar fractures). If the fractures are to receive separate fixation, the distal femoral fracture is reduced first, with anatomic restoration of the articular surface later if necessary.

COMPLICATIONS

- Nerve injury: uncommon because femoral and sciatic nerves are encased in muscle throughout length of thigh. Most occur as a result of traction or compression during surgery.
- Vascular injury: may be due to tethering of the femoral artery at the adductor hiatus. Compartment syndrome in the thigh occurs only with significant bleeding and presents as pain out of proportion, tense thigh swelling, numbness or paresthesias to the medial thigh (saphenous nerve distribution), or painful passive quadriceps stretch. Distal pulses may remain intact despite progressive nerve and muscle ischemia.
- Infection: greater risk with open versus closed intramedullary nailing. Grades I, II, and IIIa open fractures carry a low risk of infection with intramuscular nailing, whereas fractures with gross contamination, exposed bone, and extensive soft-tissue injury (grades IIIb and IIIc) have an unacceptably high risk of infection regardless of treatment method.
- Refracture: vulnerable during early callus formation and after hardware removal.
- Nonunion, delayed union: unusual. Delayed union, if healing takes longer than 6 months, is usually related to insufficient blood supply (avoid excessive periosteal stripping), uncontrolled repetitive stresses, infection, and heavy smoking. Occurrence may require dynamization of a static locked nail or reamed exchange nailing.
- Malunion: usually varus, internal rotation, and/or shortening due to muscular deforming forces. This is usually well compensated by hip and knee motion but can result in abnormal gait, leg length discrepancy, or posttraumatic arthritis.
- Fixation device failure: due to nonunion or "cycling" of the device, especially with load-bearing devices (e.g., plate).

32. DISTAL FEMUR

EPIDEMIOLOGY

- A bimodal age distribution of injury exists, with a high incidence in young adults from high energy trauma, such as motor vehicle or motorcycle accidents or falls from heights, and a second peak in the elderly from minor falls.
- As these are not as common as femoral shaft or hip fractures, fractures of the distal femur represent significant management challenges.

ANATOMY

- A distal femoral fracture is defined as any fracture involving the distal 9 cm of the femur, when measured proximally from the articular surface of the femoral condyles.
- The distal femur broadens from the cylindrical shaft to form two curved condyles separated by an intercondylar groove.
- The medial condyle extends more distally and has a more convex shape than does the lateral femoral condyle. This accounts for the 5 to 7 degrees of physiologic valgus of the femur.
- Deforming forces from muscular attachments cause characteristic displacement patterns as follows:
  - Gastrocnemius: flexes the distal fragment, causing posterior displacement and apex anterior angulation.
  - Quadriceps and hamstrings: exert proximal traction, resulting in shortening of the lower extremity.
- Thin cortices, comminution, osteopenia, and a wide medullary canal make internal fixation of the distal femur difficult, even for the experienced surgeon.

MECHANISM OF INJURY

- High energy. Younger patients sustain injury after high energy impact, most commonly vehicular trauma.
- Low energy. Elderly patients may sustain fractures through osteoporotic bone after relatively minor trauma, such as a fall onto a flexed knee. Varus or valgus stress forces with axial load and rotational components play a significant role in producing these fractures.

CLINICAL EVALUATION

- Depending on the clinical history, a full trauma evaluation may be necessary. Patients typically present nonambulatory with pain, swelling, and variable deformity in the supracondylar region of the femur.
- Gross mobility may be present at the fracture site with crepitus. Immediate assessment of neurovascular status is mandatory. The proximity of the neurovascular structures to the fracture area is an important consideration. Unusual and tense swelling in the popliteal area and the usual signs of pallor and lack of pulse suggest rupture of a major vessel; in these cases, angiography may be necessary.
- Compartment syndromes of the thigh are uncommon; they are associated with major intravascular volume loss into the voluminous compartments of the thigh. Thus, clinical suspicion must be followed by monitoring compartment pressures and assessing hemodynamic instability. Examination of the ipsilateral hip, knee, leg, and ankle are warranted, especially in the obtunded or polytraumatized patient.
- In cases in which a distal femoral fracture is associated with an overlying laceration or puncture wound, saline or methylene blue may be injected into the knee in a sterile fashion to determine continuity with the wound.

RADIOGRAPHIC EVALUATION

- Anteroposterior, lateral, and two oblique radiographs should be obtained. Traction views may be helpful; 45-degree oblique views can better delineate intercondylar

involvement. Radiographic evaluation of the entire involved lower extremity is warranted as concomitant injuries are common.
- Contralateral views may help with comparison and may serve as a template for preoperative planning.
- Computed tomography portrays the distal femur in cross-section, which helps to identify fracture lines in the frontal plane. Two- and three-dimensional reconstructions may also improve understanding of the fracture pattern in preparation for surgery.
- Magnetic resonance imaging may be of value in evaluating associated injuries to ligamentous or meniscal structures.
- Angiography is indicated with frank dislocation of the knee as 40% of such injuries are associated with vascular disruption. This occurs because the popliteal vascular bundle is tethered proximally at the adductor hiatus and distally at the soleus arch. By contrast, the incidence of vascular disruption with isolated supracondylar fractures is between 2% and 3%.

DESCRIPTIVE CLASSIFICATION

- Open versus closed
- Location: supracondylar, intercondylar, condylar involvement
- Pattern: spiral, oblique, or transverse
- Articular involvement
- Angulation: varus, valgus, or rotational deformity
- Displacement: shortening or translation
- Comminuted, segmental, or butterfly fragment

NEER CLASSIFICATION

Does not take into account associated intraarticular fractures and the possibility of articular incongruity.

Group I: Minimum displacement; impacted, linear, or slightly displaced, but stable after closed reduction; the bone is often osteoporotic and the injury usually is a trivial blow to the flexed knee.

Group IIA: Condyles displaced medially; violent force applied to the anterolateral aspect of the flexed knee; oblique fracture extending from just proximal to the lateral epicondyle to well above the medial epicondyle; the condyles are displaced medially.

Group IIB: Condyles displaced laterally; severe force applied to the lateral side of the extended limb; the shaft is displaced medially, and when the fracture is open, it penetrates the skin on the inner aspect of the thigh; spares extensor tendon.

Group III: Conjoined supracondylar and shaft fractures; high energy trauma to the anterior aspect of the flexed knee; when open, penetrates the skin superior to the patella; concomitant patellar fractures are common; associated with maximum damage to the quadriceps tendon; jagged edge of the shaft fragment poses a threat to the popliteal vessels.

SEINSHEIMER CLASSIFICATION

Addresses articular disruption.

Type 1: nondisplaced fracture or those with less than 2 mm of displacement
Type 2: fractures involving the distal metaphysis only, without intraarticular extension:
  A: two-part
  B: comminuted
Type 3: fractures involving the intercondylar notch in which one or both condyles are separate fragments:
  A: medial separate
  B: lateral separate
  C: both condyles separated from the shaft and from each other

Type 4: fractures extending through the articular surface of a femoral condyle:
- A: through medial condyle (two-part or comminuted)
- B: through lateral condyle (two-part or comminuted)
- C: complex and comminuted

ORTHOPAEDIC TRAUMA ASSOCIATION CLASSIFICATION OF DISTAL FEMORAL FRACTURES

Defines the fracture (extra- or intraarticular, comminution), indicates prognosis, and helps decide the type of treatment.

Type A: extraarticular
- A1: simple
- A2: metaphyseal wedge
- A3: metaphyseal complex

Type B: unicondylar, partial articular
- B1: lateral condyle, sagittal
- B2: medial condyle, sagittal
- B3: frontal

Type C: intercondylar/bicondylar, complete articular
- C1: articular simple, metaphyseal simple
- C2: articular simple, metaphyseal complex
- C3: multifragmentary articular fracture

TREATMENT

Nonoperative

- Closed fracture management may be undertaken with reduction by longitudinal traction and early cast brace application at 3 to 6 weeks after injury. Reduction can generally be obtained by the application of traction placed through a two-pin system—one through the supracondylar fragment and the other through the tibial tuberosity.
- Indications include nondisplaced or incomplete fractures, impacted stable fractures in elderly, osteoporotic patients, infected or severely contaminated fractures (grade IIb or IIc open injuries), advanced osteoporosis, advanced underlying medical conditions, or select gunshot injuries.
- The objective is not absolute anatomic reduction but rather restoration of the knee joint axis to a normal relationship with the hip and ankle. Good to excellent results of 84% using closed methods were reported by Neer.
- The difficulties are the inability to control the displaced intraarticular fragments and, occasionally, the tendency of the supracondylar fragments to displace posteriorly.
- Potential drawbacks include varus and internal rotational deformity, knee stiffness, and the necessity for prolonged hospitalization and bedrest.

Operative

- Indications for operative intervention include the following:
  - Absolute: open fractures, associated neurovascular injuries, ipsilateral lower extremity fractures, displaced intraarticular fractures, and irreducible fractures.
  - Relative: displaced extraarticular supracondylar fractures, periprosthetic fracture (e.g., total knee replacement), marked obesity, and pathologic fractures.
- Contraindications to operative fixation include preexisting infection, massive contamination (grade IIb or IIc injuries), marked comminution with bone loss, severe osteopenia, and hemodynamic instability from polytrauma.
- Ideally, surgery should be performed within 48 hours. If surgery is delayed by more than 8 hours, tibial pin traction should be used.
- The choice of implant is governed by operative goals. In young patients, the goal is restoration of length and axial alignment with anatomic reduction, articular congruity, stable fixation, and early functional rehabilitation. In elderly patients with osteopenia and limited functional requirements, impaction of metaphyseal fragments with small amounts of shortening or malalignment may be a reasonable trade-off for rapid fracture healing.

- 95-Degree condylar blade plate: excellent fracture control but technically demanding.
- Dynamic condylar screw: interfragmentary compression possible, but bulky at screw-plate junction, thus requiring considerable bone removal for low profile fit.
- Condylar buttress plate: used for extensive comminution or multiple intraarticular fractures. Medial plate may be necessary to prevent varus deformity.
- Locked antegrade intramedullary nail: limited use due to distal nature of fracture.
- Supracondylar nails: load sharing; less soft-tissue stripping; fracture table not required (good for multiply injured); may be used with concomitant fixation of hip fractures. Problems include possible knee sepsis, stiffness, synovial metallosis, and patellofemoral degeneration.
- Zickel supracondylar device: may be used in noncomminuted supracondylar fractures or if impaction and shortening can be accepted (e.g., in the elderly).
- Enders nails and Rush pins: not recommended.

- External fixation can be used alone or in combination with limited internal fixation as follows:
  - Grade I, II, and IIIa injuries can be managed with internal fixation after aggressive debridement and irrigation.
  - Grade IIb and IIc injuries should be managed with debridement, with or without external fixation (versus traction or splinting); serial debridements; and delayed internal fixation, allowing rapid application, minimal soft-tissue dissection, the ability to maintain length, early patient mobilization, and local wound care. Problems can include pin-tract infection, quadriceps scarring, delayed union or nonunion, and loss of reduction after device removal.
- A bone graft is recommended for any fracture that involves bone loss or severe comminution.
- This includes autogenous corticocancellous (e.g., iliac crest graft) and cancellous bone, allograft, or bone graft substitutes.
- Polymethylmethacrylate cement may be necessary in extremely osteoporotic bone to increase the fixation capability of screws.
- Supracondylar fractures after total knee replacement are uncommon. They are related to osteopenia, rheumatoid arthritis (RA), prolonged corticosteroid usage, anterior notching of the femur, and revision arthroplasty.
- Satisfactory outcomes (96% to 100%) occur with long-stem revisions and intramedullary fixation. Less successful (67%) results are recorded with plate osteosynthesis or external fixation.
- Postoperative management typically includes maintaining patients in a continuous passive motion device in the immediate postoperative period. The patient is then started on physical therapy, consisting of active range-of-motion exercises and partial weight bearing with crutches within 2 to 3 days after stable fixation. A cast brace may be used if fixation is tenuous. Weight bearing may be advanced with radiographic evidence of healing (6 to 12 weeks).

COMPLICATIONS

- Malunion. This usually results from unstable fixation or infection. Malunion with the articular surface in extension may result in relative hyperextension of the knee, whereas malunion in flexion may result in a functional loss of full extension. Varus or valgus angulation is less well tolerated. Malunion resulting in functional disability may be addressed with an osteotomy.
- Nonunion. This is infrequent due to rich vascular supply to this region and the predominance of cancellous bone.
- Posttraumatic osteoarthritis. This may result from a failure to restore articular congruity and biomechanical stability, especially in young patients. It also may reflect chondral injury at the time of trauma.
- Infection. Open fractures require meticulous debridement and copious irrigation (serial, if necessary) with intravenous antibiotics, particularly if internal fixation is anticipated. Open injuries contiguous with the knee necessitate formal washout to prevent knee sepsis.
- Loss of knee motion. This is the most common complication; it results from scarring, quadriceps damage, or articular disruption during injury. If significant, it may require lysis of adhesions or quadricepsplasty for restoration of joint motion.

33. KNEE DISLOCATIONS

EPIDEMIOLOGY

- Traumatic dislocation of the knee is an uncommon injury that may be limb-threatening; it should therefore be treated as an orthopedic emergency.
- It is extremely rare. At the Mayo Clinic, only 14 traumatic knee dislocations were observed in 2 million admissions. The largest series reported was from Los Angeles County Hospital, where over a 10-year period 53 knee dislocations were seen.

ANATOMY

- The ginglymoid (hinge joint) consists of three articulations: patellofemoral, tibiofemoral, and tibiofibular. Under normal cyclic loading, the knee may experience up to five times the body weight per step. The normal range of motion is from 10 degrees of extension to 140 degrees of flexion, with 8 to 12 degrees of rotation through the flexion-extension arc. The dynamic and static stability of the knee is conferred mainly by soft tissues (ligaments, muscles, tendons, menisci) in addition to the bony articulations.
- Significant soft-tissue injuries, including ruptures of at least three of four major ligamentous structures of the knee, are necessary for knee dislocation. The anterior and posterior cruciate ligaments are disrupted in most cases, with a varying degree of injury to the collateral ligaments, capsular elements, and menisci.
- The popliteal vascular bundle courses through a fibrous tunnel at the level of the adductor hiatus. Within the popliteal fossa, the five geniculate branches are given off, after which the vascular structures run deep to the soleus and through another fibrous canal. This tethering effect leaves the popliteal vessels vulnerable to tenting and injury, especially at the moment of dislocation. Associated fractures of the tibial eminence, tibial tubercle, fibular head or neck, and capsular avulsions are common and should be suspected.

MECHANISM OF INJURY

- High energy: motor vehicle accidents, with "dashboard" injuries involving axial loading to a flexed knee.
- Low energy: athletic injuries, falls.

CLINICAL EVALUATION

- Patients almost always present with gross knee distortion. Immediate reduction should be undertaken without waiting for radiographs in the displaced position. Of paramount importance is the arterial supply, with secondary consideration going to neurologic status.
- The extent of ligamentous injury is related to the degree of displacement, with injury occurring with displacement greater than 10% to 25% of the resting length of the ligament. Gross instability may be realized after reduction.
- A careful neurovascular examination is critical, both pre- and postreduction and serially thereafter, because vasospasm or thrombosis due to an unsuspected intimal tear may cause delayed ischemia hours or even days after reduction.

  Vascular injury—popliteal artery disruption (20% to 60%). The popliteal artery is at risk during traumatic dislocations of the knee due to the bowstring effect across the popliteal fossa secondary to proximal and distal tethering. In a cadaveric study, hyperextension of the knee induced by anterior dislocation resulted in posterior capsular tearing at 30 degrees and popliteal artery tearing at 50 degrees. Although collateral circulation may result in the presence of distal pulses and capillary refill, it is inadequate to maintain limb viability.

  Neurologic injury—peroneal nerve (10% to 35%). This is commonly associated with posterolateral dislocations, with injury varying from neurapraxia to complete transection. Primary exploration with grafting or repair is not effective; secondary exploration at 3 months also shows poor results. Bracing and/or tendon transfer may be necessary for treatment of muscular deficiencies.

RADIOGRAPHIC EVALUATION

- A knee dislocation is a potentially limb-threatening condition. Because of the high incidence of neurovascular compromise, immediate reduction is recommended before radiographic evaluation. After reduction, anteroposterior and lateral views of the knee should be obtained to assess the reduction and to evaluate associated injuries. Widened joint spaces may indicate soft-tissue interposition and the need for open reduction.
- The use of angiography in every case of knee dislocation is controversial. Vascular compromise is an indication for operative intervention. Identifying intimal tears in a neurovascularly intact limb may be unnecessary because most do not result in thrombosis and vascular occlusion. Regardless, the patient should be closely observed for at least 1 week by trained medical personnel. Until the issue is resolved, however, the current recommendation is that all knee dislocations should receive an angiogram to evaluate arterial patency.
- Magnetic resonance imaging is essential to assess the extent of soft-tissue disruption.

DESCRIPTIVE CLASSIFICATION

Based on displacement of the proximal tibia relative to the distal femur. Also should include open versus closed and reducible versus irreducible. May be classified as occult, indicating a knee dislocation with spontaneous reduction.

Anterior:	Forceful knee hyperextension beyond –30 degrees; most common (30% to 50%). Associated with posterior (and possibly anterior) cruciate ligament tear, with increasing incidence of popliteal artery disruption with increasing degree of hyperextension.
Posterior:	Posteriorly directed force against proximal tibia of flexed knee (25%); "dashboard" injury. Accompanied by anterior and posterior ligament disruption and popliteal artery compromise with increasing proximal tibial displacement.
Lateral:	Valgus force (13%). Medial supporting structures disrupted, often with tears of both cruciate ligaments.
Medial:	Varus force (3%). Lateral and posterolateral structures disrupted.
Rotational:	Varus/valgus with rotatory component (4%). Usually results in buttonholing of the femoral condyle through the articular capsule.

TREATMENT

Nonoperative Treatment

- Immediate closed reduction is essential, even in the field and especially in the compromised limb. Direct pressure on the popliteal space should be avoided both during and after reduction. Reduction maneuvers are as follows:
  - Anterior: axial limb traction combined with anteriorly directed force on the distal femur.
  - Posterior: axial limb traction combined with extension and anteriorly directed force on the proximal tibia.
  - Medial/lateral: axial limb traction combined with lateral/medial translation of the tibia.
  - Rotatory: axial limb traction combined with derotation of the tibia.
- The posterolateral dislocation may be "irreducible" due to buttonholing of the medial femoral condyle through the medial capsule, resulting in a dimple sign over the medial aspect of the limb.
- The knee should be splinted at 20 to 30 degrees of flexion. The knee must be perfectly reduced in the cast or splint. After adequate soft-tissue healing (6 to 12 weeks), range-of-motion exercises may be instituted.

Operative Treatment

- Indications for operative treatment of knee dislocation include the following:
  - Unsuccessful closed reduction.
  - Residual soft-tissue interposition.
  - Open injuries.
  - Vascular injuries.
- Vascular injuries require external fixation and vascular repair with a reverse saphenous vein graft from the contralateral leg; amputation rates as high as 86% have been reported when a delay of more than 8 hours occurs with documented vascular compromise to limb. A fasciotomy should be performed at the time of vascular repair for limb ischemia times greater than 6 hours.
- Ligamentous repair is controversial. The current literature favors acute repair of lateral ligaments, followed by early motion and functional bracing. The timing of surgical repair depends on the condition of both the patient and the limb. Meniscal injuries should also be addressed at the time of surgery.
- The role of cruciate reconstruction in the acute setting remains controversial. Insulated medial collateral ligament injuries generally will heal without surgery.

COMPLICATIONS

- Limited range of motion: most common, related to scar formation and capsular tightness. This reflects the balance between sufficient immobilization to achieve stability versus mobilization to restore motion. If severely limiting, lysis of adhesions may be undertaken to restore range of motion.
- Ligamentous laxity and instability: redislocation uncommon, especially after ligamentous reconstruction and adequate immobilization.
- Vascular compromise: may result in atrophic skin changes, hyperalgesia, claudication, and muscle contracture. Recognition of popliteal artery injury is of paramount importance, particularly between 24 to 72 hours after the initial injury when a late thrombosis related to intimal injury may be overlooked.
- Nerve traction injury: results in sensory and motor disturbances; portends a poor prognosis, as explorations in the acute (<24 hours), subacute (1 to 2 weeks), and long-term (3 months) settings have yielded poor results. Bracing or muscle tendon transfers may be necessary to improve function.

34. PATELLA

PATELLAR FRACTURES

Epidemiology

- Represent 1% of all skeletal injuries.
- Male-to-female ratio of 2:1.
- Occur in all age groups, but primarily found between 20 and 50 years of age.
- Bilateral injuries uncommon.
- Must also suspect ipsilateral femoral shaft or distal femoral fracture, proximal tibia fracture, or posterior dislocation of the hip with high energy injuries.

Anatomy

- The patella is the largest sesamoid bone in the body.
- The quadriceps tendon inserts on the superior pole and the patellar ligament originates from the inferior pole.
- Seven articular facets are found.
- The medial and lateral extensor retinacula are strong longitudinal expansions of the quadriceps; they insert directly onto the tibia. If these remain intact in the presence of a patella fracture, then active extension will be preserved.
- The patella increases the mechanical advantage and leverage of the quadriceps tendon, aids in nourishment of the femoral articular surface, and protects the femoral condyles from direct trauma.
- The blood supply arises from the geniculate arteries, which form an anastomosis circumferentially around the patella.

Mechanism of Injury

- *Direct.* Trauma to the patella may produce incomplete, simple, stellate, or comminuted fracture patterns. Displacement is typically minimal due to preservation of the medial and lateral retinacular expansions. Abrasions over the area or open injuries are common. Active knee extension may be observed.
- *Indirect.* This results from secondary to forcible quadriceps contraction while the knee is in a semiflexed position (e.g., in a "stumble" or "fall"). The intrinsic strength of the patella is exceeded by the pull of the musculotendinous and ligamentous structures, with continued tearing of the medial and lateral retinacular structures with continued injury. A transverse fracture pattern with variable inferior pole comminution is most commonly seen with this mechanism. The degree of displacement of the fragments suggests the degree of retinacular disruption. Active knee extension is usually lost.
- *Combined direct/indirect mechanisms.* These may be caused by trauma in which the patient experiences direct and indirect trauma to the knee, such as in a fall from a height. Fracture fragments are usually considerably separated.

Clinical Evaluation

- Patients typically present with limited or no ambulatory capacity with pain, swelling, and tenderness of the involved knee. Defects may be palpable.
- Ruling out open fractures is important because they constitute surgical emergencies; to do so may require instillation of saline or methylene blue to determine communication with overlying lacerations.
- Active knee extension should be evaluated to determine injury to the retinacular expansions. This may be aided by decompression of a hemarthrosis or by an intra-articular injection of lidocaine.
- Associated lower extremity injuries may be present in the setting of high energy trauma. The physician must carefully evaluate the ipsilateral hip, femur, tibia, and ankle, with appropriate radiographic assessment if indicated.

Radiographic Evaluation

- Anteroposterior and lateral views of the knee should be obtained. Axial (sunrise) views of the bilateral patellae should be obtained.

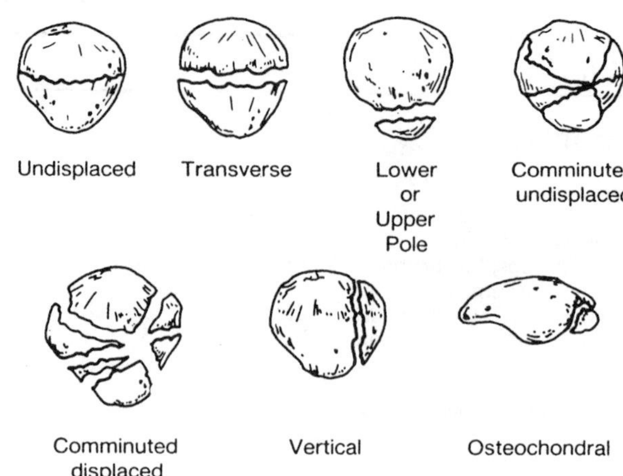

FIG. 34.1. Classification of patellar fractures. (From Heckman JD, Bucholz RW, eds. *Rockwood, Green, and Wilkins' fractures in adults*, 5th ed. Philadelphia: Lippincott Williams & Wilkins, 2001, with permission.)

Anteroposterior view. The bipartite patella may be mistaken for a fracture (1%). The bipartite fragment usually occurs in the superolateral position and has smooth margins; it is bilateral in 50% of patients.

Lateral view. Displaced fractures usually are obvious.

Axial view (sunrise). Osteochondral or vertical marginal fractures may be identified.

- Arthrograms, computed tomography, or magnetic resonance imaging are usually unnecessary but may further delineate fracture patterns, marginal fractures, or free osteochondral fragments.

DESCRIPTIVE CLASSIFICATION (FIG. 34.1)

- Open versus closed
- Displacement
- Pattern: stellate, comminuted, transverse, vertical (marginal), polar
- Osteochondral

ORTHOPAEDIC TRAUMA ASSOCIATION CLASSIFICATION OF PATELLAR FRACTURES

Type A: extraarticular
- A1: avulsion
- A2: isolated body fracture

Type B: partial articular
- B1: vertical, lateral
- B2: vertical, medial
- B3: multifragmentary (stellate)

Type C: complete articular, disrupted extensor mechanism
- C1: transverse
- C2: transverse plus second fragment
- C3: complex

Treatment

Nonoperative Treatment

- Indications include nondisplaced or minimally displaced (2 to 3 mm) fractures with minimal articular disruption (1 to 2 mm). This requires an intact extensor mechanism.

- A cylinder cast is required for 4 to 6 weeks. Early weight bearing is encouraged and should be advanced to full weight bearing with crutches as tolerated by the patient. After radiographic evidence of healing, progressive active flexion and extension strengthening exercises with a hinged knee brace initially locked in extension for ambulation should begin.

Operative Treatment
Treatment with open reduction and internal fixation includes the following:

- Indications for open reduction and internal fixation include >2 mm articular incongruity, >3 mm fragment displacement, or open fracture.
- Multiple methods of operative fixation exist, including tension banding with parallel longitudinal Kirschner wires or cancellous lag screws. Retinacular disruption should be repaired at the time of surgery.
- Postoperatively, the patient should be placed in a splint for 3 to 6 days until the skin has healed. Physical therapy should be instituted early. The patient should perform active assisted range-of-motion exercises and should progress to partial and full weight bearing by 6 weeks.
- Continuous passive motion devices may be used early if patient can tolerate passive range of motion.
- Severely comminuted or marginally repaired fractures may necessitate immobilization for 3 to 6 weeks.

Treatment with patellectomy is as follows:

- Partial patellectomy:
  - Indications for partial patellectomy include the presence of a large salvageable fragment in the presence of smaller comminuted polar fragments with which restoring the articular surface or achieving stable fixation is impossible.
  - The quadriceps or patellar tendons must be reattached without creating a patella baja or alta.
  - Reattachment of the patellar tendon close to the articular surface will prevent patellar tilt.
- Total patellectomy:
  - Total patellectomy is reserved for cases with extensive and severe comminution.
  - Advantages include a shorter period of immobilization, a less complicated operative procedure, and an earlier return to work.
  - However, peak torque of the quadriceps is reduced by 50%, making this only rarely indicated.
  - Repair of medial and lateral retinacular injuries at the time of patellectomy is essential.
- Postoperatively, the knee should be immobilized in a long-leg cast at 10 degrees of flexion for 3 to 6 weeks.

Complications

- Postoperative infection: uncommon; related to open injuries that may necessitate serial debridement. Relentless infection may require excision of nonviable fragments and plastic repair of the extensor mechanism.
- Fixation failure: increased incidence in osteoporotic bone or with failure to achieve compression at the fracture site.
- Refracture (1% to 5%): secondary to decreased inherent strength at the fracture site.
- Nonunion (2%): most patients retain good function, although partial patellectomy may be a consideration for painful nonunion. Consider revision osteosynthesis in more active, younger patients.
- Avascular necrosis (proximal fragment): associated with greater degrees of initial fracture displacement. Treatment consists of observation only, with spontaneous revascularization occurring within 2 years.
- Posttraumatic osteoarthritis: present in over 50% of patients in long-term studies. Intractable patellofemoral pain may require Maquet tibial tubercle advancement.

- Loss of knee range of motion: secondary to prolonged immobilization or postoperative scarring.
- Painful retained hardware: may necessitate removal for adequate relief of symptoms.
- Loss of extensor strength and an extensor lag: approximately 5 degrees on average; rarely is clinically significant.
- Patellar instability.

PATELLAR DISLOCATION

Epidemiology

Patellar dislocation is more common in females, due to physiologic laxity, and in patients with hypermobility and connective tissue disorders (e.g., Ehlers-Danlos or Marfan syndromes).

Anatomy

- The "Q-angle" is defined as the angle subtended by an axis drawn from the anterior inferior iliac spine through the center of the patella and a second axis from the center of the patella to the tibial tubercle. The Q-angle ensures that the resultant vector of pull with quadriceps action is laterally directed; this lateral moment is normally counterbalanced by patellofemoral, patellotibial, and retinacular structures and by patellar engagement within the trochlear groove.
- Dislocations are associated with patella alta, congenital abnormalities of the patella and trochlea, hypoplasia of the vastus medialis, and a hypertrophic lateral retinaculum.

Mechanism of Injury

- Lateral: forced internal rotation of the femur on an externally rotated and planted tibia with the knee in flexion. Associated with a 5% risk of osteochondral fractures.
- Medial instability: rare and usually iatrogenic, congenital, traumatic, or associated with atrophy of the quadriceps musculature.
- Intraarticular: uncommon but may occur after knee trauma in adolescent boys. The patella is avulsed from the quadriceps tendon and rotated around the horizontal axis, with the proximal pole lodged in the intercondylar notch.
- Superior: occurs in elderly individuals from forced hyperextension injuries to the knee with the patella locked on an anterior femoral osteophyte.

Clinical Evaluation

- Patients with unreduced patellar dislocations will present with a hemarthrosis, an inability to flex the knee, and a displaced patella on palpation.
- Lateral dislocations may also present with medial retinacular pain.
- Patients with reduced or chronic patellar dislocation may demonstrate a positive "apprehension test," in which a laterally directed force applied to the patella with the knee in extension reproduces the sensation of impending dislocation, causing pain and quadriceps contraction to limit patellar mobility.

Radiographic Evaluation

- Anteroposterior and lateral views of the knee should be obtained. In addition, an axial (sunrise) view of bilateral patellae should be taken (Fig. 34.2). Various axial views have been described by several authors as follows:
  - **Hughston** (55 degrees of flexion): sulcus angle, patellar index.
  - **Merchant** (45 degrees of flexion): sulcus angle, congruence angle.
  - **Laurin** (20 degrees of flexion): patellofemoral index, lateral patellofemoral angle.
- Assessment of patella alta or baja is based on the lateral radiograph of the knee as the following explains:
  - *Blumensaat line.* Lower pole of the patella should lie on a line projected anteriorly from the intercondylar notch on the lateral radiograph with knee flexed to 30 degrees.

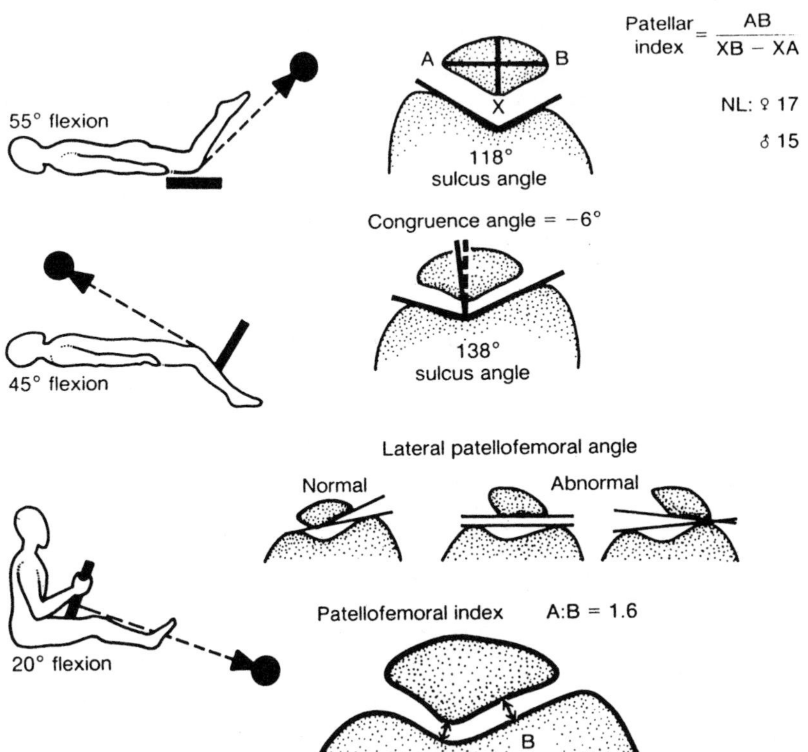

FIG. 34.2. A representation of the Hughston (55-degree), Merchant (45-degree), and Laurin (20-degree) patella views. (From Rockwood CA Jr, Green DP, Bucholz RW, Heckman JD, eds. *Rockwood and Green's fractures in adults*, 4th ed. Vol. 2. Philadelphia: Lippincott-Raven, 1996:2038, with permission.)

Insall-Salvati ratio. The ratio of the length of the patellar ligament (LL; from the inferior pole of the patella to the tibial tubercle) to the patellar length (LP; the greatest diagonal length of the patella) should be 1.0. A ratio of 1.2 indicates patella alta, whereas 0.8 indicates patella baja.

DESCRIPTIVE CLASSIFICATION

- Reduced versus unreduced
- Congenital versus acquired
- Acute (traumatic) versus chronic (recurrent)
- Lateral, medial, intraarticular, superior

Treatment

Nonoperative Treatment

- Reduction and extension casting or bracing may be undertaken with or without arthrocentesis for comfort.
- The patient may ambulate in locked extension for 3 weeks, at which time progressive flexion can be instituted with physical therapy for quadriceps strengthening. After a total of 6 to 8 weeks, the patient may be weaned from the brace as tolerated.

- Surgical intervention for acute dislocations is not warranted except in those cases of displaced intraarticular fractures exclusive of the medial border or with recurrent dislocations. Intraarticular dislocations may require reduction under anesthesia.
- Functional taping with moderate success has been described in physical therapy literature.

Operative

- No single procedure corrects all patellar malalignment problems—the patient's age, diagnosis, level of activity, and the condition of the patellofemoral articulation must be taken into consideration.
- Patellofemoral instability must be addressed by correction of all malalignment factors.
- Degenerative articular changes influence the selection of the realignment procedure.
- Surgical interventions include the following:
  - Lateral release: indicated for patellofemoral pain with lateral tilt, lateral retinacular pain with lateral patellar position, and lateral patellar compression syndrome. It may be performed arthroscopically or as an open procedure.
  - Medial plication: may be performed at the time of lateral release to centralize the patella.
  - Proximal patellar realignment: medialization of the proximal pull of the patella indicated when a lateral release/medial plication fails to centralize the patella. The release of tight proximal lateral structures and the reinforcement of the pull of medial supporting structures, especially the vastus medialis obliquus, are performed in an effort to decrease lateral patellar tracking and to improve the congruence of the patellofemoral articulation. Indications include recurrent patellar dislocations that have failed following nonoperative therapy, as well as acute dislocations in young and athletic patients, especially with medial patellar avulsion fractures or radiographic lateral subluxation/tilt after closed reduction.
  - Distal patellar realignment: reorientation of the patellar ligament and tibial tubercle indicated when an adult patient experiences recurrent dislocations and patellofemoral pain with malalignment of the extensor mechanism. It is contraindicated in patients with open physes and normal Q-angles. It is designed to advance and medialize the tibial tubercle, thus correcting patella alta and normalizing the Q-angle.

Complications

- Redislocation. This has a statistically significant lower risk in patients older than 20 years at the time of first episode. Recurrent dislocation is an indication for surgical intervention.
- Loss of range of motion of the knee. Prolonged immobilization may result in loss of range of motion. Surgical intervention may lead to scarring with resultant arthrofibrosis. This emphasizes the need for aggressive physical therapy to increase quadriceps tone, to maintain patellar alignment, and to maintain knee range of motion.
- Patellofemoral pain. This may result from retinacular disruption at the time of dislocation or due to chondral injury.

35. TIBIAL PLATEAU

EPIDEMIOLOGY

- Fractures of the tibial plateau constitute 1% of all fractures; they comprise 8% of fractures seen in the elderly.
- Isolated injuries to the lateral plateau account for 70% to 80% of tibial plateau fractures, in comparison to 10% to 23% isolated medial plateau involvement and 10% to 30% with bicondylar lesions.
- One percent to 3% of these fractures are open injuries.

ANATOMY

- The tibia is the major weight-bearing bone of the leg, accounting for 85% of the transmitted load.
- The tibial plateau is composed of the articular surfaces of the medial and lateral tibial plateaus, upon which are the cartilaginous menisci. The medial plateau is larger and is concave in both the sagittal and coronal axes. The lateral plateau extends higher and is convex in both the sagittal and coronal planes.
- The normal tibial plateau has a 10-degree posteroinferior slope. The two plateaus are separated from one another by the intercondylar eminence, which is nonarticular and which serves as the tibial attachment of the cruciate ligaments. Three bony prominences exist 2 to 3 cm distal to the tibial plateau. The tibial tubercle is located anteriorly, upon which the patellar ligament inserts. Medially, the pes anserinus serves as an attachment for the medial hamstrings. Laterally, the Gerdy tubercle affords the insertion of the iliotibial band.
- The medial articular surface and its supporting medial condyle are stronger than their lateral counterparts. As a result, fractures of the lateral plateau are more common.
- Medial plateau fractures are associated with more violent injuries and more commonly have associated soft-tissue injuries, such as disruptions of the lateral collateral ligament complex, lesions of the peroneal nerve, and damage to the popliteal vessels.

MECHANISM OF INJURY

- Fractures of the tibial plateau occur in the setting of violent varus or valgus forces coupled with axial loading. Motor vehicle accidents account for the majority of these ("bumper injuries") in the young, but elderly patients with osteopenic bone may experience them after a fall.
- The direction and magnitude of the generated force, the age of the patient, bone quality, and the amount of knee flexion at the moment of impact determine fracture fragment size, location, and displacement as follows:
  - Young patients with strong rigid bone typically develop split fractures and have a high rate of associated ligamentous disruption, although whether an intact collateral ligament on one side of the knee is necessary for a fracture of the contralateral plateau is controversial.
  - Older patients with decreased bone strength and rigidity incur depression and split-depression fractures and have a lower rate of ligamentous injury.
  - If a severe axial force is exerted on a fully extended knee, a bicondylar split fracture results.

CLINICAL EVALUATION

- A neurovascular examination is essential, especially with high energy trauma. The trifurcation of the popliteal artery is tethered posteriorly between the adductor hiatus proximally and the soleus complex distally. The peroneal nerve is tethered laterally as it courses around the fibular neck.
- Frequently, a hemarthrosis occurs in the setting of a markedly swollen, painful knee upon which the patient is unable to bear weight. Aspiration may reveal marrow fat.

- Direct trauma is usually evident upon examination of the overlying soft tissues; open injuries must be ruled out. Intraarticular instillation of saline or methylene blue may be necessary to evaluate possible communication with overlying lacerations.
- Compartment syndrome must be ruled out, especially with Schatzker type V or VI fractures.
- Assessment for ligament injury is essential.

Associated Injuries

- Meniscal tears occur in up to 50% of tibial plateau fractures.
- Associated ligamentous disruption of the cruciates or collaterals occur in up to 30% of tibial plateau fractures.
- Young patients, whose strong subchondral bone resists depression, are at the highest risk of collateral or cruciate ligament rupture.
- Fractures involving the medial tibial plateau are associated with higher incidences of peroneal nerve or popliteal neurovascular lesions due to higher energy mechanisms; that many of these represent knee dislocations that have spontaneously reduced has been postulated.
- Peroneal nerve injuries are caused by stretching (neurapraxia); these generally resolve with time.
- Arterial injuries frequently represent traction-induced intimal injuries presenting as thrombosis; only rarely do they present as transection injuries secondary to laceration or avulsion.

RADIOGRAPHIC EVALUATION

- Anteroposterior lateral views supplemented by 40-degree internal (lateral plateau) and external rotation (medial plateau) oblique projections should be obtained.
- Stress views are preferably obtained under sedation or anesthesia and with fluoroscopic image intensification; these are occasionally useful for the detection of collateral ligament ruptures.
- Computed tomography with two- or three-dimensional reconstruction has supplanted linear tomography for delineating the degree of fragmentation or the depression of the articular surface, as well as for preoperative planning.
- Magnetic resonance imaging is useful for evaluating injuries to the menisci, the cruciate and collateral ligaments, and the soft-tissue envelope.
- Arteriography should be performed if diminution of the distal pulses is found. High energy mechanisms, unexplained compartment syndromes, severely displaced fracture-dislocation patterns, and Schatzker type IV to VI lesions should raise suspicion of possible vascular compromise.

SCHATZKER CLASSIFICATION (FIG. 35.1)

Type I: lateral plateau, split fracture
Type II: lateral plateau, split depression fracture
Type III: lateral plateau, depression fracture
Type IV: medial plateau fracture
Type V: bicondylar plateau fracture
Type VI: plateau fracture with metaphyseal-diaphyseal dissociation

ORTHOPAEDIC TRAUMA ASSOCIATION CLASSIFICATION OF TIBIAL PLATEAU FRACTURES

Type A: extraarticular fractures (no articular surface involved)
Type B: partial articular fracture
- B1: pure split
- B2: pure depression
- B3: split depression

Type C: complete articular fracture
- C1: articular simple, metaphyseal simple
- C2: articular simple, metaphyseal multifragmentary
- C3: articular and metaphyseal multifragmentary

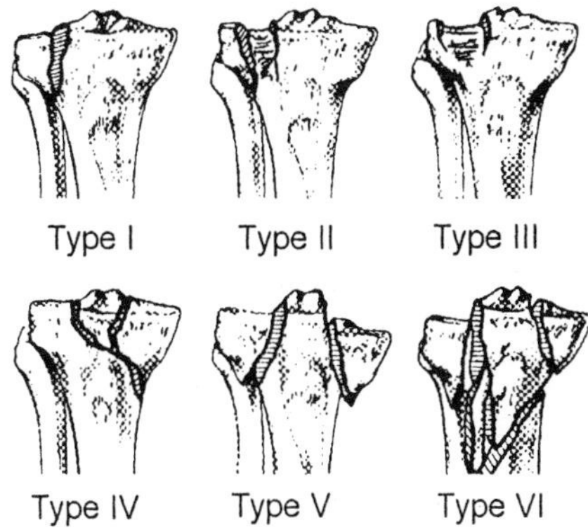

FIG. 35.1. Schatzker classification of tibial plateau fractures. (From Hansen S, Swiontkowski M. *Orthopaedic trauma protocols*. New York: Raven Press, 1993:315, with permission.)

TREATMENT

The goal of treatment is to obtain a stable, aligned, mobile, and painless joint and to minimize the risk of posttraumatic arthritis.

Nonoperative Treatment

- Nonoperative treatment is used for nondisplaced or minimally displaced fractures, especially in patients with significant comorbid diseases or advanced osteoporosis.
- It may also be used with selected gunshot wounds and severely contaminated or infected fractures.
- Reduction is by distal supramalleolar skeletal traction and ligamentotaxis.
- The limb is immobilized in a fracture brace, and weight bearing is prohibited.
- If displacement is unlikely, beginning early passive range-of-motion exercises promotes cartilage healing and prevents loss of motion.
- If the fracture is unstable because of excessive comminution or advanced osteoporosis, skeletal traction and early passive range of motion may be appropriate.
- The goal of nonsurgical treatment is not anatomic reduction but restoration of axial alignment and knee motion. Up to 7 degrees of varus/valgus malalignment may be accepted.

Operative

- Surgical indications are as follows:
  - Displacement: amount of displacement necessary for operative intervention is controversial—up to 1 cm on the lateral side accepted. Joint irregularities <1.5 mm are not associated with increased contact pressure, although depression >3 mm is associated with a significant increase in contact pressure.
  - Instability: >10 degrees with an extended knee (relative).
  - Open fractures.
  - Compartment syndrome.
  - Vascular injury: requires operative treatment.
  - Critically ill from comorbid trauma or with compromised soft tissues: approached with percutaneous or bridging external fixation or skeletal traction rather than with cast immobilization (relative).
  - Arthroscopy: may be used to evaluate the articular surfaces, menisci, and integrity of the cruciate ligaments. It may also be used for evacuation of a hemarthrosis and particulate debris and meniscal procedures, as well as for arthroscopic-assisted reduction and fixation. It has a limited role in the evaluation of rim pathology, as well as limited utility in the management of complicated fractures.
  - Ruptured collateral ligament combined with a plateau fracture: repaired at the time of surgery.

  - Avulsed anterior cruciate ligament with a large bony fragment: also repaired. If the fragment is minimal or if the ligament has an intrasubstance tear, reconstruction should be delayed.
- Surgery in isolated injuries should proceed only after a full appreciation of the personality of the fracture is achieved. This delay will also allow swelling to subside and local skin conditions to improve.
- Type I to IV fractures can be fixed with percutaneous screws or lateral "L" plates. If satisfactory closed reduction (<1 mm articular step-off) cannot be achieved with closed techniques, open reduction and internal fixation are indicated.
- The meniscus should never be excised to facilitate exposure.
- Depressed fragments can be elevated en masse from below by using a bone tamp and working through the split component or a cortical window. The metaphyseal defect should be filled with cancellous autograft or allograft.
- Type V and VI fractures are best managed with a ring fixator or hybrid fixator to preserve the surrounding soft tissues. Limited internal fixation can be added to restore the articular surface. Postoperative non–weight bearing with continuous passive motion and active range of motion is encouraged.
  - Schatzker types I to III: partial weight bearing is started at 4 to 8 weeks and is advanced with radiographic evidence of healing, with progression to weight bearing as tolerated at 12 weeks.
  - Schatzker types IV to VI: partial weight bearing is begun at 8 to 12 weeks with individualized advancement.

COMPLICATIONS

- Knee stiffness: common, related to trauma from injury and surgical dissection, extensor retinacular injuries, scarring, and postoperative immobility.
- Infection: often related to ill-timed incisions through compromised soft tissues with extensive dissection for implant placement. May require delayed primary or flap closure to achieve tension-free approximation.
- Compartment syndrome: uncommon but devastating complication involving the tight fascial compartments of the leg. Emphasizes the need for high clinical suspicion; serial neurovascular examinations, particularly in the unconscious or obtunded patient; aggressive evaluation, including compartment pressure measuring if necessary; and expedient treatment, consisting of emergent fasciotomies of all compartments of the leg.
- Malunion/nonunion: most common in Schatzker type VI at the metaphyseal-diaphyseal junction; related to comminution, unstable fixation, implant failure, or infection. Nonunion uncommon due to predominance of well-vascularized cancellous bone.
- Posttraumatic osteoarthritis: may result from residual articular incongruity or chondral damage at the time of injury.
- Peroneal nerve injury: most common with trauma to the lateral aspect of the leg where the peroneal nerve courses in proximity to the fibular head and lateral tibial plateau.
- Popliteal artery laceration.
- Avascular necrosis of small articular fragments: may result in loose bodies within the knee articulation.

36. TIBIAL/FIBULAR SHAFT

EPIDEMIOLOGY

- Fractures of the tibial and fibular shaft are the most common long-bone fractures, accounting for almost 500,000 cases per year in the United States.
- In the early 1990s, fractures of the tibia and fibula accounted for 77,000 hospitalizations per year, accounting for 569,000 hospital days with an average length of stay of 7.4 days and 825,000 office visits to physicians.

ANATOMY

- The tibia is a long tubular long bone with a triangular cross-section. It has a subcutaneous anteromedial border and is bounded by four tight fascial compartments.
- Its blood supply is from the following:
  - The nutrient artery arises from the posterior tibial artery, entering the posterolateral cortex distal to the origination of the soleus muscle, at the oblique line of the tibia. Once the vessel enters the intramedullary canal, it gives off three ascending branches and one descending branch. These give rise to the endosteal vascular tree, which anastomoses with periosteal vessels arising from the anterior tibial artery.
  - The anterior tibial artery is particularly vulnerable to injury as it passes through a hiatus in the interosseus membrane.
  - The peroneal artery has an anterior communicating branch to the dorsalis pedis artery. It may therefore be occluded despite an intact dorsalis pedis pulse.
  - The distal third is supplied by periosteal anastomoses around the ankle with branches entering the tibia through ligamentous attachments.
  - A watershed area may be found at the junction of the middle and distal thirds; this is controversial.
  - If the nutrient artery is disrupted, reversal of flow through the cortex occurs with the periosteal blood supply becoming more important. This emphasizes the importance of preserving periosteal attachments during fixation.
- The fibula is responsible for 6% to 17% of weight-bearing load. The common peroneal nerve courses around the neck of the fibula, which is nearly subcutaneous in this region (Fig. 36.1); it is therefore especially vulnerable to direct blows or traction injuries at this level.

MECHANISM OF INJURY

Direct

- High energy (e.g., motor vehicle accidents)
  - Transverse, comminuted, displaced fractures.
  - High incidence of soft-tissue injury.
- Penetrating (e.g., gunshot)
  - Injury pattern: variable.
  - Low velocity missiles (handguns): bone or soft-tissue damage not as problematic as when caused by high energy (motor vehicle accidents) or high velocity (shotguns, assault weapons) mechanisms.
- Bending: three or four point (e.g., ski boot injuries)
  - Short oblique or transverse fractures, possible butterfly fragment.
  - Crush.
  - Highly comminuted or segmental patterns associated with extensive soft-tissue compromise.
  - Must rule out compartment syndrome and open fractures.
- Fibular shaft: typically results from direct trauma to the lateral aspect of the leg.

Indirect

- Torsional mechanisms
  - Twisting with foot fixed, falls from low heights.
  - Spiral nondisplaced fractures, minimal comminution associated with minimal soft-tissue damage.

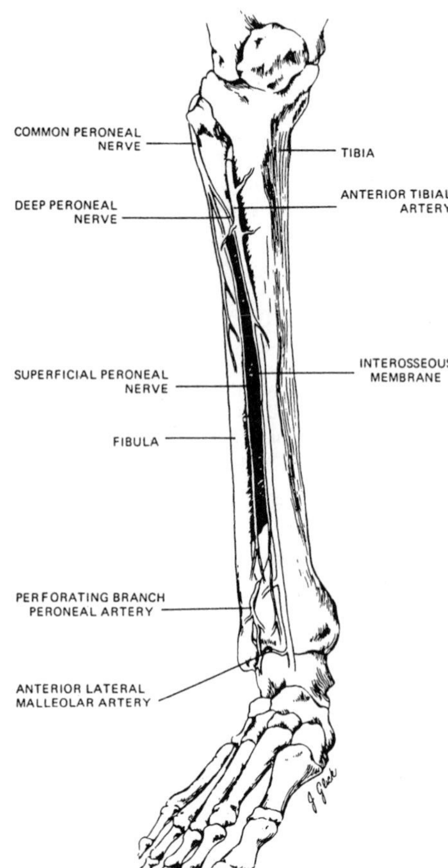

FIG. 36.1. The anatomy of the tibial and fibular shaft. (From Rockwood CA Jr, Green DP, Bucholz RW, Heckman JD, eds. *Rockwood and Green's fractures in adults*, 4th ed. Vol. 2. Philadelphia: Lippincott-Raven, 1996: 2124, with permission.)

- Stress fractures
  - In military recruits, most commonly occurs at the metaphyseal/diaphyseal junction, with reaction being most marked at the posteromedial cortex.
  - In ballet dancers, most commonly occurs in the middle third; insidious in onset; overuse injuries.
  - Radiographic findings may be delayed several weeks.

CLINICAL EVALUATION

- Evaluate neurovascular status. Dorsalis pedis and posterior tibial artery pulses must be evaluated and documented, especially in open fractures where vascular flaps may be necessary. Common peroneal nerve integrity must be documented.
- Assess soft-tissue injury. Fracture blisters may contraindicate open reduction.
- Monitor for compartment syndrome. Sensory loss is the first sign of impending compartment syndrome. Four compartment fasciotomies should be performed for pressures above 30 mm Hg.
- Deep posterior compartment pressures may be elevated in the face of a soft superficial posterior compartment.

RADIOGRAPHIC EVALUATION

- Radiographic evaluation must include a full knee and ankle series and entire tibia (anteroposterior and lateral views; oblique views if necessary to characterize fracture pattern).
- Postreduction radiographs should include the knee and ankle for preoperative planning and alignment.
- Computed tomography and magnetic resonance imaging usually are not necessary.
- Obtain an angiogram if arterial injury is suspected.

CLASSIFICATION

Poor sensitivity, reproducibility, and interobserver reliability have been reported for present classification schemes.

DESCRIPTIVE CLASSIFICATION

- Open versus closed
- Anatomic location: proximal, middle, or distal third
- Fragment number and position: comminution, butterfly fragments
- Configuration: transverse, spiral, oblique
- Angulation: varus/valgus, anterior/posterior
- Shortening
- Displacement: percentage of cortical contact
- Rotation
- Associated injuries

ORTHOPAEDIC TRAUMA ASSOCIATION CLASSIFICATION OF TIBIAL FRACTURES (FIG. 36.2)

Type A: simple
- A1: spiral
- A2: oblique (>30 degrees)
- A3: transverse (<30 degrees)

Type B: wedge (butterfly)
- B1: spiral
- B2: bending
- B3: fragmented

Type C: complex (comminuted)
- C1: spiral
- C2: segmented
- C3: irregular

TREATMENT

Acceptable Reduction

- Less than 5 degrees of varus/valgus angulation.
- Less than 10 degrees of anterior/posterior angulation; <5 degrees preferred.
- Less than 10 degrees of rotational deformity, with external rotation better tolerated than internal rotation.
- Less than 1 cm of shortening; 5 mm of distraction may delay healing 8 to 12 months.
- More than 50% cortical contact.

Nonoperative Treatment

- Reduction followed by application of a long-leg cast with progressive weight bearing is most commonly used for isolated, closed, low-energy fractures with minimal displacement and comminution.
- Traction is rarely indicated because it may distract the fracture site and precludes ambulation.

(text continues on 240)

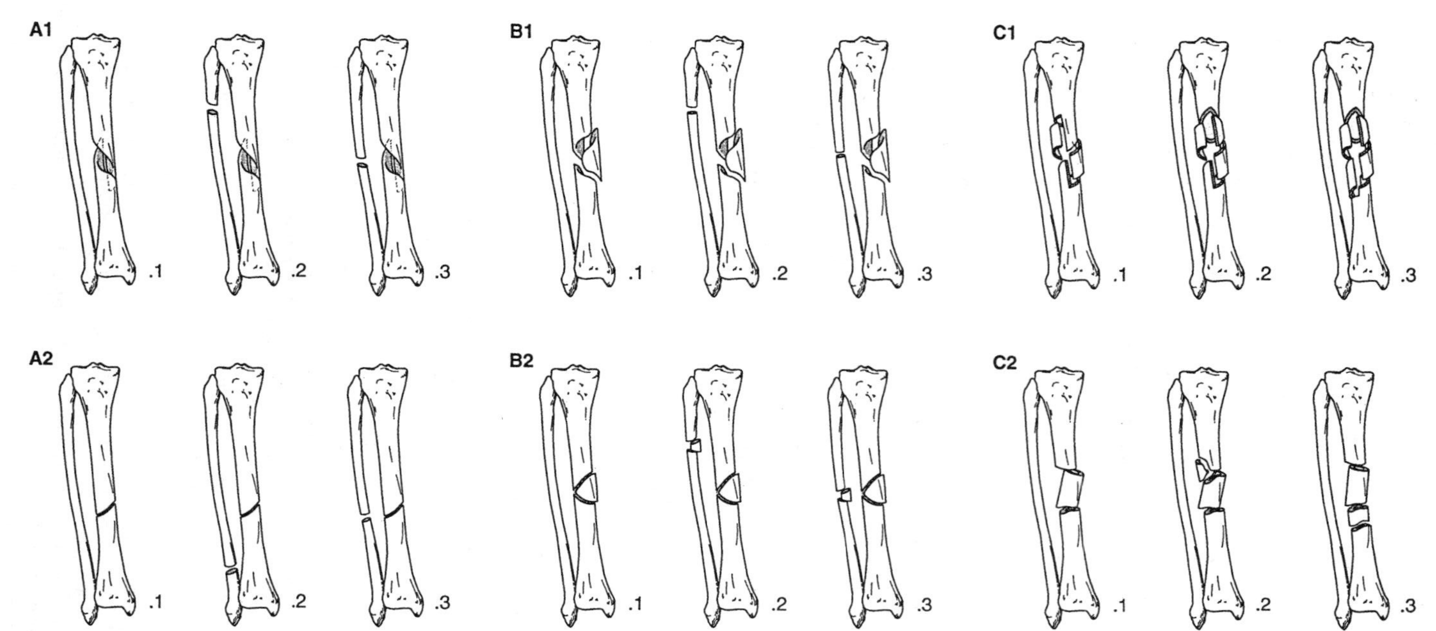

FIG. 36.2. The Orthopaedic Trauma Association (OTA) classification of tibial diaphyseal fractures. (From Heckman JD, Bucholz RW, eds. *Rockwood, Green, and Wilkins' fractures in adults*, 5th ed. Philadelphia: Lippincott Williams & Wilkins, 2001, with permission.)

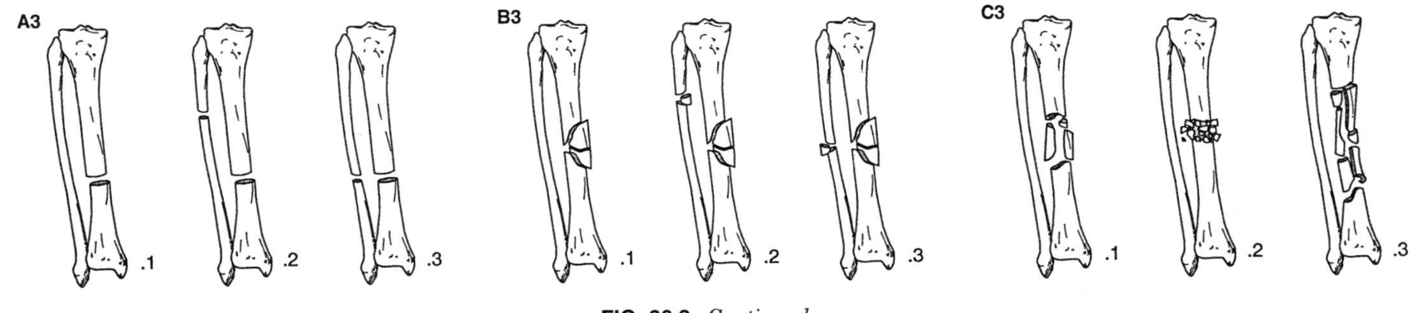

FIG. 36.2. *Continued.*

- The cast is applied with the knee in 0 to 5 degree of flexion to allow for weight bearing with crutches as soon as tolerated by patient, with advancement to full weight bearing by second to fourth week.
- After the initial swelling subsides, the cast may be exchanged for a patellar-bearing cast or fracture brace.
- Union rates as high as 97% have been reported, although delayed weight bearing is related to delayed or nonunion.

Time to Union

- Average 16 ± 4 weeks: highly variable, depending on fracture pattern and soft-tissue injury.
- Delayed union: defined as >20 weeks.
- Nonunion: when clinical and radiographic signs demonstrate that the potential for union is lost, including sclerotic ends at the fracture site and a persistent gap unchanged for several weeks; usually apparent by 36 weeks.

Tibial Stress Fracture

- Treatment consists of cessation of the offending activity.
- A short-leg cast may be necessary; with partial weight bearing, ambulation is usually sufficient to heal the fracture in 6 to 10 weeks.

Fibular Shaft Fracture

- Treatment consists of weight bearing as tolerated; although a long-leg cast is not required for healing, it may be used initially to minimize pain.
- Nonunion is uncommon due to the extensive muscular attachments.

Operative Treatment

Fasciotomy

Evidence of compartment syndrome is an indication for emergent fasciotomies of all muscle compartments of the leg (anterior, lateral, superficial, and deep posterior) through one or multiple incision techniques. After operative fixation of the fracture, the fascial openings should not be reapproximated.

External Fixation

- Primarily used to treat open fractures but also indicated in unstable closed fractures and in closed fractures complicated by compartment syndrome, concomitant head injury, burns, or impaired sensation.
- Partial weight bearing encouraged soon after wound healing.
- Allows easy access to soft tissues and provides fairly rigid fixation of the fracture site.
- Union rates of up to 90%, with an average of 3.6 months to union.
- Ten percent to 15% incidence of pin-tract infections.

Plates and Screws

- Generally reserved for fractures extending into the metaphysis or epiphysis.
- Success rates as high as 97%.
- Complication rates of infection, wound breakdown, and mal- or nonunion increased with higher energy injury patterns.

Flexible Nails (Enders, Rush Rods)

- Multiple curved intramedullary pins exert a spring force to resist angulation and rotation, with minimal damage to the medullary circulation.
- Recommended only in stable fractures with >25% cortical continuity to prevent angulation and shortening.
- Union rates of up to 94% reported.
- Rarely used in United States due to predominance of unstable fracture patterns and success with interlocking nails.

Intramedullary Nailing

- Intramuscular nailing carries the advantages of preservation of periosteal blood supply and significant reduction of soft-tissue damage. In addition, it carries the biomechanical advantages of ability to control alignment, translation, and rotation. It is therefore recommended for most fracture patterns.
- The decision to use a locked versus unlocked nail is as follows:
  Locked nail: provides rotational control; effective in preventing shortening in comminuted fractures and those with significant bone loss; interlocking screws can be removed at a later time to dynamize the fracture site and to encourage healing.
  Unlocked nail: allows impaction at the fracture site with weight bearing but has difficulty controlling rotation.
- The choice of a reamed versus an unreamed nail is as follows:
  Reamed nail: for closed fractures; allows excellent intramedullary splinting of the fracture and use of a larger, stronger nail.
  Unreamed nail: designed to preserve the intramedullary blood supply in open fractures where the periosteal supply has been destroyed; currently used in grades I, II, and occasionally in IIIA fractures; its disadvantage is that it is significantly weaker than the larger reamed nail; full weight bearing is not advised.

Tibia Fracture with an Intact Fibula

- Treatment consists of long-leg casting with early non–weight bearing and close observation to halt any varus tendency.
- Some recommend immediate intramedullary nailing; others suggest immediate fibular osteotomy with removal of 2.5 cm of bone.
- A significant incidence of varus malunion, particularly in patients older than 20 years of age, occurs.

COMPLICATIONS

- Malunion: includes any deformity outside the acceptable range.
- Nonunion: associated with high velocity injuries, open fractures (especially Gustilo grade III), infection, intact fibula, inadequate fixation, and increased displacement.
- Infection.
- Soft-tissue loss: delaying wound coverage for greater than 7 to 10 days in Gustilo II and III injuries is associated with greater rates of infection. Local rotational flaps or free flaps may be needed for adequate coverage.
- Stiffness at the knee and/or ankle.
- Reflex sympathetic dystrophy (Sudek atrophy): most common in patients unable to bear weight early and with prolonged cast immobilization. Characterized by initial pain and swelling followed by atrophy of limb that is associated radiographically by spotty demineralization of the foot, distal tibia, and equinovarus ankle. Treated by elastic compression stockings, weight bearing, sympathetic blocks, and foot orthoses accompanied by aggressive physical therapy.
- Compartment syndrome: anterior is most common due to volume. Highest pressures at the time of open or closed reduction. Deep posterior compartment syndrome may be missed due to uninvolved overlying superficial compartment. May require fasciotomy. Muscle death occurs after 6 to 8 hours.
- Neurovascular injury: vascular compromise uncommon except with high velocity, markedly displaced, often open fractures. Most commonly occurs as the anterior tibial artery traverses the interosseous membrane of the proximal leg. May require a saphenous interposition graft. Common peroneal nerve vulnerable to direct injuries to the proximal fibula and fractures with significant varus angulation. Overzealous traction can result in distraction injuries to the nerve; inadequate cast molding/padding may result in neuropraxia.
- Fat embolism.
- Claw toe deformity: associated with scarring of extensor tendons or ischemia of posterior compartment muscles.

37. PILON

EPIDEMIOLOGY

- Pilon fractures account for 7% to 10% of all tibia fractures.
- Most pilon fractures are a result of high energy mechanisms; thus, concomitant injuries are common and should be ruled out.

ANATOMY

- The ankle is a complex joint consisting of the tibiofibular, tibiotalar, and talofibular articulations.
- Distally, the tibia flares out as the cortical diaphyseal bone changes to cancellous metaphyseal bone overlying the articular surface. This is similar to the tibial plateau in that primarily cancellous bone is found within a thin cortical shell.
- The articular surface, or tibial plafond, is concave in both the anteroposterior and mediolateral planes. It is wider anteriorly than posteriorly and longer laterally than medially. This is designed to accommodate the wedge-shaped talus, conferring intrinsic stability to the tibiotalar articulation, especially in weight bearing.
- Medially, the plafond is continuous with the medial malleolus and is articulated with the medial aspect of the talus.
- A thin soft-tissue envelope, with a precarious microcirculation, surrounds the distal tibia.

MECHANISM OF INJURY

In addition to the radiographically evident bony disruption, the compressive nature of the injury also results in significant articular damage to the plafond and talus. The severity of the damage to the bearing surfaces and the fragile soft-tissue envelope are important factors for long-term outcome.

- Axial compression: fall from a height
  - The force is axially directed through the talus into the tibial plafond, causing impaction of the articular surface, which may be associated with significant comminution. If the fibula remains intact, the ankle is forced into varus with impaction of the medial plafond. Plantarflexion or dorsiflexion of the ankle at the time of injury results in primarily posterior or anterior plafond injury, respectively.
- Shear: skiing accident
  - This mechanism is primarily torsion combined with a varus or valgus stress. It produces two or more large fragments and minimal articular comminution.
  - Usually, an associated fibular fracture, which is usually transverse or short oblique, is present. These injuries are unstable.
- Combined compression and shear
  - These fracture patterns demonstrate components of both compression and shear. The vector of these two forces determines the fracture pattern.
  - Because of their high energy nature, these fractures can be expected to have specific associated injuries as follows:
    - Calcaneus, tibial plateau, pelvis, and vertebral fractures.
    - Severe damage to the thin poorly vascularized subcutaneous tissues around the ankle, with ensuing massive swelling and skin necrosis.

CLINICAL EVALUATION

- Most pilon fractures are associated with high energy trauma; thus, a full trauma evaluation and survey are typically necessary.
- Patients typically present nonambulatory with variable gross deformity of the involved distal tibia.
- Evaluation includes assessment of neurovascular status and evaluation of any associated injuries.

- The tibia is nearly subcutaneous in this region; therefore, fracture displacement or excess skin pressure may convert a closed injury into an open one.
- Swelling is often massive and rapid, necessitating serial neurovascular examinations and assessment of skin integrity, necrosis, and fracture blisters.
- Meticulous assessment of soft-tissue damage is of paramount importance. Significant damage occurs to the thin soft-tissue envelope surrounding the distal tibia as the forces of impact are dissipated. This may result in inadequate healing of surgical incisions with wound necrosis and skin sloughs if not treated appropriately. Some advise waiting 7 to 10 days to allow soft-tissue healing to occur before planning surgery.

RADIOGRAPHIC EVALUATION

- Anteroposterior, lateral, mortise, and 45-degree oblique radiographs should be obtained.
- Computed tomography with coronal and sagittal reconstructions is extremely helpful in evaluation of the fracture pattern and articular surface.
- Careful preoperative planning with a strategically planned sequence of reconstruction is essential; radiographs of the contralateral side may be useful as a template for adequate preoperative planning.

RUEDI-ALLGOWER CLASSIFICATION (FIG. 37.1)

- Based on the severity of comminution and the displacement of the articular surface.
- Most commonly used classification.
- Prognosis correlated with increasing grade.

  Type 1: No significant articular incongruity; cleavage fractures without displacement of bony fragments.

  Type 2: Significant articular incongruity with minimal impaction or comminution.

  Type 3: Significant articular comminution with metaphyseal impaction.

MAST CLASSIFICATION

Combination of the Lauge-Hansen classification of ankle fractures and the Ruedi-Allgower classification.

Type A: Malleolar fractures with significant posterior lip involvement (Lauge-Hansen supination external rotation, type 4 fracture (SER-IV) injury).

Type B: Spiral fractures of the distal tibia with extension into the articular surface.

Type C: "Central impaction injuries" as a result of talar impaction, either with or without fibula fracture; subtypes 1, 2, and 3 correspond to the Ruedi-Allgower classification.

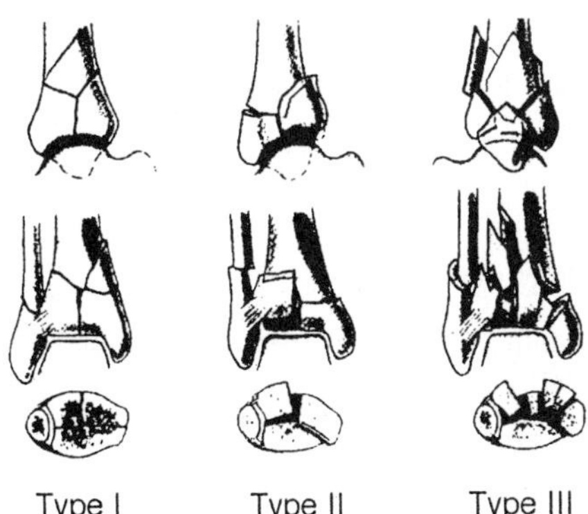

FIG. 37.1. Ruedi-Allgower classification of distal tibial (pilon) fractures. (From Muller ME, Narzarian S, Koch P, et al. *Manual of internal fixation,* 2nd ed. New York: Springer-Verlag, 1979:279, with permission.)

ORTHOPAEDIC TRAUMA ASSOCIATION CLASSIFICATION OF DISTAL TIBIA FRACTURES

Based on increasing degree of articular involvement.

Type A: extraarticular distal tibia fracture
- A1: metaphyseal simple
- A2: metaphyseal wedge
- A3: metaphyseal complex

Type B: partial articular distal tibia fracture
- B1: pure split
- B2: split depression
- B3: multifragmentary depression

Type C: complete articular distal tibia fracture
- C1: articular simple, metaphyseal simple
- C2: articular simple, metaphyseal multifragmentary
- C3: articular multifragmentary

TREATMENT

Decisions on treatment are based on many factors, including age and functional status of the patient; severity of injury to bone, cartilage, and soft-tissue envelope; degree of comminution and osteoporosis; and the capabilities of the surgeon.

Nonoperative Treatment

Long-leg cast for 6 weeks, followed by fracture brace and range-of-motion exercises:

- Manipulation is unlikely to result in reduction of intraarticular fragments.
- Loss of reduction is common.
- Inability to monitor soft-tissue status and swelling is a major disadvantage.
- This treatment is used primarily for nondisplaced fracture patterns or severely debilitated patients.

Severely Comminuted Fractures

- Deficiencies in articular cartilage and subchondral bone result in articular incongruity, rendering reconstruction of the articular surface virtually impossible. Posttraumatic arthritis is inevitable in cases of severe comminution, regardless of the form of treatment. The fibula should receive early open reduction and internal fixation to preserve length.
- The foot may be placed in 5-pound calcaneal pin traction until the soft tissues are healed and a cast or fracture brace can be applied. Alignment may be relatively preserved if the central articular surface is not severely impacted. Traction may be used provisionally while awaiting surgery as the soft tissues are allowed to heal.

Operative Treatment

Timing of Surgery

Displaced fractures should undergo some form of operative reduction and fixation if the articular surface is amenable to reconstruction. Surgery should be delayed to allow for optimization of soft-tissue status, including a diminution of swelling about the ankle, resolution of fracture blisters, and the sloughing of compromised soft tissues. Associated fibular fractures may initially be addressed with open reduction and internal fixation to maintain length as soft-tissue issues are addressed.

Internal Versus External Fixation

The goals of operative fixation of pilon fractures include the following:

- Maintenance of fibular length and stability with initial open reduction and internal fixation if necessary to restore length;
- Restoration of the tibial bearing surface;
- Bone grafting of any metaphyseal defects;
- Buttressing of the medial tibia.

The choice of fixation of the articular surface to the tibial shaft depends on the degree of metaphyseal comminution and soft-tissue injury.

- Internal fixation: may be used for fractures with no comminution and minimal soft-tissue injury. A low profile anterior or medial buttress plate may be used for definitive fixation.
- External fixation: may be used in patients with significant soft-tissue compromise or open fractures. Reduction is maintained via distraction and ligamentotaxis. If adequate reduction is obtained, external fixation may be used as definitive treatment.
  - *External fixation as a medial buttress in combination with internal fixation.* The external fixator maintains the medial buttress effect without the need for extensive medial dissection.
  - *Hybrid external fixation.* Reduction is enhanced by using small pins with or without olives to restore the articular surface and to maintain bony stability. It is especially good when internal fixation of any kind is contraindicated.
  - *Articulating versus nonarticulating external fixation.* Nonarticulating (rigid) external fixation is most commonly used, with theoretically no ankle motion, thus allowing healing of the articular surface. Articulating external fixation allows motion in the sagittal plane, thus preventing ankle varus and shortening; its application is limited, but it theoretically results in improved chondral lubrication and nutrition due to ankle motion and may be used when soft-tissue integrity is the primary indication for external fixation.
  - *Calcaneal pin.* Distraction across the tibiotalar joint via calcaneal traction with external fixation may be useful in avoiding joint stiffness in patients in whom ankle motion is strictly contraindicated.

The following treatments are controversial:

- Some advocate crossing the ankle and subtalar joint with a triangular frame to protect the soft tissues.
- Others recommend a ring fixator or hybrid frame that does not cross the ankle and that allows early range of motion.

Arthrodesis

Few advocate performing this procedure acutely. It is best done after comminution has consolidated and soft tissues have recovered. It is generally performed as a salvage procedure after other treatments have failed and posttraumatic arthritis has ensued.

Postoperative Management

- Initial placement in a splint or traction in neutral dorsiflexion with careful monitoring of soft tissues.
- Early motion when wounds and fixation allow.
- Non–weight bearing for 12 to 16 weeks, then progression to full weight bearing with radiographic evidence of healing.

COMPLICATIONS

- Soft-tissue slough, necrosis, and hematomas: due to initial trauma combined with improper handling of soft tissues. Must avoid excessive stripping and closing under tension. Secondary closure, skin grafts, or flaps may be required for adequate closure.
- Nonunion: results from significant comminution and bone loss, as well as from hypovascularity and infection.
- Malunion: common with nonanatomic reductions, inadequate buttressing followed by collapse, or premature weight bearing.
- Infection: acutely associated with open injuries and soft-tissue devitalization. Late infectious complications may manifest as osteomyelitis, malunion, or nonunion.
- Posttraumatic arthritis: more frequent with increasing severity of intraarticular comminution; emphasizes the need for anatomic restoration of the articular surface.
- Tibial shortening: due to fracture comminution, metaphyseal impaction, or a failure to restore length by fibular fixation initially.

38. ANKLE

EPIDEMIOLOGY

- The true incidence of ankle fractures is unknown because of the variety of physicians treating ankle injuries and the imprecise definition.
- Ankle injuries account for significant morbidity in the United States, with direct correlation to athletic participation, which accounts for a high proportion of ankle fractures, and trends in fashion footwear, with its incidence in women paralleling the use of high-heeled shoes.

ANATOMY

- The ankle is a complex hinge joint composed of articulations among the fibula, tibia, and talus in close association with a complex ligamentous system.
- The distal tibial articular surface is referred to as the "plafond," which, together with the medial and lateral malleoli, form the mortise, a constrained articulation with the talar dome.
- The plafond is concave in both the coronal and sagittal planes and is wider anteriorly to allow for congruency with the wedge-shaped talus. This provides for intrinsic stability, especially in weight bearing.
- The talar dome is trapezoidal, with the anterior aspect 2.5 mm wider than the posterior talus. The body of the talus is almost entirely covered by articular cartilage.
- The medial malleolus articulates with the medial facet of the talus and divides into an anterior and a posterior colliculus, which serve as attachments for the superficial and deep deltoid ligaments, respectively.
- The lateral malleolus represents the distal aspect of the fibula and provides lateral support to the ankle. No articular surface exists between the distal tibia and fibula, although some motion occurs between the two. Some intrinsic stability is provided between the distal tibia and fibula just proximal to the ankle where the fibula sits between a broad anterior tubercle and a smaller posterior tubercle of the tibia. The distal fibula has articular cartilage on its medial aspect extending from the level of the plafond distally to a point halfway down its remaining length.
- The syndesmotic ligament complex (Fig. 38.1) exists between the distal tibia and fibula, resisting axial, rotational, and translational forces to maintain the structural integrity of the mortise. It is composed of four ligaments:
  - Anterior tibiofibular ligament.
  - Posterior tibiofibular ligament: thicker and stronger than the anterior counterpart. Because of this, torsional or translational forces that rupture the anterior tibiofibular ligament may cause an avulsion fracture of the posterior tibial tubercle, leaving the posterior tibiofibular ligament intact.
  - Transverse tibiofibular ligament (inferior to posterior tibiofibular).
  - Interosseous ligament (distal continuation of the interosseous membrane).
- The deltoid ligament provides ligamentous support to the medial aspect of the ankle. It is separated into superficial and deep components as follows:
  - Superficial portion—comprised of three ligaments that originate on the anterior colliculus but that add little to ankle stability.
    - Tibionavicular ligament: suspends the spring ligament and prevents inward displacement of the talar head.
    - Tibiocalcaneal ligament: prevents valgus displacement.
    - Superficial tibiotalar ligament.
  - Deep portion—an intraarticular ligament (deep tibiotalar) that originates on the intercollicular grove and the posterior colliculus of the distal tibia and that inserts on the entire nonarticular medial surface of the talus. Its fibers are transversely oriented, and it is the primary medial stabilizer against lateral displacement of the talus.
- The fibular collateral ligament is made up of three ligaments that, with the distal fibula, provide lateral support to the ankle (Fig. 38.2). The lateral ligamentous complex is not as strong as the medial complex (Fig. 38.3).

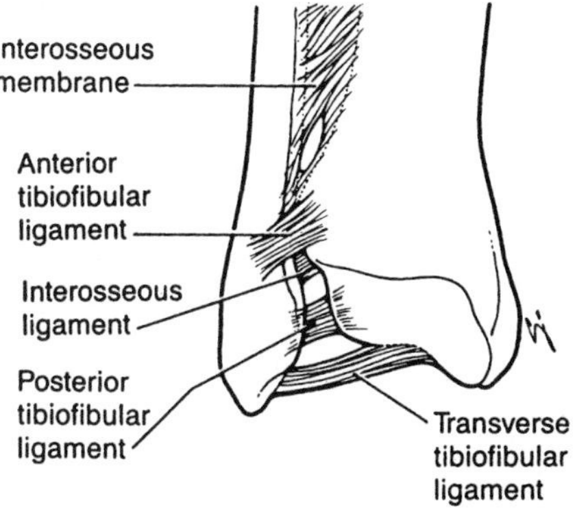

FIG. 38.1. The syndesmotic ligaments of the ankle. (From Rockwood CA Jr, Green DP, Bucholz RW, Heckman JD, eds. *Rockwood and Green's fractures in adults*, 4th ed. Vol. 2. Philadelphia: Lippincott-Raven, 1996: 2206, with permission.)

Anterior talofibular ligament: the weakest of the lateral ligaments; prevents anterior subluxation of the talus primarily in plantarflexion; rupture of this ligament results in a positive anterior drawer test.

Posterior talofibular ligament: strongest of the lateral ligaments; prevents posterior and rotatory subluxation of the talus.

Calcaneofibular ligament: lax in neutral dorsiflexion due to the relative valgus orientation of the calcaneus; stabilizes the subtalar joint and limits inversion; rupture of this ligament will thus cause a positive talar tilt test.

- Biomechanics are as follows:

  The normal range of motion of the ankle in dorsiflexion is 30 degrees; in plantarflexion, 45 degrees. Motion analysis studies reveal that minimums of 10 degrees of dorsiflexion and of 20 degrees of plantarflexion are required for normal gait.

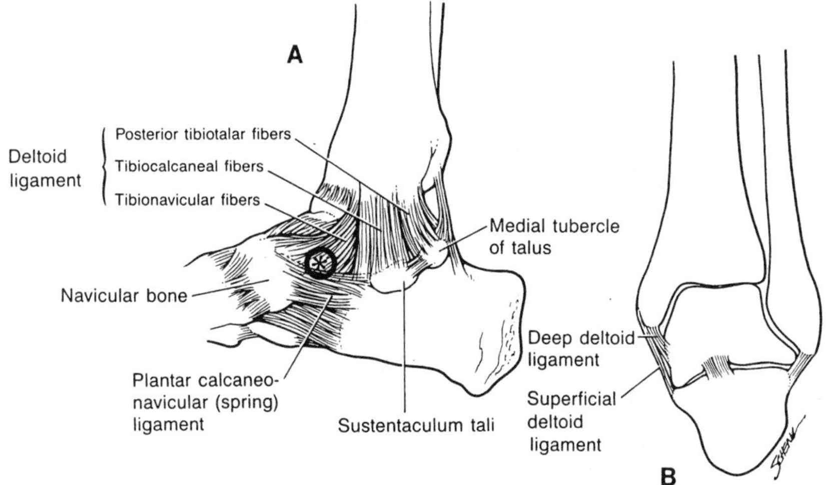

FIG. 38.2. Medial collateral ligaments. **A.** Bands of the superficial deltoid ligament. The asterisk represents the head of the talus. **B.** Position of the deep deltoid ligament. (From Rockwood CA Jr, Green DP, Bucholz RW, Heckman JD, eds. *Rockwood and Green's fractures in adults*, 4th ed. Vol. 2. Philadelphia: Lippincott-Raven, 1996:2207, with permission.)

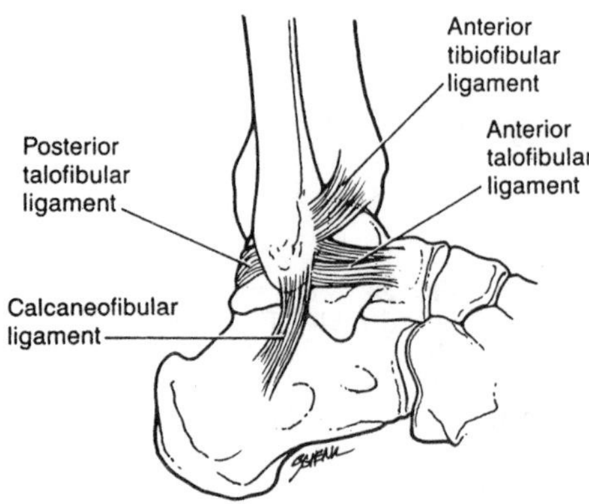

FIG. 38.3. Lateral collateral ligaments with adjacent tibiofibular ligament. (From Rockwood CA Jr, Green DP, Bucholz RW, Heckman JD, eds. *Rockwood and Green's fractures in adults*, 4th ed. Vol. 2. Philadelphia: Lippincott-Raven, 1996:2207, with permission.)

The axis of flexion of the ankle runs between the distal aspect of the two malleoli, which are externally rotated 20 degrees compared with the knee axis.

A lateral talar shift of 1 mm will decrease surface contact by 40%; a 3-mm shift results in >60% decrease.

Disruption of the syndesmotic ligaments may result in decreased tibiofibular overlap.

- Syndesmotic disruption associated with lateral disruption may be associated with a 2- to 3-mm lateral talar shift even with an intact deep deltoid ligament. A further lateral talar shift implies medial compromise.

MECHANISM OF INJURY

The pattern of ankle injury depends on many factors, including mechanism (axial vs. rotational loading); chronicity (recurrent ankle instability may result in chronic ligamentous laxity and distorted ankle biomechanics); patient's age; bone quality; comorbidity (related to soft-tissue issues); position of the foot at time of injury; and the magnitude, direction, and rate of loading. Specific mechanisms and injuries are discussed below under the Classification.

CLINICAL EVALUATION

- Patients may have a variable presentation, ranging from an antalgic gait to nonambulatory in significant pain and discomfort, with swelling, tenderness, and variable deformity.
- Neurovascular status should be carefully documented and should be compared with the contralateral side.
- The extent of soft-tissue injury should be evaluated, with particular attention to possible open injuries and blistering. The quality of surrounding tissues should also be noted.
- The entire length of the fibula should be palpated for tenderness because associated fibular fractures may be found proximally as high as the proximal tibiofibular articulation. A "squeeze test" may be performed approximately 5 cm proximal to the intermalleolar axis to assess possible syndesmotic injury.
- Stress testing (anterior/posterior, inversion/eversion, external rotation) is usually of limited yield in the acute setting in the face of a swollen, painful, recently injured ankle. If it is undertaken, comparison should be made to the contralateral ankle with the foot in neutral dorsiflexion and plantarflexion.
- A dislocated ankle should be reduced and splinted immediately (before radiographs if clinically evident) to prevent pressure or impaction injuries to the talar dome and to preserve neurovascular integrity.

RADIOGRAPHIC EVALUATION

- Anteroposterior, lateral, and mortise views of the ankle should be obtained.
  - Anteroposterior view (Fig. 38.4):
    - Tibiofibular overlap: <10 mm is abnormal and implies syndesmotic injury.
    - Tibiofibular clear space: >5 mm is abnormal and implies syndesmotic injury.
    - Talar tilt: a difference in width of the medial and lateral aspects of the superior joint space; >2 mm is abnormal and indicates medial or lateral disruption.
  - Lateral view:
    - The dome of the talus should be centered under the tibia and should be congruous with the tibial plafond.
    - Posterior tibial tuberosity fractures and the direction of fibular injury can be identified.
    - Avulsion fractures of the talus by the anterior capsule may be identified.
  - Mortise view (Fig. 38.5):
    - Taken with the foot in 15 to 20 degrees of internal rotation to offset the intermalleolar axis.
    - Medial clear space: >4 mm is abnormal and indicates lateral talar shift.
    - Talar tilt: a line drawn parallel to the distal tibial articular surface and a second line drawn parallel to the talar surface should be parallel. More than 2 degrees of angulation is indicative of talar tilt.
    - Talocrural angle: the angle subtended between the intermalleolar line and a line parallel to the distal tibial articular surface should be between 8 and 15 degrees. A smaller angle indicates fibular shortening.
    - Tibiofibular overlap: <1 cm indicates syndesmotic disruption.
    - Talar shift: >1 mm is abnormal.
- Arthrography historically was used before the advent of magnetic resonance imaging to evaluate ligamentous disruption.

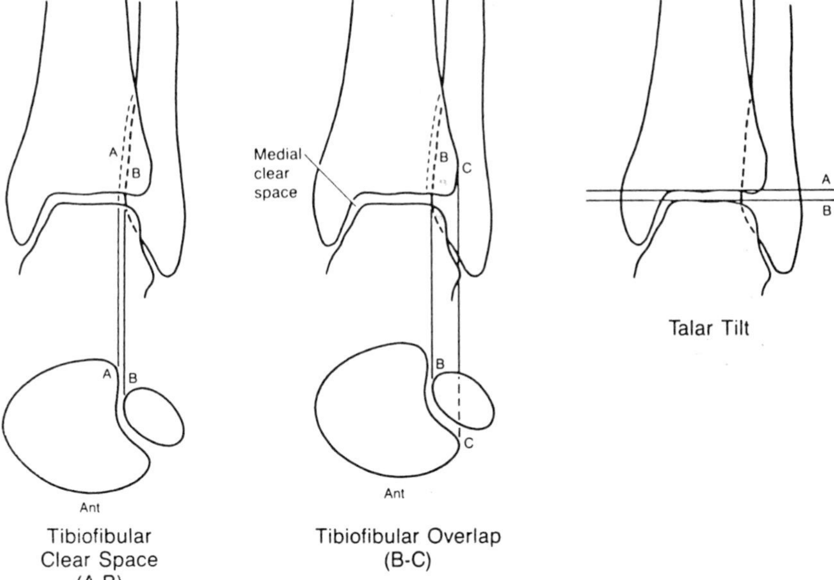

FIG. 38.4. Anteroposterior view of the ankle. **A.** X-ray of normal ankle. **B.** Parameters measured from anteroposterior x-ray: *A-B*, tibiofibular clear space; *B-C*, tibiofibular overlap. (From Rockwood CA Jr, Green DP, Bucholz RW, Heckman JD, eds. *Rockwood and Green's fractures in adults*, 4th ed. Vol. 2. Philadelphia: Lippincott-Raven, 1996:2220, with permission.)

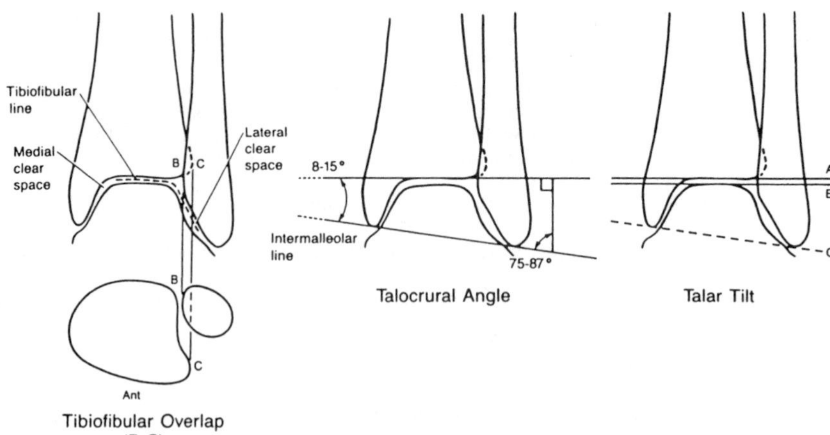

FIG. 38.5. Mortise view of the ankle. **A.** X-ray of a normal ankle. **B.** Parameters measured from the mortise x-ray: *B-C*, tibiofibular overlap. (From Rockwood CA Jr, Green DP, Bucholz RW, Heckman JD, eds. *Rockwood and Green's fractures in adults*, 4th ed. Vol. 2. Philadelphia: Lippincott-Raven, 1996:2222, with permission.)

- Computed tomography is useful in the evaluation of complex or comminuted fractures, especially of the distal tibia when plain radiographs are not able to delineate fully the fracture extent, or in adolescents to demonstrate a possible triplane fracture.
- Magnetic resonance imaging is useful in characterizing subtle fractures, such as osteochondral or stress fractures, or the extent of soft-tissue injuries, such as those involving tendons, ligaments, or the capsule.
- A bone scan is useful in chronic ankle injuries, such as osteochondral injuries, stress fractures, infection, or reflex dystrophies.

LAUGE-HANSEN CLASSIFICATION (FIG. 38.6)

- Four patterns, based on "pure" injury sequences, each subdivided into stages of increasing severity.

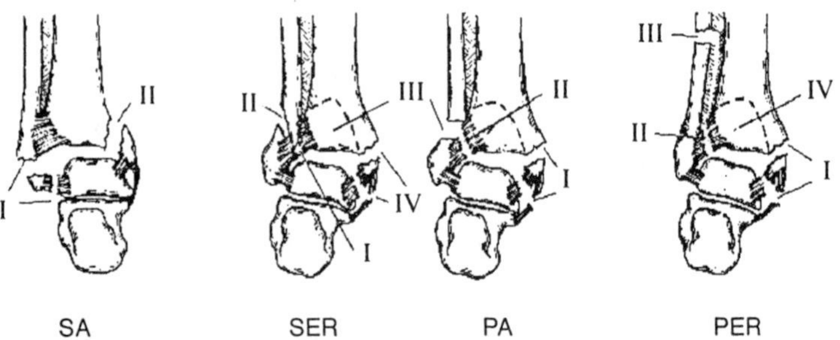

FIG. 38.6. Lauge-Hansen classification of ankle fractures. Abbreviations: PA, pronation-abduction; PER, pronation-external rotation; SA, supination-adduction; SER, supination-external rotation. (From Browner BD, Jupiter JB, Levine AM, et al. *Skeletal trauma*. Philadelphia: W.B. Saunders, 1992:1891, with permission.)

- Based on cadaveric studies.
- Patterns may not always reflect clinical reality.
- System takes into account the position of the foot at the time of injury and the direction of the deforming force.

Supination-Adduction (SA)

- Accounts for 10% to 20% of malleolar fractures.
- The only type associated with medial displacement of the talus.

  Stage I: Produces either a transverse avulsion-type fracture of the fibula distal to the level of the joint or a rupture of the lateral collateral ligaments.

  Stage II: Results in a vertical medial malleolus fracture.

Supination-External Rotation (SER)

Accounts for 40% to 75% of malleolar fractures.

Stage I: Produces disruption of the anterior tibiofibular ligament with or without an associated avulsion fracture at its tibial or fibular attachment.

Stage II: Results in the typical spiral fracture of the distal fibula, which runs from anteroinferior to posterosuperior.

Stage III: Produces either a disruption of the posterior tibiofibular ligament or a fracture of the posterior malleolus.

Stage IV: Produces either a transverse avulsion-type fracture of the medial malleolus or a rupture of the deltoid ligament.

Pronation-Abduction (PA)

Accounts for 5% to 20% of malleolar fractures.

Stage I: Results in either a transverse fracture of the medial malleolus or a rupture of the deltoid ligament.

Stage II: Produces either a rupture of the syndesmotic ligaments or an avulsion fracture at their insertion sites.

Stage III: Produces a transverse or short oblique fracture of the distal fibula at or above the level of the syndesmosis; this results from a bending force that causes medial tension and lateral compression of the fibula, producing lateral comminution or a butterfly fragment.

Pronation-External Rotation (PER)

Accounts for 5% to 20% of malleolar fractures.

Stage I: Produces either a transverse fracture of the medial malleolus or a rupture of the deltoid ligament.

Stage II: Results in disruption of the anterior tibiofibular ligament with or without an avulsion fracture at its insertion sites.

Stage III: Results in a spiral fracture of the distal fibula at or above the level of the syndesmosis running from anterosuperior to posteroinferior.

Stage IV: Produces either a rupture of the posterior tibiofibular ligament or an avulsion fracture of the posterolateral tibia.

DANIS-WEBER CLASSIFICATION (FIG. 38.7)

Based on the level of the fibular fracture: the more proximal, the greater the risk of syndesmotic disruption and associated instability. Three types of fractures have been described:

Type A: involves a fracture of the fibula below the level of the tibial plafond; an avulsion injury that results from supination of the foot that may be associated with an oblique or vertical fracture of the medial malleolus. This is equivalent to the Lauge-Hansen supination-adduction injury.

Type B: an oblique or spiral fracture of the fibula caused by external rotation occurring at or near the level of the syndesmosis. Fifty percent have an associated disruption of the anterior syndesmotic ligament, whereas the posterior syndesmotic

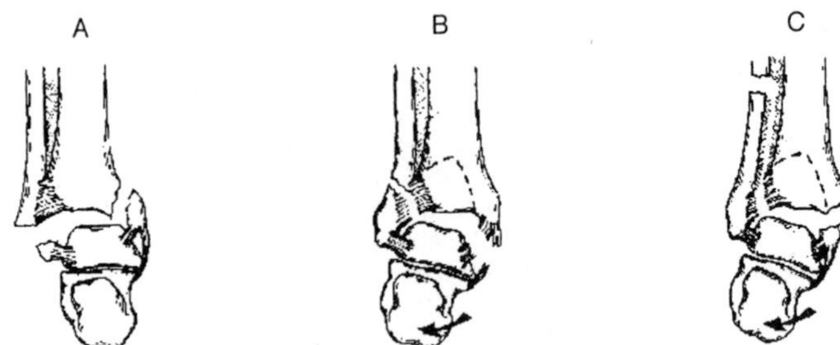

FIG. 38.7. Danis-Weber classification of ankle fractures. (From Browner BD, Jupiter JB, Levine AM, et al. *Skeletal trauma.* Philadelphia: W.B. Saunders, 1992:1891, with permission.)

ligament remains intact and attached to the distal fibular fragment. An associated injury to the medial structures or the posterior malleolus may be found. This is equivalent to the Lauge-Hansen supination-eversion injury.

Type C: involves a fracture of the fibula above the level of the syndesmosis, causing disruption of the syndesmosis almost always with associated medial injury. This category includes Maisonneuve-type injuries and corresponds to Lauge-Hansen pronation eversion or pronation abduction stage III injuries.

TILE CLASSIFICATION

Categorizes fracture types according to level and characteristics of the injury on the lateral side of the joint and takes into account joint instability.

Type I: due to an adduction-inversion force producing a lateral injury below the syndesmosis; corresponds to Lauge-Hansen supination-adduction type and Danis-Weber type A.
- Stable: fracture of fibula below syndesmosis or rupture of the lateral ligament complex; intact syndesmosis.
- Unstable: disruption of anterior capsule, displacement of fibular avulsion fracture, and varus subluxation of the talus in the mortise; concomitant axial loading causes a vertical fracture of the medial malleolus with crunching of medial talar and tibial articular cartilage; further force causes a posteromedial tibial fracture.

Type II: due to an external rotation-abduction force producing a lateral injury at or above the syndesmosis; corresponds to Lauge-Hansen SER, pronation-abduction, and PER types and Danis-Weber types B and C; an isolated fracture of the medial malleolus or rupture of the deltoid ligament may also occur.
- Stable: fracture of fibula at or above syndesmosis with disruption of the anterior tibiofibular ligament (or bony equivalent).
- Unstable: unstable posterior syndesmotic ligament complex (ligament or bony equivalent); with disruption of the medial structures, results in gross instability.

ORTHOPAEDIC TRAUMA ASSOCIATION CLASSIFICATION OF ANKLE FRACTURES (FIG. 38.8)

Based primarily on fracture level in relation to the syndesmosis.

Type A: infrasyndesmotic lesion
- A1: infrasyndesmotic lateral malleolus, isolated
- A2: infrasyndesmotic lateral malleolus with associated medial malleolar fracture
- A3: infrasyndesmotic lateral malleolus with associated posteromedial tibial fracture

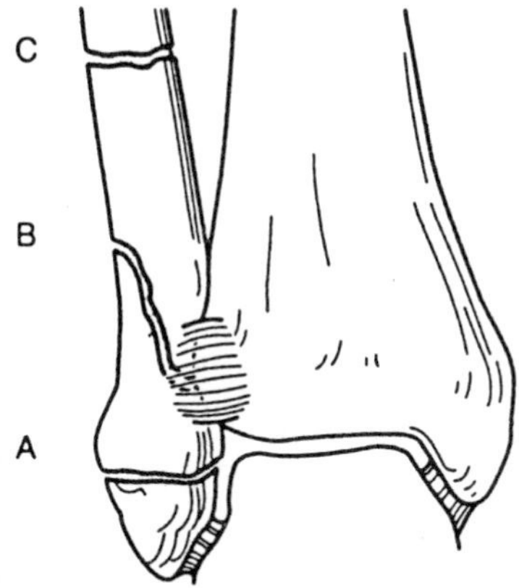

FIG. 38.8. Orthopaedic Trauma Association classification of ankle fractures. (From Heckman JD, Bucholz RW, eds. *Rockwood, Green, and Wilkins' fractures in adults*, 5th ed. Philadelphia: Lippincott Williams & Wilkins, 2001, with permission.)

Type B: transsyndesmotic lesion
- B1: transsyndesmotic lateral malleolus, isolated
- B2: transsyndesmotic lateral malleolus with associated medial lesion
- B3: transsyndesmotic lateral malleolus with medial lesion and fracture of the posterolateral rim of the tibia (Volkmann)

Type C: suprasyndesmotic lesion
- C1: simple diaphyseal fibular fracture
- C2: complex (multifragmentary) diaphyseal fibular fracture with associated medial injury
- C3: proximal fibular fracture with associated medial injury

CLASSIFICATION OF FRACTURE VARIANTS

Maisonneuve Fracture

- Originally described as an ankle injury with a fracture of the proximal third of the fibula.
- An external rotation-type injury of the ankle; important to distinguish from direct-trauma fractures.
- Most resemble Lauge-Hansen PER type with a fibula pattern from anterosuperior to posteroinferior.

Curbstone Fracture

Avulsion fracture of the posterior tibia produced by a tripping mechanism.

LeForte-Wagstaffe Fracture

Anterior fibular tubercle avulsion fracture by the anterior tibiofibular ligament, usually associated with Lauge-Hansen SER type fracture patterns.

Tillaux-Chaput Fracture

Avulsion of anterior tibial margin by the anterior tibiofibular ligament; tibial counterpart of LeForte-Wagstaffe fracture.

Collicular Fractures

- Anterior colliculus fracture: the deep portion of the deltoid remains intact.
- Posterior colliculus fracture: the fragment is usually nondisplaced because of stabilization by the posterior tibial and the flexor digitorum longus tendons; classically one sees a "supramalleolar spike" very clearly on an external rotation view.

Chip Avulsion

Small avulsions of either colliculus.

Pronation-Dorsiflexion Fracture

Displaced fracture of the anterior articular surface; considered a pilon variant when a significant articular fragment is found.

TREATMENT

The goal of treatment is to restore the ankle joint anatomically. Fibular length and rotation must be restored to obtain an anatomic reduction.

Emergency Room Treatment

- After a careful clinical evaluation is performed as outlined above, an attempt at reduction should be performed for displaced fractures.
- Dislocated ankles should be reduced before radiographic evaluation.
- Open wounds and abrasions should be cleansed and dressed in a sterile fashion as dictated by the degree of injury. Fracture blisters should be left intact and should be dressed with a well-padded sterile dressing.
- After reduction, a posterior splint with a U-shaped component should be placed to maintain stability and comfort.
- Postreduction radiographs should be obtained for reassessment of the fracture. The limb should be aggressively elevated with or without the use of ice.

Nonoperative Treatment

- Indications for nonoperative treatment include the following:
  - Nondisplaced stable fracture patterns with an intact syndesmosis.
  - Displaced fractures for which stable anatomic reduction is achieved.
  - An unstable or multiple trauma patient in whom operative treatment is contraindicated due to the condition of the patient or the limb.
- If anatomic reduction is achieved with closed manipulation, a bulky dressing and a posterior splint with a U-shaped component may be used for the first few days while swelling subsides.
- The patient is then placed in a long-leg cast to maintain rotational control for 4 to 6 weeks with serial radiographic evaluation to ensure maintenance of reduction and healing. If adequate healing is demonstrated, the patient can be placed in a short-leg cast or fracture brace.
- Weight bearing is restricted until fracture healing is demonstrated. Alternatively, if the fracture pattern is very stable, a short-leg cast for 4 to 6 weeks may be used initially instead of the long-leg cast.

Operative Treatment

- Open reduction and internal fixation is indicated for the following:
  - Failure to achieve or to maintain closed reduction.
  - Displaced or unstable fractures that result in talar displacement or widening of the mortise by 2 mm.
  - Fractures that require abnormal foot positioning to maintain reduction (e.g., extreme plantarflexion).
  - Open fractures.
- Open reduction and internal fixation should be carried out as soon as the patient's general medical condition, swelling about the ankle, and soft-tissue status allow. Swelling, blisters, and soft-tissue issues usually stabilize within 1 to 7 days following injury with elevation, ice, and compressive dressings; but occasionally, a closed fracture with severe soft-tissue injury or massive swelling may require reduction and stabilization with traction on an elevated frame or with external fixation to allow soft-tissue management before definitive fixation.
- Lateral malleolar fractures distal to the syndesmosis may be stabilized using a lag screw or Kirschner wires with tension banding. With more proximal fibular injuries, restoration of fibular length and rotation is essential for obtaining an accurate reduction. This is most often accomplished using a combination of lag screws and a one-third tubular plate. Fractures up to the midshaft should be stabilized, but

more proximal fractures can be ignored unless significantly displaced, in which case plate fixation may be indicated.

- Management of medial malleolar fractures is controversial. In general, with a deltoid rupture, the talus follows the fibula. Theoretically, anatomic restoration of the fibula restores the talus to its physiologic position, thus obviating the need for medial operative repair. Indications for operative fixation of the medial malleolus include concomitant syndesmotic injury, 2-mm widening of the medial clear space after fibular reduction, inability to obtain adequate fibular reduction, or persistent medial instability despite fibular fixation. Medial malleolar fractures can usually be held with cancellous screws or a figure-of-eight tension band.
- Indications for fixation of posterior malleolus fractures include involvement of >25% of the articular surface, >2 mm displacement, or persistent posterior subluxation of the talus. Fixation may be achieved by indirect reduction and placement of an anterior to posterior lag screw or a posterior to anterior lag screw through a separate incision.
- Fibula fractures above the syndesmosis may require syndesmotic stabilization. After fixation of the medial and lateral malleoli is achieved, the syndesmosis should be stressed intraoperatively by a lateral pull on the fibula with a bone hook or by stressing the ankle in external rotation. Syndesmotic instability can then be recognized clinically and under image intensification. The syndesmotic screw is placed 1.5 to 2.0 cm above the plafond from the fibula to the tibia. Controversy exists as to the number of purchased cortices (three or four) and the size of the screw (3.5 mm or 4.5 mm). The screw is placed with the ankle in maximum dorsiflexion, and the reduction is held with a large-pointed reduction clamp.
- After fracture fixation, the limb is placed in either a short-leg cast or a bulky cotton dressing incorporating a plaster splint. Progression to weight bearing is based on the fracture pattern, stability of fixation, patient compliance, and philosophy of the surgeon.

Open Fractures

- These fractures require immediate irrigation and debridement in the operating room.
- Stable fixation is an important prophylaxis against infection; it also helps soft-tissue healing. Leaving plates and screws exposed is permissible, but efforts should be made to cover hardware.
- Tourniquet use should be avoided.
- Surgical incisions should be closed with or without the use of drains; injury wounds should be left open.
- Antibiotic prophylaxis should be continued postoperatively.
- Serial debridements may be required for removal of necrotic, infected, or compromised tissues.

COMPLICATIONS

- Nonunion: rare; usually involves the medial malleolus when treated closed and associated with residual fracture displacement, interposed soft tissue, or associated lateral instability resulting in shear stresses across the deltoid ligament. May be treated with open reduction and internal fixation or electrical stimulation. Excision of the fragment may be necessary if not amenable to internal fixation and the patient is symptomatic.
- Malunion: lateral malleolus shortened and malrotated; a widened medial clear space and large posterior malleolar fragment are most predictive of poor outcome. The medial malleolus may heal in an elongated position, resulting in residual instability.
- Wound problems: edge necrosis (3%); decreased risk with minimal swelling, no tourniquet, and good soft-tissue technique. Fractures that are operated on in the presence of fracture blisters or abrasions have more than twice the average complication rate.

- Infection: Less than 2% of closed fractures; leave implants alone if stable, even with deep infection. May require serial debridements with possible arthrodesis as a salvage procedure.
- Posttraumatic arthritis: either secondary to damage at the time of injury, due to altered mechanics, or as a result of inadequate reduction. Rare in anatomically reduced fractures, with increasing incidence with articular incongruity.
- Reflex sympathetic dystrophy: rare; may be minimized by anatomic restoration of the ankle and early return to function.
- Compartment syndrome of foot: immediate postoperative period; rare.
- Tibiofibular synostosis: associated with the use of a syndesmotic screw; usually asymptomatic.

39. FOOT

FRACTURES OF THE HINDFOOT

Talus

Epidemiology

- Second in frequency (to calcaneal fractures; see below) among all tarsal fractures.
- Incidence markedly increased with the use of motor vehicles in the 1900s, due to the vehicle operator "slamming" his or her foot on the brakes in an attempt to avoid an accident.

Anatomy

- The body of the talus is covered superiorly by the trochlear articular surface through which the body weight is transmitted. The anterior aspect is wider than the posterior aspect, which confers intrinsic stability to the ankle.
- Medially and laterally the articular cartilage extends plantar-ward to articulate with the medial and lateral malleoli, respectively. The inferior surface of the body forms the articulation with the posterior facet of the calcaneus.
- The neck of the talus is roughened by ligamentous attachments and the vascular foramina. It deviates medially 15 to 20 degrees and is the area most vulnerable to fracture.
- The talar head has continuous articular facets for the navicular anteriorly, the spring ligament inferiorly, the sustentacular tali posteroinferiorly, and the deltoid ligament medially.
- Two bony processes exist. The lateral process is wedge-shaped and articulates with the posterior calcaneal facet inferomedially and the lateral malleolus superolaterally. The posterior process has a medial and lateral tubercle separated by a groove for the flexor hallucis longus tendon.
- An os trigonum is present in up to 50% of normal feet. It arises from a separate ossification center just posterior to the lateral tubercle of the posterior talar process.
- Sixty percent of the talus is covered by articular cartilage. No muscles originate from, or insert into, the talus. The vascular supply is dependent on fascial structures to reach the talus; therefore, capsular disruptions may result in osteonecrosis.
- The vascular supply to the talus consists of the following:
  - Artery to the sinus tarsi (peroneal and dorsalis pedis arteries);
  - Artery of the tarsal canal (posterior tibial artery);
  - Deltoid artery (posterior tibial artery), which supplies the medial body;
  - Capsular and ligamentous vessels and intraosseous anastomoses.

Mechanism of Injury

- This injury is most commonly associated with motor vehicle accidents or fall from heights with a component of hyperdorsiflexion of the ankle. The talar neck fractures as it impacts the anterior margin of the tibia.
- "Aviator astragalus" is a fracture of the talar neck historically resulting from the rudder bar of a crashing airplane, impacting the plantar aspect of the foot.

Clinical Evaluation

- Patients typically present with extreme pain to weight bearing on the affected extremity.
- Range of motion is typically painful, and it may elicit crepitus.
- Diffuse swelling of the hindfoot may be present, with tenderness to palpation of the talus and subtalar joint.
- A neurovascular examination should be performed.

Radiographic Evaluation (Fig. 39.1)

- Anteroposterior, mortise, and lateral radiographs of the ankle and anteroposterior, lateral, and oblique views of the foot should be obtained. Overpenetration of the foot may be necessary to visualize the tarsal bones adequately, although osseous detail in the forefoot may be obscured.

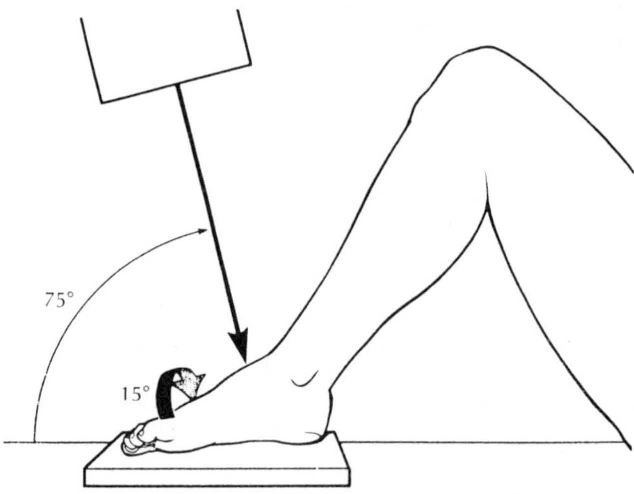

FIG. 39.1. The correct position of the foot for x-ray evaluation of the talar neck is shown. (From Rockwood CA Jr, Green DP, Bucholz RW, Heckman JD, eds. *Rockwood and Green's fractures in adults*, 4th ed. Vol. 2. Philadelphia: Lippincott-Raven, 1996:2298, with permission.)

- The Canale view provides the optimum view of the neck. With the ankle in maximum equinus, the foot is placed on a cassette and is pronated 15 degrees; and the radiographic source is directed cephalad 15 degrees from the vertical.
- Computed tomography or tomograms may be obtained to characterize the fracture further and to assess articular involvement.
- Technetium-99m bone scans or magnetic resonance imaging may be useful for evaluating possible occult talar fractures.

ANATOMIC CLASSIFICATION

- Lateral process fractures
- Posterior process fractures
- Talar head fractures
- Talar body fractures
- Talar neck fractures

HAWKINS CLASSIFICATION OF TALAR NECK FRACTURES (FIG. 39.2)

Type I: nondisplaced
Type II: associated subtalar subluxation or dislocation
Type III: associated subtalar and ankle dislocation
Type IV: Canale and Kelley—type III with associated talonavicular subluxation or dislocation

ORTHOPAEDIC TRAUMA ASSOCIATION (OTA) CLASSIFICATION OF TALAR FRACTURES

Type A: extraarticular
A1: extraarticular, neck
A2: extraarticular, avulsions
Type B: partial articular
B1: partial articular, lateral half body
B2: partial articular, medial half body
B3: partial articular, coronal

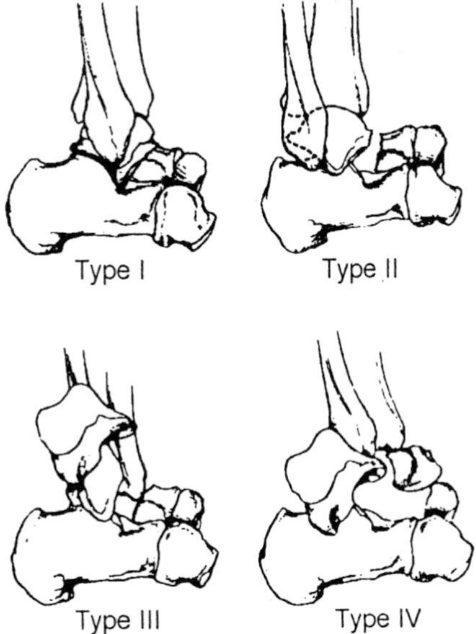

FIG. 39.2. Hawkins classification of talar neck fractures. (From Mann RA, Coughlin MJ. *Surgery of the foot and ankle,* 6th ed. St. Louis, MO: Mosby-Year Book, 1993:1550–1551, with permission.)

Type C: articular
  C1: articular, simple
  C2: articular, complex (multifragmentary)

Treatment
Fractures of the talar neck and body represent a continuum and may be considered together.

Nondisplaced fractures (Hawkins type I):

- Fractures that appear nondisplaced on plain radiographs may show unrecognized comminution or articular step-off on tomograms or computed tomography. Fractures must truly be nondisplaced with no evidence of subtalar incongruity to be considered a type I fracture.
- Treatment consists of a short-leg cast for 8 to 12 weeks. The patient should remain non–weight bearing for 6 weeks until clinical and radiographic evidence of fracture healing are present.

Displaced fractures (Hawkins types II to IV):

- Immediate closed reduction should be obtained with emergent open reduction and internal fixation for all open or irreducible fractures.
- If anatomic reduction is obtained, the patient may be placed in a short-leg cast with treatment as per nondisplaced fractures.
- If open reduction is necessary, all major fragments should be salvaged. Primary arthrodesis should be avoided at all costs.
- Surgical approaches include the following:
  1. *Anteromedial.* This approach may be extended from a limited capsulotomy in the anterior-posterior tibial tendon interval to a wide exposure with malleolar osteotomy. Extreme care must be taken to preserve the saphenous vein and nerve and, more importantly, the deltoid artery.
  2. *Posterolateral.* This approach provides access to posterior process or body fractures and nondisplaced neck or body fractures. The interval is between the peroneus brevis and the flexor hallucis longus (FHL). The sural nerve must be protected. Displacing the FHL from its groove in the posterior process is usually necessary to facilitate exposure.

3. *Anterolateral.* This approach allows visualization of the sinus tarsi, lateral neck, and comminution in the subtalar joint. Inadvertent damage to the artery of the tarsal sinus can occur through this approach.
4. *Combined anteromedial-anterolateral.* A combined anteromedial and anterolateral approach can be used to achieve an anatomic reduction for comminuted fractures.

- Interfragmentary compression screws may be used with every attempt made at anatomic reduction.
- For internal fixation, two interfragmentary lag screws (4.0-mm cancellous or 3.5-mm cortical) are placed perpendicular to the fracture line. Areas of significant comminution and bone loss should be grafted.
- A short-leg cast should be placed postoperatively for 8 to 12 weeks and should be non–weight bearing.
- The *Hawkins sign* refers to subchondral osteopenia in the vascularized non–weight-bearing talus at 6 to 8 weeks; although this tends to indicate talar viability, the presence of this sign does not rule out osteonecrosis.

Lateral process fractures

- These are intraarticular fractures of the subtalar or ankle joint that occur most frequently when the foot is dorsiflexed and inverted. An increase in incidence has occurred with the rise in popularity of snowboarding.
- Less than 2 mm displacement requires a short-leg cast for 6 weeks and non–weight bearing for at least 4 weeks.
- More than 2 mm displacement requires open reduction and internal fixation (ORIF) (2.0- or 2.7-mm screws or Kirschner wires) in the lateral approach.
- Comminuted fractures require excision of nonviable fragments.

Posterior process fractures

- These comprise the posterior 25% of the articular surface, involving the medial and lateral tubercles. Fractures may occur in a severe ankle inversion injury whereby the posterior talofibular ligament avulses the lateral tubercle or by forced equinus and direct compression.
- Nondisplaced or minimally displaced fractures require a short-leg cast for 6 weeks and non–weight bearing for at least 4 weeks.
- Displaced fractures require open reduction and internal fixation if large fragments are present or primary excision if small fragments are present; the posterolateral approach may be used.

Talar head fractures

- These are due to plantarflexion and longitudinal compression along the axis of the forefoot. Comminution is not uncommon; one must also suspect navicular injury and talonavicular disruption.
- Nondisplaced fractures require a short-leg walking cast molded to preserve the longitudinal arch, as well as partial weight bearing, for 6 weeks. Arch support in the shoe is used to splint the talonavicular articulation for 3 to 6 months.
- Displaced fractures require ORIF, with primary excision of small fragments; either an anterior or anteromedial approach is used.

Complications

- Infection: can be avoided for the most part with early open reduction and internal fixation with soft-tissue coverage for open injuries.
- Osteonecrosis: rate of osteonecrosis related to displacement of fracture:
  Hawkins I: 0 to 13%
  Hawkins II: 20% to 50%
  Hawkins III: 20% to 100%

Bone scans are unreliable in diagnosing osteonecrosis, although magnetic resonance imaging may be clinically useful.

- Posttraumatic arthritis: occurs in 40% to 90% of cases; typically related to articular incongruity or chondral injury at the time of fracture. May be evident in either the ankle or subtalar joints.

- Delayed union and nonunion: delay in union >6 months occurs in <15% of cases. May be treated by rigid open reduction and bone grafting.
- Open fracture: complicates up to 15% to 20% of injuries and reflects the often high energy mechanisms that produce these fractures. Copious irrigation and meticulous debridement are necessary to prevent infectious complications.
- Skin slough: may occur secondary to prolonged dislocation, with pressure necrosis on the overlying soft tissues. When severe, may result in pressure erosions, compromising soft-tissue integrity and causing possible infectious complications.
- Interposition of long flexor tendons: may prevent adequate closed reduction and may necessitate open reduction and internal fixation. Alternatively, malreduction may result in aberrant foot biomechanics, resulting in impingement of, or abrasions to, surrounding tendons with consequent symptoms.
- Compartment syndrome of the foot: uncommon. However, pain on passive extension of the toes must raise clinical suspicion of possible evolving or present compartment syndrome of the foot, particularly in a patient in whom symptoms are out of proportion to the apparent injury. Emergent fasciotomy is indicated for avoidance of potentially disastrous complications of neurovascular compromise and muscle death.

Calcaneus

Epidemiology

- The calcaneus, or os calcis, is the most frequently fractured tarsal bone.
- Despite extensive clinical experience with this injury, its major socioeconomic impact in regard to the time lost from work and recreation, and recent advances in imaging and operative treatment, the results of this fracture are often poor.

Anatomy

- The anterior half of the superior articular surface contains three facets that articulate with the talus. The posterior facet is the largest and constitutes the major weight-bearing surface. The middle facet is located anteromedially on the sustentaculum tali. The anterior facet is often confluent with the middle facet.
- Between the middle and posterior facets lies the interosseous sulcus (calcaneal groove) that, with the talar sulcus, forms the sinus tarsi.
- The sustentaculum tali supports the neck of the talus medially; it is attached to the talus by the interosseus talocalcaneal and deltoid ligaments and contains the middle articular facet on its superior aspect. The flexor hallucis longus tendon passes beneath the sustentaculum tali medially.
- The peroneal tendons pass between the calcaneus and the lateral malleolus laterally.
- The Achilles tendon attaches to the posterior tuberosity.
- Associated injuries that must be suspected include the following:
  - Bilateral calcaneal fractures are present in 5% to 10% of cases.
  - In 10% of cases, compression fractures of the lumbar spine are present.
  - Concomitant injuries of the lower extremities are present in 26% of cases.

Mechanism of Injury

- *Axial loading.* Falls from a height are responsible for most intraarticular fractures; they occur as the talus is driven down into the calcaneus, which is composed of a thin cortical shell surrounding cancellous bone. In motor vehicle accidents, calcaneal fractures may occur when the accelerator or brake pedal impacts the plantar aspect of the foot.
- *Twisting forces.* These may be associated with extraarticular calcaneus fractures, in particular, fractures of the anterior and medial processes or the sustentaculum. In diabetics, an increased incidence of tuberosity fractures is due to avulsion by the triceps surae.

Clinical Evaluation

- Patients typically present with moderate to severe heel pain, associated with tenderness, swelling, and heel widening and shortening. Ecchymosis around the heel extending to the arch is highly suggestive of a calcaneal fracture. Blistering may be present; it occurs due to massive swelling, usually within the first 36 hours after the injury. Open fractures are rare but, when present, occur medially.

- Careful evaluation of soft tissues and neurovascular status is essential. Compartment syndrome of the foot must be ruled out because it occurs in 10% of calcaneal fractures and it may result in clawing of the lesser toes.

Radiographic Evaluation

- Anteroposterior and lateral radiographs of the foot should be obtained. Overpenetration may result in enhanced detail of the tarsal bones, although osseous detail of the forefoot may be compromised.
- A dorsoplantar (anteroposterior) radiograph shows calcaneocuboid extension or a lateral wall bulge and subluxation of the talonavicular articulation.
- Lateral radiograph shows the following:
  - Bohler tuber joint angle: represented by the supplement (180-degree measured angle) of two lines—a line from the highest point of the anterior process to the highest point of the posterior articular surface and a line drawn between the same point on the posterior articular surface and the most superior point of the tuberosity. Normally this angle is between 25 and 40 degrees; flattening of this angle indicates collapse of the posterior facet.
  - Gissane (crucial) angle: formed by the confluence of two struts, one extending along the posterior facet and the other anteriorly to the beak of the calcaneus; an increase in this angle indicates collapse of the posterior facet (Fig. 39.3).
- The Harris axial view is as follows:
  - Taken with the foot in maximum dorsiflexion and the beam angled at 45 degrees cephalad.
  - Allows visualization of the subtalar joint involvement and comminution, calcaneal loss of height and widening, angulation of the tuberosity fragment, impingement of the lateral fragment on the peroneal space and lateral malleolus, and overriding of the superomedial fragment on the posterolateral fragment.
- Broden views are as follows:
  - Taken with the patient supine with the leg internally rotated 30 to 40 degrees and the ankle in neutral dorsiflexion. The beam is centered over the lateral malleolus; views are taken at 40, 30, 20, and 10 degrees cephalad, showing the posterior facet as it moves posterior (10 degrees) to anterior (40 degrees).
  - Allow for visualization of the posterior facet.
  - Are most useful intraoperatively to assess reduction.
  - Are not as effective as computed tomography preoperatively.
- With computed tomography, 3- to 5-mm slices are necessary for adequate analysis.
  - A coronal view is taken perpendicular to the posterior facet; it demonstrates the articular surface of the posterior facet, the sustentaculum tali, the shape of the heel, and peroneal and flexor hallucis longus tendons.

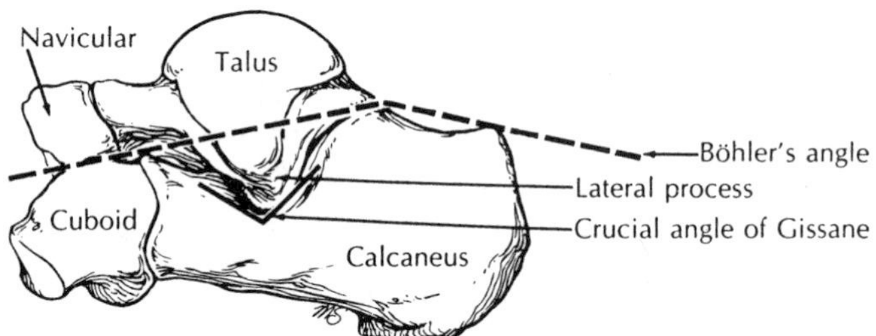

FIG. 39.3. Lateral view of the calcaneus demonstrating Bohler tuber angle (*dotted line*) and the crucial angle of Gissane. (From Rockwood CA Jr, Green DP, Bucholz RW, Heckman JD, eds. *Rockwood and Green's fractures in adults*, 4th ed. Vol. 2. Philadelphia: Lippincott-Raven, 1996:2326, with permission.)

- A transverse view is taken perpendicular to the coronal views; it demonstrates the calcaneocuboid joint, the anteroinferior aspect of the posterior facet, and the sustentaculum tali.

CLASSIFICATION OF EXTRAARTICULAR FRACTURES

- Anterior process fractures: may occur due to strong plantar flexion and inversion, which tightens the bifurcate and interosseous ligaments and leads to an avulsion fracture; alternatively, may occur with forefoot abduction with calcaneocuboid compression. Often confused with lateral ankle sprain; seen on lateral or lateral oblique views.
- Tuberosity fractures: may be due to avulsion by the Achilles tendon, especially in diabetics or osteoporotic women, or, rarely, may result from direct trauma; seen on lateral radiographs.
- Medial process fractures: vertical shear fracture due to loading of the heel in valgus; seen on axial radiograph.
- Sustentacular fractures: occur with heel loading accompanied by severe foot inversion. Often confused with medial ankle sprain; seen on axial radiograph.
- Body fractures not involving the subtalar articulation: due to axial loading. Significant comminution, widening, and loss of height may occur along with a reduction in the Bohler angle without posterior facet involvement.

ESSEX-LOPRESTI CLASSIFICATION OF INTRAARTICULAR FRACTURES (FIG. 39.4)

Primary Fracture Line

The posterolateral edge of the talus splits the calcaneus obliquely through the posterior facet. The fracture line exits anterolaterally at the crucial angle or as far distally as the calcaneocuboid joint. Posteriorly, the fracture moves medially, producing two main fragments: the sustentacular (anteromedial) and the tuberosity (posterolateral).

- The anteromedial fragment is rarely comminuted; it remains attached to the talus by deltoid and interosseous talocalcaneal ligaments.

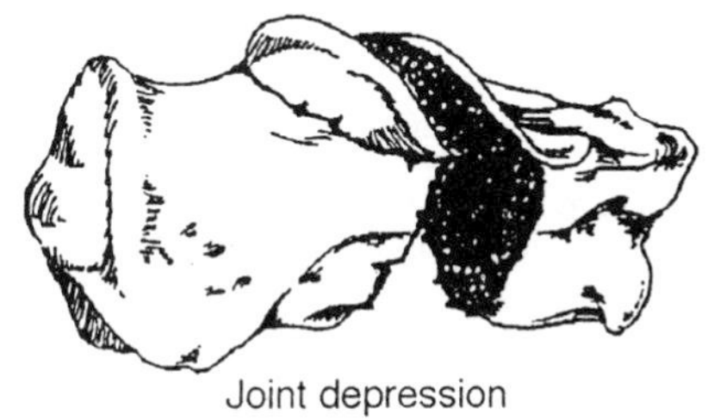

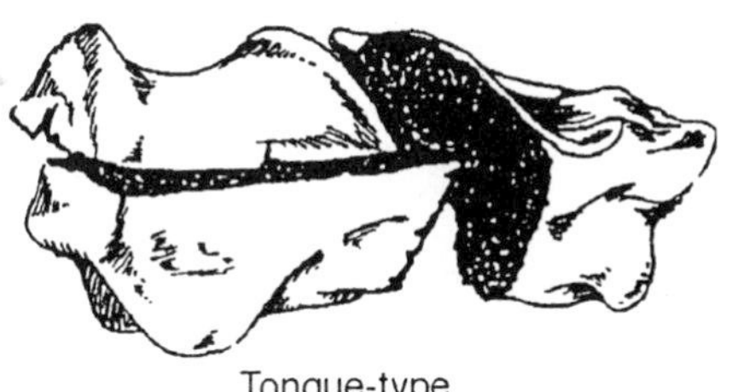

FIG. 39.4. Primary and secondary fracture patterns in intraarticular calcaneal fractures. (From Spivak JM, DiCesare PE, Feldmar DS, et al. *Orthopaedics: a study guide*. New York: McGraw Hill, 1999:564.)

- The posterolateral fragment usually displaces superolaterally with variable comminution, resulting in incongruity of the posterior facet and shortening and widening.

Secondary Fracture Line
With continued compressive forces additional comminution occurs, creating a free lateral piece of posterior facet separate from the tuberosity fragment.

- *Tongue fracture.* Secondary fracture line appears beneath the facet and exits posteriorly.
- *Joint depression fracture.* Secondary fracture line exits just behind the posterior facet.

Continued axial force causes the sustentacular fragment to slide medially, causing heel shortening and widening. As this occurs, the tuberosity fragment will rotate into varus. The posterolateral aspect of the talus will force the free lateral piece of the posterior facet down into the tuberosity fragment, rotating it as much as 90 degrees. This causes lateral wall blowout, which may extend as far anteriorly as the calcaneocuboid joint. As the lateral edge of the talus collapses further, additional comminution of the articular surface will occur.

SOUER AND REMY CLASSIFICATION

Based on the number of bony fragments determined on Broden, lateral, and Harris axial views.

First degree: nondisplaced intraarticular fractures
Second degree: secondary fracture lines resulting in a minimum of three additional pieces, with the posterior main fragment breaking into lateral, middle, and medial fragments
Third degree: highly comminuted

SANDERS CLASSIFICATION (FIG. 39.5)

- Classification based on the number and location of articular fragments as observed by computed tomography and found on the coronal image that shows the widest surface of the inferior facet of the talus.
- The posterior facet of the calcaneus is divided into three fracture lines (A, B, and C, corresponding to lateral, middle, and medial fracture lines, respectively, on the coronal image).
- Thus, a total of four potential pieces can result: lateral, central, medial, and sustentaculum tali.

Type I: all nondisplaced fractures regardless of the number of fracture lines
Type II: two-part fractures of the posterior facet; subtypes IIA, IIB, IIC based on the location of the primary fracture line
Type III: three-part fractures in which a centrally depressed fragment exists; subtypes IIIAB, IIIAC, IIIBC
Type IV: four-part articular fractures; highly comminuted

OTA CLASSIFICATION OF CALCANEAL FRACTURES

Type A: extraarticular
A1: extraarticular, avulsion
Type B: isolated body
B1: isolated body, nondisplaced
B2: isolated body, displaced
B3: isolated body, with associated fracture into calcaneocuboid articulation
Type C: articular
C1: articular, two-part
C2: articular, three-part
C3: articular, four plus parts

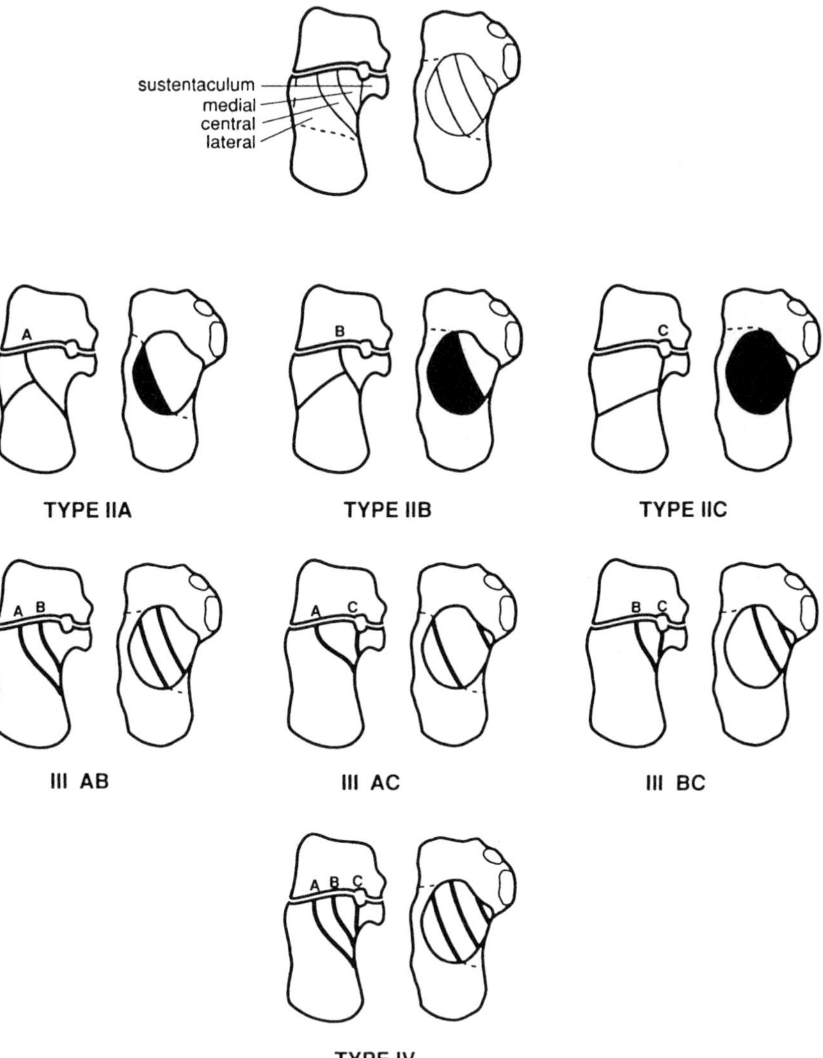

FIG. 39.5. Classification of intraarticular fractures of the calcaneus as seen on coronal **(left)** and transverse **(right)** computed tomographies of the subtalar joint. Type I (not shown) are nondisplaced; type II have two parts; type III have three parts; and type IV are comminuted. (From Sanders R, Fortin P, DiPasquale T, et al. Operative treatment in 120 displaced intraarticular calcaneal fractures. *Clin Orthop* 1993;290: 87–95, with permission.)

Treatment

Despite adequate reduction and treatment, fractures of the os calcis may be severely disabling injuries, with variable prognoses and degrees of functional debilitation accompanied by chronic pain issues. Treatment remains controversial with no clear indication for operative versus nonoperative treatment.

Nonoperative treatment

- Most appropriate for extraarticular fractures and for fractures that are extremely comminuted in osteopenic bone.
- Some advocate no reduction with elevation, compression, and early active motion because cast immobilization may lead to stiffness. The patient may progress to full weight bearing by 4 to 8 weeks after injury with the expectation that pain may persist for over 6 months.
- The Essex-Lopresti maneuver for tongue-type fractures with little articular comminution is closed reduction with a percutaneous Steinmann pin, followed by short-leg casting with incorporation of the pin and non–weight bearing for 4 to 6 weeks. The cast is then replaced (with removal of the pin) until radiographic healing occurs usually at 8 to 12 weeks after injury. Progressive weight bearing and active range of motion are then encouraged.

Operative treatment

- Goals include the following:
  1. Restoration of congruity of the subtalar articulation.
  2. Restoration of the Bohler angle.
  3. Restoration of the normal width of the calcaneus.
- Restoring calcaneal height, maintaining the normal calcaneocuboid articulation, and neutralizing the varus deformity of the fracture are also desirable.
- Open reduction and internal fixation are generally performed through a lateral L-shaped incision; care should be taken not to damage the sural nerve both proximally and distally.
- The posterior facet is reduced and stabilized with lag screws into the sustentaculum tali. The calcaneocuboid joint and the lateral wall are reduced. The length of the heel is regained with neutralization of varus deformity. A lateral thin plate (typically H or Y configuration) is then used as a buttress with possible bone grafting to restore bone stock.
- Primary subtalar or triple arthrodesis is not recommended and should not be necessary with restoration of the subtalar and calcaneocuboid articulations.
- Postoperative management includes the following:
  - Early supervised subtalar range-of-motion exercises.
  - Non–weight bearing for 8 to 12 weeks.
  - Full weight bearing by 3 months.

Complications

- Wound dehiscence: most common at the angle of incision. Avoidance requires meticulous soft-tissue technique, with adequate drainage and minimization of skin trauma during closure. Its appearance may be treated with wet to dry dressing changes, skin grafting, or a muscle flap if necessary.
- Calcaneal osteomyelitis: may be avoided by allowing soft-tissue edema to resolve preoperatively.
- Posttraumatic osteoarthritis (subtalar or calcaneocuboid): reflects articular damage in addition to fracture displacement and comminution; thus, may occur even in the presence of an anatomic reduction; may be treated with injections and orthoses or may ultimately require subtalar or triple arthrodesis.
- Increased heel width: expected, even with open reduction and internal fixation. May result in lateral impingement on the peroneal tendons or the fibula. It is aggravated by increased residual lateral width, and it may be treated by wall resection or hardware removal.
- Chronic pain: may occur despite nonoperative or operative treatment; may be debilitating; many are unable to return to gainful employment.

FRACTURES OF THE MIDFOOT

Midtarsal Joint (Chopart Joint)

Epidemiology

Injuries to the midfoot, which are relatively uncommon, occur as a result of high energy trauma, such as vehicular trauma, or low energy mechanisms, such as twisting injuries in athletics or dancing.

Anatomy

- The midtarsal joint consists of the calcaneocuboid and talonavicular joints, which act in concert with the subtalar joint during inversion and eversion of the foot.
- The Chopart joint is more mobile with the heel in pronation and is relatively fixed with the heel in supination. The cuboid acts as a linkage across three naviculocuneiform joints, allowing only minimal motion. The configuration of multiple constrained joints is what minimizes susceptibility to injury.
- Ligamentous attachments include the plantar calcaneonavicular (spring) ligament, bifurcate ligament, dorsal talonavicular ligament, dorsal calcaneocuboid ligament, dorsal cuboideonavicular ligament, and long plantar ligament.

Mechanism of Injury

- High energy trauma: most common; may result from direct impact due to motor vehicle accidents or from a combination of axial loading and torsion, such as during impact after a fall or a jump from a height.
- Low energy injuries: may result in a sprain during athletic or dance activities.

Clinical Evaluation

- Patient presentation is variable, ranging from an antalgic gait with swelling and tenderness on the dorsum of the midfoot to nonambulatory in significant pain with gross swelling, ecchymosis, and variable deformity.
- Stress maneuvers consist of forefoot abduction, adduction, flexion, and extension and may result in reproduction of pain and instability.
- A careful neurovascular examination should be performed. In cases of extreme pain and swelling, serial examinations may be warranted to evaluate the possibility of compartment syndrome of the foot.

Radiographic Evaluation

- Anteroposterior, lateral, and oblique radiographs of the foot should be obtained. Comparison views of the uninjured contralateral foot may be obtained.
- Stress views may help to delineate subtle injuries.
- Computed tomography may aid in characterizing fracture-dislocation injuries with articular comminution.
- Magnetic resonance imaging may be used to evaluate ligamentous injury.

CLASSIFICATION

Medial Stress Injury (30%)

- This is an inversion injury with adduction of the midfoot on the hindfoot.
- Flake fractures of the dorsal margin of the talus or navicular and of the lateral margin of the calcaneus or the cuboid may indicate a sprain.
- In more severe injuries, the midfoot may be completely dislocated or an isolated talonavicular dislocation may occur. A medial swivel dislocation is one in which the talonavicular joint is dislocated, the subtalar joint is subluxed, and the calcaneocuboid joint is intact.

Longitudinal Stress Injury (41%)

- Force is transmitted through the metatarsal heads proximally along the rays, with resultant compression of the midfoot between the metatarsals and the talus with the foot plantarflexed.
- Longitudinal forces pass between the cuneiforms and fracture the navicular, typically in a vertical pattern.

Lateral Stress Injury (17%)

- This so-called "nutcracker fracture" is a characteristic fracture of the cuboid as the forefoot is driven laterally, causing crushing of the cuboid between the calcaneus and the bases of the fourth and fifth metatarsals.
- This is most commonly an avulsion fracture of the navicular with a comminuted compression fracture of the cuboid.
- In more severe trauma, the talonavicular joint subluxes laterally and the lateral column of the foot collapses due to comminution of the calcaneocuboid joint.

Plantar Stress Injury (7%)

- Plantarly directed forces may result in sprains to the midtarsal region with avulsion fractures of the dorsal lip of the navicular, talus, or anterior process of the calcaneus.

Treatment

Nonoperative treatment

- Sprain: nonrigid dressings with protected weight bearing for 4 to 6 weeks; prognosis is excellent.
- Nondisplaced fracture: treated with short-leg casting with initial non–weight bearing for 6 weeks.

Operative treatment

- High energy mechanisms resulting in displaced fracture patterns often require open reduction and internal fixation (e.g., with Kirschner wires) and/or external fixation.
- Prognosis is often poor, depending on degree of intraarticular incongruity.
- Bone grafting of the cuboid may be necessary in lateral stress injuries.
- Severe crush injuries with extensive comminution may require arthrodesis to restore the longitudinal arch of the foot.

Complications

Posttraumatic osteoarthritis: may occur as a result of residual articular incongruity or chondral injury at the time of trauma. If severe and debilitating, it may require arthrodesis for adequate relief of symptoms.

Tarsal Navicular

Epidemiology

Isolated fractures of the navicular occur uncommonly; they may be diagnosed only after ruling out concomitant injuries to the midtarsal joint complex.

Anatomy

- The talocalcaneonavicular complex demonstrates ball-and-socket type joint motion, although the socket rotates about the ball in this case.
- The tarsal navicular articulates with the talus proximally, the cuneiforms distally, and the cuboid laterally.

Mechanism of Injury

- Direct: trauma to the dorsomedial aspect of the foot.
- Indirect: axial compression along the medial aspect of the foot or capsular avulsion during ankle injury.
- Stress fractures: may occur in athletes who run and jump, with increased risk in patients with cavus foot/calcaneal navicular coalition.

Clinical Evaluation

- Patients typically present with a painful foot that may demonstrate dorsomedial swelling and point tenderness.
- Physical examination should include assessment of the ipsilateral ankle and foot with careful palpation of all bony structures to rule out associated injures.
- Pain is usually along the dorsomedial or medial arch, possibly leading to the misdiagnosis of anterior tibial tendonitis in cases of navicular stress fractures.

Radiographic Evaluation

- Anteroposterior, lateral, and oblique views of the foot should be obtained.
- Magnetic resonance imaging or technetium-99m scan may be obtained if a fracture is not apparent by plain radiography but is suspected.
- Computed tomography may be performed to characterize the fracture.

ANATOMIC CLASSIFICATION

The fracture is typically in the sagittal plane (partial vs. complete).

Cortical Avulsion Fractures (47%)

- Excessive flexion or eversion of the midfoot, resulting in a dorsal lip avulsion of the navicular by the talonavicular capsule and the anterior fibers of the deltoid ligament.
- Symptomatic, small, nonarticular fragments may be excised. Large fragments (>25% articular surface) may be reattached with a compression screw.

Body Fractures (29%)

These are high energy injuries.

Tuberosity Fractures (20% to 25%)

- Forced eversion injury causing avulsion of the tuberosity by the posterior tibial tendon insertion or deltoid ligament.
- Often part of the "nutcracker fracture"; therefore, concomitant midtarsal injury must be ruled out.
- Must rule out the presence of accessory navicular injury, which is bilateral in 64% of cases.
- If symptomatic, small fragments can be excised and the posterior tibial tendon reattached; larger fragments generally require open reduction and internal fixation with a lag screw, especially if posterior tibial tendon function is compromised.

Stress Fractures

- These fractures occur primarily in young athletes.
- They frequently require a bone scan or magnetic resonance imaging for diagnosis.
- The fracture line is usually sagittally oriented in the middle third and may be complete or incomplete.
- Due to an increased incidence of persistent problems with pain and healing, screw fixation with autologous bone grafting should be used with all comminuted and complete fractures.

SANGEORZAN CLASSIFICATION (FIG. 39.6)

Type I: Transverse fracture line in the coronal plane, minimal comminution; dorsal displacement of the free fragment; the medial border of the foot appears intact on the anteroposterior radiograph.

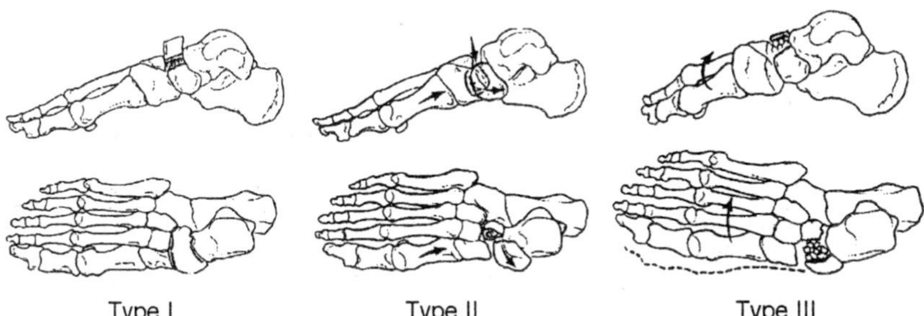

FIG. 39.6. Sangeorzan classification of navicular body fractures. (From Sangeorzan BJ, Benirscke SK, Mosca V, et al. Displaced intraarticular fractures of the tarsal navicular. *J Bone Joint Surg Am* 1989;71A:1504–1510, with permission.)

Type II: Most common; fracture line from dorsolateral to plantar-medial with talonavicular joint disruption; dorsomedial displacement of the fracture fragment.
Type III: Comminuted fracture pattern with naviculocuneiform joint disruption; associated fractures may exist (cuboid, anterior calcaneus, calcaneocuboid joint).

Reduction of at least 60% of the joint surface on both anteroposterior and lateral views is necessary to prevent talonavicular joint subluxation after healing.

OTA CLASSIFICATION OF NAVICULAR FRACTURES (FIG. 39.7)

Type A: extraarticular
- A1: extraarticular avulsion
- A2: extraarticular, coronal body split
- A3: extraarticular, multifragmentary body

Type B: partial articular (talonavicular joint)
- B1: partial articular, sagittal lateral half
- B2: partial articular, sagittal medial half
- B3: partial articular, horizontal fracture

Type C: articular, talonavicular and naviculocuneiform
- C1: articular, both surfaces, multifragmentary
  - C1.1: nondisplaced
  - C1.2: displaced

Treatment

Nonoperative treatment

Indicated for incomplete lesions; short-leg cast (non–weight bearing) for 4 to 6 weeks, followed by a gradual return to activities over the subsequent 6 weeks.

Operative treatment

- Indicated for complete or displaced fractures.
- Open reduction and internal fixation with a lag screw (dorsomedial incision), followed by a short-leg cast (partial weight bearing) for 6 weeks and an additional 4 weeks of partial weight bearing.

Complications

- Osteonecrosis: increased risk with significantly displaced, markedly comminuted, or inadequate immobilization. May result in a collapse of the navicular, with need for bone grafting and internal fixation.
- Posttraumatic osteoarthritis: may occur as a result of articular incongruity, chondral damage, or free osteochondral fragments from articular comminution.

Cuboid

Epidemiology

- Isolated injury to the cuboid may occur with athletic or dance participation or in high energy injuries.
- Patients with Ehlers-Danlos syndrome have increased incidences of dislocation and fracture–dislocation of the cuboid.

Anatomy

- The cuboid articulates with the calcaneus proximally, the navicular and lateral cuneiform medially, and the lateral two metatarsals distally.
- Its plantar aspect forms a portion of the roof of the peroneal groove through which the peroneus longus tendon runs; thus, scarring and irregularity of the peroneal groove caused by cuboid fracture may compromise function of the peroneus longus tendon.

Mechanism of Injury

- Direct: uncommon; trauma to the dorsolateral aspect of the foot may result in fractures of the cuboid.

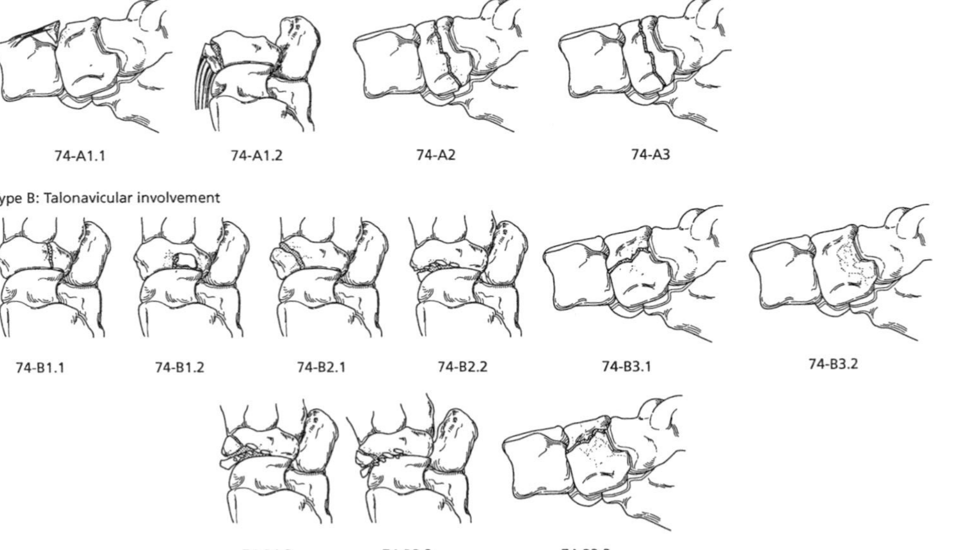

FIG. 39.7. A–C. OTA classification for navicular fractures. The initial differentiation is by articular involvement. Type A is extraarticular; B is mainly uniarticular involvement; and C signifies multiarticular multifragmented involvement. Further subdivision is by fracture pattern. (From OTA Committee for Coding and Classification. Fracture and dislocation compendium. *J Orthop Trauma* 1996;10[Suppl 1]:114–118, with permission.)

- Indirect: accounts for most cuboid fractures.
  - "Nutcracker injury": torsional stress or forefoot abduction may result in impaction of the cuboid between the calcaneus and the lateral metatarsals.
  - Extreme plantarflexion: may cause isolated sprain or dislocation of calcaneocuboid joint in high velocity trauma, dance injuries, or patients with Ehlers-Danlos syndrome.
- Stress fractures: may occur in athletic individuals.

Clinical Evaluation

- Patients typically present with pain, swelling, and point tenderness to palpation of the dorsolateral aspect of the foot.
- Palpation of all bony structures of the foot should be performed to rule out associated injuries.
- Pain on the lateral aspect of the foot may be confused with symptoms of peroneal tendonitis in cases of stress fractures of the cuboid.

Radiographic Evaluation

- Anteroposterior, lateral, and oblique views of the foot should be obtained.
- Technetium-99m bone scanning or magnetic resonance imaging may be useful for diagnosing a stress fracture.

OTA CLASSIFICATION OF CUBOID FRACTURES (FIG. 39.8)

Type A: extraarticular
- A1: extraarticular, avulsion
- A2: extraarticular, coronal
- A3: extraarticular, multifragmentary

Type B: partial articular, single joint (calcaneocuboid or cubotarsal)
- B1: partial articular, sagittal
- B2: partial articular, horizontal

Type C: articular, calcaneocuboid and cubotarsal involvement
- C1: articular, multifragmentary
  - C1.1: nondisplaced
  - C1.2: displaced

Treatment

Nonoperative treatment

With minimal impaction or nondisplaced fractures, a short-leg cast for 6 weeks with progressive weight bearing is indicated.

Operative treatment

Displaced fractures may require open reduction and internal fixation with Kirschner wires or screws; severe comminution and residual displacement may necessitate calcaneocuboid arthrodesis for proper foot alignment and minimization of late complications.

Complications

- Osteonecrosis: may complicate severely displaced fractures or those with significant comminution.
- Posttraumatic osteoarthritis: may occur as a result of articular incongruity, chondral damage, or free osteochondral fragments from articular comminution.
- Nonunion: may occur with significant displacement and inadequate immobilization or fixation. If severely symptomatic, it may necessitate open reduction and internal fixation with bone grafting.

Tarsometatarsal (Lisfranc) Joint

Epidemiology

Very uncommon, accounting for only 16 cases in a review of approximately 82,500 fractures over a 15-year period in one series.

Anatomy

- In the anteroposterior plane, the base of the second metatarsal is recessed between the medial and lateral cuneiforms. This limits translation of the metatarsals in the frontal plane.
- In the coronal plane, the middle three metatarsal bases are trapezoidal in shape, forming a transverse arch that prevents plantar displacement of the metatarsal bases. The second metatarsal base is the keystone in the transverse arch of the foot.
- Only slight motion occurs across the tarsometatarsal joints, with 10 to 20 degrees of dorsal-plantar motion at the fifth metatarsocuboid joint and progressively less motion medially except for the first metatarsocuneiform (20 degrees plantarflexion from neutral).
- The ligamentous support begins with the strong ligaments linking the bases of the second through fifth metatarsals. The most important ligament is the Lisfranc ligament, which attaches the medial cuneiform to the base of the second metatarsal.
- Ligamentous, bony, and soft-tissue support provides intrinsic stability across the plantar aspect of Lisfranc joint; conversely, the dorsal aspect of this articulation is not reinforced by structures of similar strength.
- No ligamentous connection is found between the base of the first and second metatarsals.
- The dorsalis pedis artery dives between the first and second metatarsals at the Lisfranc joint and thus may be damaged during injury or at the time of reduction.

Mechanism of Injury

The three most common mechanisms include the following:

- Twisting: forceful abduction of the forefoot on the tarsus resulting in fracture of the base of the second metatarsal and a shear or crush fracture of the cuboid. Historically seen in equestrian accidents when a rider fell from a horse with a foot engaged in a stirrup. Commonly seen today in motor vehicle accidents (Fig. 39.9).
- Axial loading of a fixed foot: may be seen with extrinsic axial compression applied to the heel, such as a heavy object striking the heel of a kneeling patient, or in extreme ankle equinus with axial loading of the body weight, such as a missed step off a curb or a landing from a jump during a dance maneuver.
- Crushing mechanisms: common in industrial-type injuries to the Lisfranc joint, with frequently associated sagittal plane displacement, soft-tissue compromise, and compartment syndrome.

Clinical Evaluation

- Patients present with variable foot deformity, pain, swelling, and tenderness on the foot dorsum.
- A careful neurovascular examination is essential as frank dislocation of the Lisfranc joint may be associated with impingement upon or partial or complete laceration of the dorsalis pedis artery. In addition, dramatic swelling of the foot is common with high energy mechanisms; compartment syndrome of the foot must be ruled out on the basis of serial neurovascular examination or with compartment pressure monitoring, if necessary.
- Stress testing may be performed by gentle passive forefoot abduction and pronation with the hindfoot firmly stabilized in the examiner's other hand. Alternatively, pain can typically be reproduced by gentle supination and pronation motions of the forefoot.

Radiographic Evaluation

- Standard anteroposterior, lateral, and oblique films are usually diagnostic.
- The medial border of the second metatarsal should be co-linear with the medial border of the middle cuneiform on the anteroposterior view.
- The medial border of the fourth metatarsal should be co-linear with the medial border of the cuboid on the oblique view.
- Dorsal displacement of the metatarsals on the lateral view is indicative of ligamentous compromise.

(*text continues on page 276*)

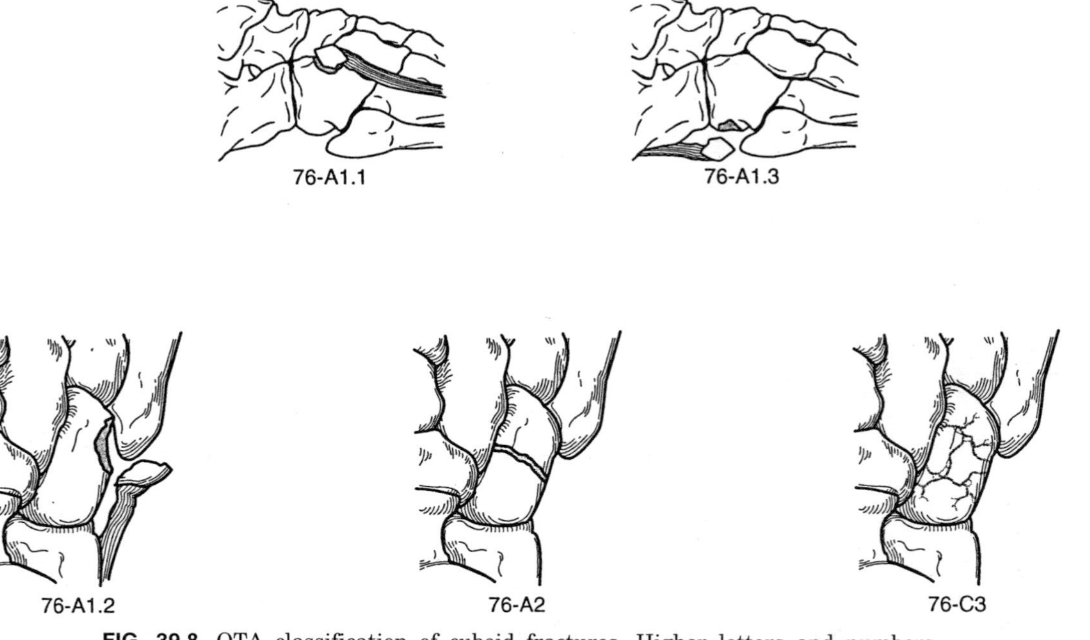

FIG. 39.8. OTA classification of cuboid fractures. Higher letters and numbers denote more significant injury. Type A: extraarticular, no joint involvement. (From OTA Committee for Coding and Classification. Fracture and dislocation compendium. *J Orthop Trauma* 1996;10[Suppl 1]:123–126, with permission.)

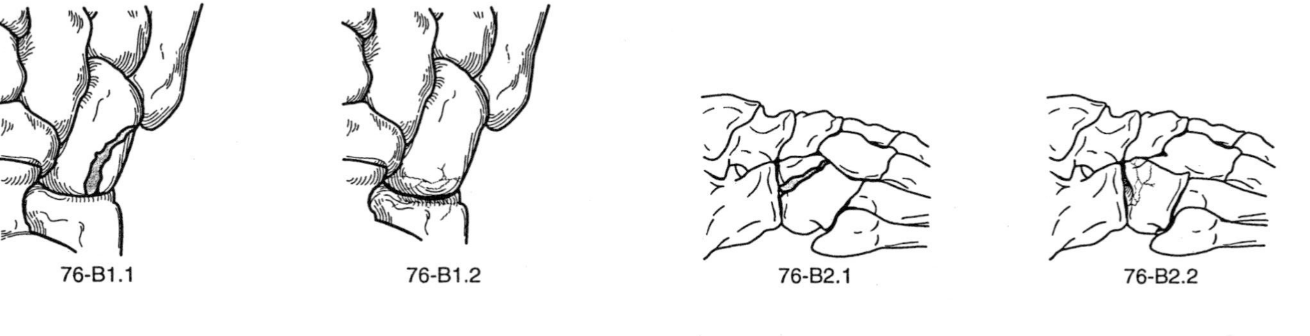

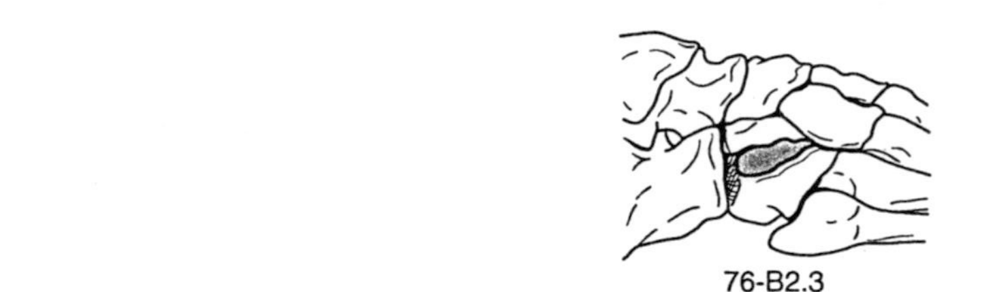

FIG. 39.8. *Continued*. Type B: partial articular. 1, calcaneal-cuboid; 2, cuboid-tarsal.

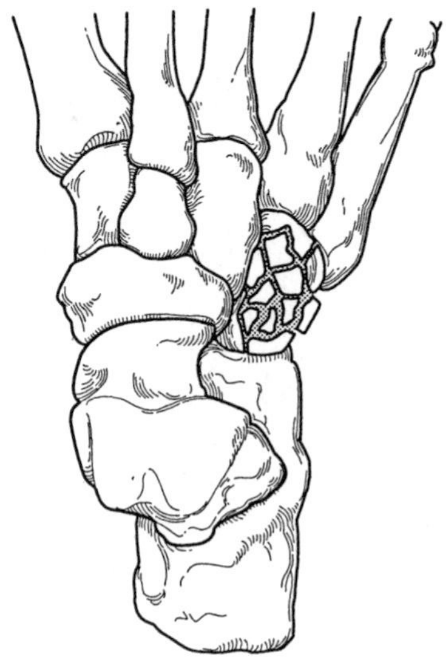

FIG. 39.8. *Continued.* Type C: articular, both joints.

- Flake fractures around the base of the second metatarsal are indicative of disruption of the Lisfranc joint.
- If clinically indicated, stress views should be obtained under regional or general anesthesia. The forefoot is held in abduction for the anteroposterior view and in plantar flexion for the lateral view.

GENERAL CLASSIFICATION (FIG. 39.10)

Classification schemes for Lisfranc injuries guide the clinician in defining the extent and pattern of injury, although they are of little prognostic value.

OUENU AND KUSS CLASSIFICATION

Based on commonly observed patterns of injury.

Homolateral: all five metatarsals displaced in the same direction
Isolated: one or two metatarsals displaced from the others
Divergent: displacement of the metatarsals in both the sagittal and coronal planes

MYERSON CLASSIFICATION (FIG. 39.11)

Based on commonly observed patterns of injury with regard to treatment.

Total incongruity: lateral and dorsoplantar
Partial incongruity: medial and lateral
Divergent: partial and total

Treatment

Nonoperative treatment

- Injury may be accompanied by massive swelling and may require a 2- to 3-day period of neurovascular monitoring for compartment syndrome; monitoring should be followed by splinting, strict bedrest, and aggressive elevation.

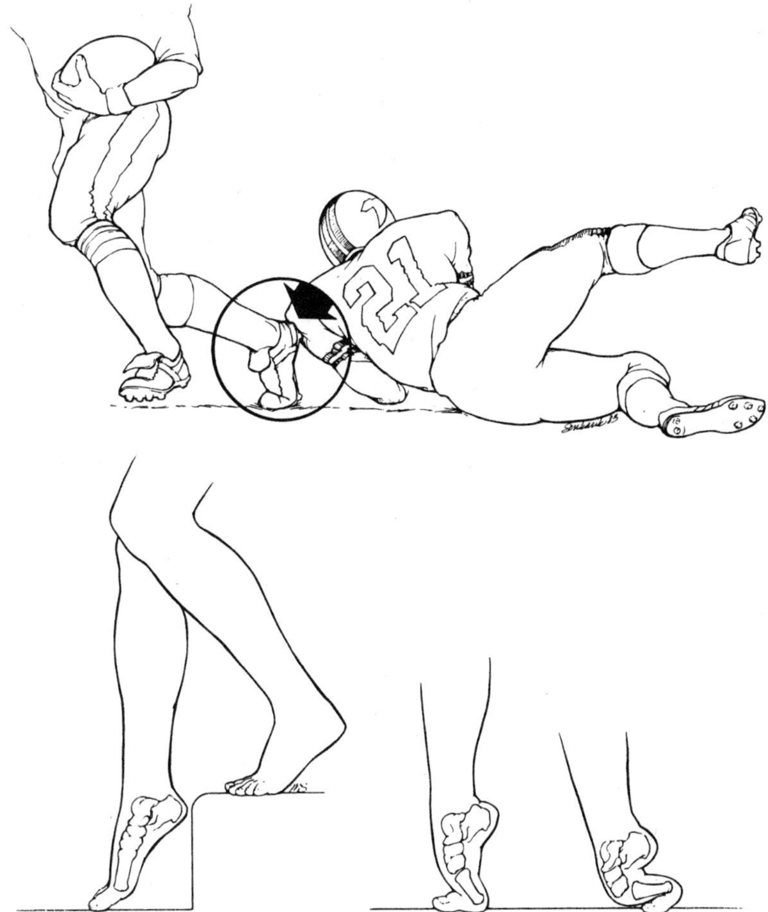

FIG. 39.9. Top: An axial load applied directly to the heel, when the foot is fixed to the ground in equinus, can produce a tarsometatarsal injury. **Bottom:** The common mechanism of Lisfranc joint collapse when, with the ankle in extreme equinus, the body weight produces an axial load on the joint complex. (From Rockwood CA Jr, Green DP, Bucholz RW, Heckman JD, eds. *Rockwood and Green's fractures in adults*, 4th ed. Vol. 2. Philadelphia: Lippincott-Raven, 1996:2365, with permission.)

- Nondisplaced or minimally displaced injuries may be amenable to casting for 6 weeks.

Operative treatment

- Operative treatment should be considered when displacement of the tarsometatarsal joint is >2 mm. This may consist of closed reduction with pin fixation, although some argue for open reduction and internal fixation regardless of displacement, even if an anatomic reduction can be obtained. Open reduction and internal fixation should be pursued for cases with >2-mm residual displacement or >15-degree tarsometatarsal angulation.
- Relative indications include the following:
  1. Severe displacement of metatarsal bases.
  2. Entrapment of bony fragments in the joint.

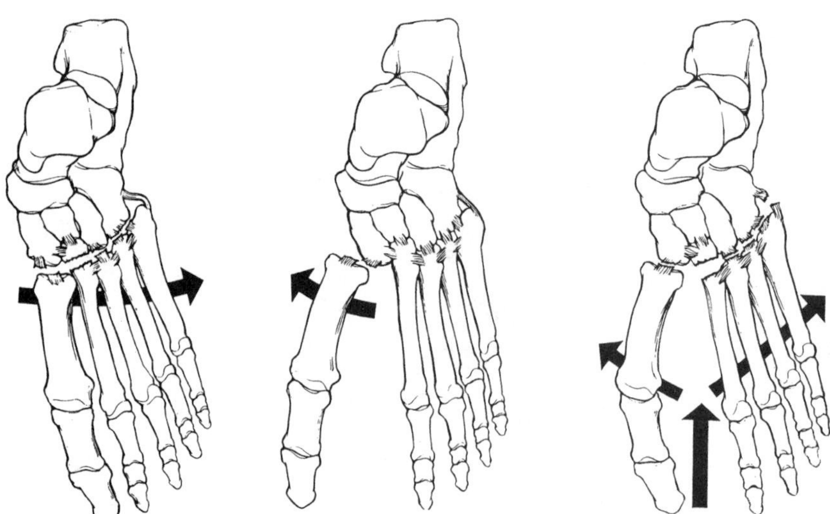

FIG. 39.10. The three commonly occurring patterns of tarsometatarsal joint dislocation: **(left)** homolateral, **(center)** isolated, and **(right)** divergent. (From Rockwood CA Jr, Green DP, Bucholz RW, Heckman JD, eds. *Rockwood and Green's fractures in adults*, 4th ed. Vol. 2. Philadelphia: Lippincott-Raven, 1996:2366, with permission.)

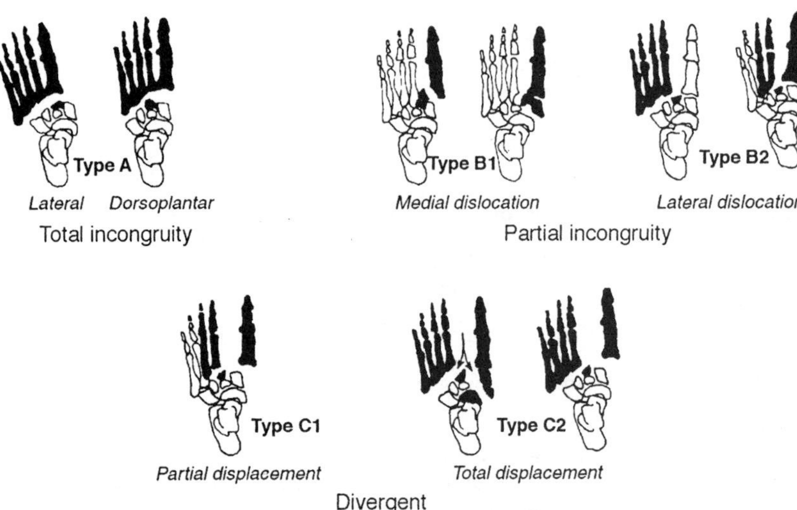

FIG. 39.11. Myerson classification of Lisfranc fracture-dislocations. (From Myerson MS, Fisher RT, Burgess AR, et al. Fracture-dislocations of the tarsometatarsal joints: end results correlated with pathology and treatment. *Foot Ankle* 1986; 6:225–242, with permission.)

3. Entrapment of soft tissue in the joint, especially the anterior tibial tendon (complex dislocation).

- The key to reduction is correction of the fracture-dislocation of the second metatarsal base. Clinical results suggest that accuracy and maintenance of reduction are of utmost importance and correlate directly with the overall outcome.
- Stiffness due to open reduction and internal fixation is not of significant concern because of the already limited motion of the tarsometatarsal joints.

Complications
The main complication of a Lisfranc injury is posttraumatic arthritis. This can usually be addressed through the use of a well-molded firm arch support with a long steel shank in the shoe. Recalcitrant cases may require arthrodesis for symptomatic relief.

FRACTURES OF THE FOREFOOT

Metatarsals

Epidemiology
The true incidence of metatarsal shaft fractures is unknown due to the variety of physicians treating such injuries.

Anatomy
- Displaced fractures of the metatarsals result in the disruption of the major weight-bearing complex of the forefoot.
- Disruptions produce an alteration in the normal distribution of weight in the forefoot, leading to problems of metatarsalgia and transfer lesions (intractable plantar keratoses).

Mechanism of Injury
- Direct trauma: most commonly occurs when a heavy object is dropped on the forefoot.
- Twisting: occurs with the body torque when toes are fixed, such as when a person catches their toes in a narrow opening with continued ambulation.
- Avulsion: particularly at the base of the fifth metatarsal.
- Stress fractures: especially at the necks of the second and third metatarsals and the proximal fifth metatarsal.

Clinical Examination
- Patients typically present with pain, swelling, and tenderness over the site of fracture.
- Evaluation of neurovascular status, as well as of soft-tissue injury and ambulatory capacity, is important.

Radiographic Evaluation
- Anteroposterior, lateral, and oblique views of the foot should be obtained. Decreasing the beam intensity (thus underpenetrating the tarsal bones of the hindfoot) to enhance osseous detail of the forefoot may be necessary.
- A technetium-99m bone scan may aid in the diagnosis of an occult stress fracture.

ANATOMIC CLASSIFICATION

First Metatarsal Injuries

- Larger and stronger than lesser metatarsals; less frequently injured.
- Injuries usually related to direct trauma (often open and/or comminuted).
- Anatomic reduction and fixation important due to its importance in weight bearing.

Second, Third, and Fourth Metatarsal Injuries

- Indirect twisting mechanisms: result in spiral pattern. Must be wary of a Lisfranc injury with involvement of the base of the second metatarsal.
- Stress fractures.

Fifth Metatarsal Injuries

- Direct trauma: most injuries.
- Dancer fracture: spiral fracture of the distal fifth metatarsal shaft due to an inversion force applied to the foot when the dancer falls from the demi-pointe position.

OTA CLASSIFICATION OF METATARSAL SHAFT FRACTURES (FIG. 39.12)

Type A: extraarticular
- A1: proximal, extraarticular
- A2: diaphyseal, simple
- A3: distal, extraarticular

Type B: partial articular
- B1: proximal, partial articular
- B2: diaphyseal, wedge
- B3: distal, partial articular

Type C: articular
- C1: proximal, articular
- C2: diaphyseal, complex (multifragmentary)
- C3: distal, articular

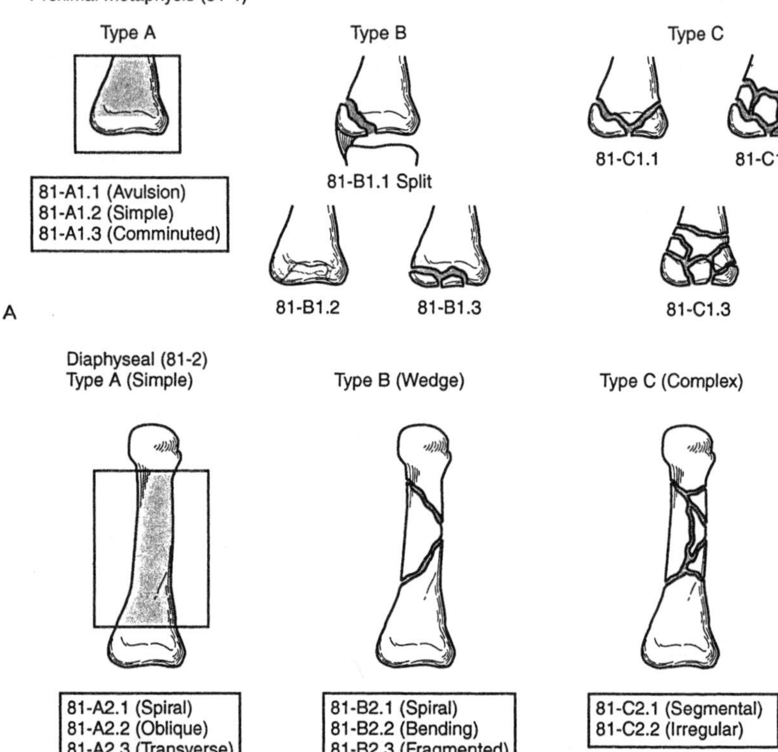

FIG. 39.12. A–C. OTA classification for metatarsal fractures. Modifiers are used to specify the metatarsal involved and follow the classification number: *T*, great; *N*, index; *M*, middle; *R*, ring; *L*, little. (From OTA Committee for Coding and Classification. Fracture and dislocation compendium. *J Orthop Trauma* 1996;10[Suppl 1]:127–131, with permission.)

Treatment
Anatomic reduction is important for maintaining normal length, rotation, and declination of the ray.

Nonoperative treatment
Nondisplaced fractures may be treated in a short-leg walking cast for 2 to 4 weeks with early ambulation encouraged.

Operative treatment

- First and fifth metatarsals: provide stability and protection to the second, third, and fourth metatarsals; therefore, an aggressive approach to open reduction and internal fixation for displaced fractures is recommended.
  Anatomic reduction is crucial for the first metatarsal.
  Displacement of a fifth metatarsal fracture often requires open reduction and internal fixation to prevent deformity of the lateral border of the foot, which may compromise shoe wearing.
- Displaced fractures (2 to 4 mm of shortening or elevation): best managed with open reduction and internal fixation to prevent the development of painful plantar keratoses or dorsal calluses; fixation may be accomplished with intramedullary Kirschner wire fixation or a one-fourth tubular plate.
- Displaced stress fractures: treat like an acute injury.
- Special fractures: base of the fifth metatarsal.
  1. Avulsion (pseudo-Jones fracture):
     Mechanism of injury is acute inversion with plantar flexion of the foot with avulsion caused by peroneus brevis or lateral plantar aponeurosis—controversial. Occasionally, it may occur as a stress fracture.
     These are metaphyseal and often nondisplaced; they typically experience rapid union.
     This fracture may be treated with a walking cast or a walking boot in cases of minimal displacement (<2 mm).
     Open reduction with internal fixation is indicated in delayed unions or nonunions, fractures with significant displacement, and those involving the articular surface of the cuboid/fifth metatarsal joint.
  2. Jones fracture
     This is a fracture of the proximal shaft of the fifth metatarsal at the metaphyseal/diaphyseal junction.
     The mechanism of injury is an inversion stress injury to the foot. The fracture is due to the dense ligamentous attachments between the base of the fifth metatarsal and the base of the fourth metatarsal and cuboid that limit the degree of "give" and that predispose to fracture in the metaphyseal-diaphyseal region.

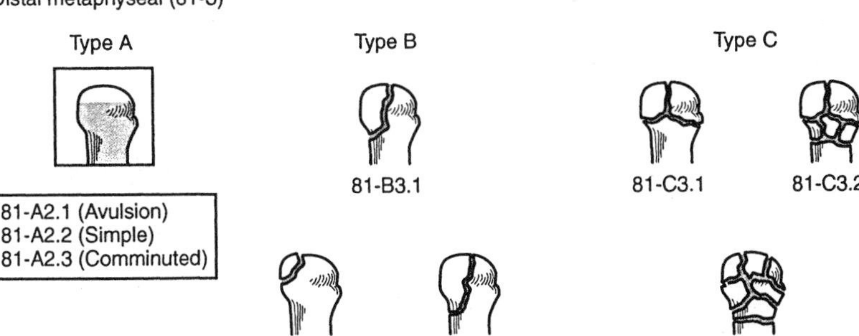

FIG. 39.12. *Continued.*

These often begin as stress fractures that progress to acute displaced fractures.
Treatment consists of application of a short-leg cast with non–weight bearing for 6 weeks, followed by progressive weight bearing.
Some recommend immediate open reduction and internal fixation with a malleolar screw.
Complications include delayed union and nonunion, with an incidence of 67% with displaced fractures; in these cases, open reduction and internal fixation with possible bone grafting are recommended.

Metatarsophalangeal Joints

Mobility of the metatarsophalangeal joints is essential for forefoot comfort in normal gait; attempts should thus be made to salvage any motion at this level.

First Metatarsophalangeal Joint

Epidemiology

- Injuries to the first metatarsophalangeal joint are relatively common, especially in athletic activities or ballet.
- The incidence in American football and soccer has risen due to the use of forgiving artificial playing surfaces and of lighter, more flexible shoe wear that permits enhanced motion at the metatarsophalangeal level.

Anatomy

- Condylar articulation with 75-degree dorsiflexion and 35-degree plantarflexion.
- Ligamentous constraints: dorsal capsule reinforced by the extensor hallucis longus tendon; plantar plate (capsular ligament) reinforced by the flexor hallucis longus tendon, flexor hallucis brevis tendon, and medial and lateral collateral ligaments.

Mechanism of Injury

- "Turf toe" (Fig. 39.13) is a sprain of the first metatarsophalangeal joint. It reflects a hyperextension injury to the first metatarsophalangeal joint as the ankle is in equinus, causing temporary subluxation with stretching on the plantar capsule and plate.
- This may result in articular injury, especially to the dorsal metatarsal head, with progressive hallux rigidus and valgus.
- In ballet dancers, injury may occur as a dancer "falls over" a maximally extended first metatarsophalangeal joint, injuring the dorsal capsule. Forced abduction may result in lateral capsular injury with possible avulsion from the base of the proximal phalanx.

Clinical Evaluation

- Patients typically present with pain, swelling, and tenderness of the first metatarsophalangeal joint.
- Pain may be reproduced with range of motion of the first metatarsophalangeal joint, especially at terminal dorsiflexion or plantarflexion.
- Chronic injuries may present with decreased range of motion.

Radiographic Evaluation

Anteroposterior, lateral, and oblique views of the foot may demonstrate capsular avulsion or chronic degenerative changes indicative of long-standing injury.

BOWERS AND MARTIN CLASSIFICATION

Grade I: strain at the proximal attachment of the volar plate from the first metatarsal head
Grade II: avulsion of the volar plate from the metatarsal head
Grade III: impaction injury to the dorsal surface of the metatarsal head with or without an avulsion or chip fracture

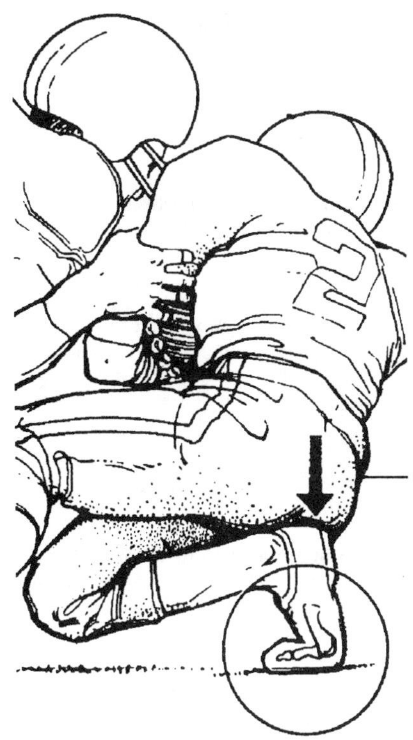

FIG. 39.13. Hyperextension mechanism of the "turf toe" injury. (From Rodeo SA, O'Brien S, Warren RF, et al. Turf toe: an analysis of metatarsophalangeal joint sprains in professional football players. *Am J Sports Med* 1990;18: 280–285, with permission.)

Treatment

- Rest, ice, compression, elevation, and nonsteroidal antiinflammatory medications are used.
- Protective taping with gradual return to full activity is employed; the patient may temporarily wear a hard-soled shoe with a rocker bottom for comfort.
- Pain usually subsides after 3 weeks of treatment, but an additional 3 weeks is usually necessary to regain strength and motion for return to competitive activity.
- Injections with cortisone and lidocaine are contraindicated.

Complications

Hallux rigidus and degenerative arthritis complicate chronic injuries and may prevent return to competitive activity.

Dislocation of the First Metatarsophalangeal Joint

Epidemiology

- This is a rare injury related to high energy trauma.
- Concomitant foot injuries should be considered.

Anatomy

Intrinsic stability of the first metatarsophalangeal articulation is provided by the congruity of the concave proximal phalanx and the convex metatarsal head, as well as by the strong ligamentous attachments.

Mechanism of Injury

- Most commonly high energy trauma, such as a motor vehicle accident, in which forced hyperextension of the joint occurs with gross disruption of the plantar capsule and plate.
- Commonly associated with other injuries to the foot.

Clinical Evaluation

- Most are dorsal dislocations with the proximal phalanx cocked up and displaced dorsally and proximally, producing a dorsal prominence and shortening of the toe.
- Neurovascular examination of the toe is essential as tenting of the dorsal skin may occur, often impairing distal capillary refill.

Radiographic Evaluation

- Anteroposterior, lateral, and oblique views of the forefoot demonstrate dorsal and proximal displacement of the base of the proximal phalanx on the metatarsal head.
- Occasionally, small avulsion fractures of the base of the proximal phalanx are seen.
- Sesamoids of the flexor tendons must be inspected for fracture because this occurrence may affect closed reduction.

JAHSS CLASSIFICATION

Based on integrity of the sesamoid complex.

Type I:	Volar plate is avulsed off the first metatarsal head; proximal phalanx displaced dorsally; intersesamoid ligament remains intact and lies over the dorsum of the metatarsal head.
Type IIA:	Intersesamoid ligament is ruptured.
Type IIB:	Longitudinal fracture of either sesamoid is seen.

Treatment

- *Type I fracture.* Closed reduction may be attempted initially. However, if it is irreducible by closed means, it requires open reduction.
- *Type IIA and IIB fractures.* These are easily reduced by closed means (longitudinal traction with or without hyperextension of the first metatarsophalangeal joint).
- After reduction, the patient should be placed in a short-leg walking cast with a toe extension for 3 to 4 weeks to allow for capsular healing.
- Displaced avulsion fractures of the base of the proximal phalanx should be fixed with either lag screws or a tension band technique. Small osteochondral fractures may be excised; larger fragments require reduction with Kirschner wires, compression screws, or Herbert screws.

Complications

- Posttraumatic osteoarthritis: may reflect chondral damage at the time of injury or may arise due to abnormal resultant laxity with subsequent degenerative changes.
- Recurrent dislocation: uncommon; may occur in patients with connective tissue disorders.

Fractures and Dislocations of the Lesser Metatarsophalangeal Joints

Epidemiology

- "Stubbing" injuries are very common.
- Incidence is higher for the fifth metatarsophalangeal joint as its lateral position renders it vulnerable.

Anatomy

Stability of the metatarsophalangeal joints is conferred by the articular congruity between the metatarsal head and the base of the proximal phalanx, the plantar capsule, the transverse metatarsal ligament, the flexor and extensor tendons, and the intervening lumbrical muscles.

Mechanism of Injury
- Dislocations are usually the result of low energy "stubbing" injuries and are most commonly displaced dorsally.
- Avulsion or chip fractures may occur by the same mechanism.
- Comminuted intraarticular fractures may occur by direct trauma, usually from a heavy object dropped onto the foot dorsum.

Clinical Evaluation
- Patients typically present with pain, swelling, tenderness, and variable deformity of the involved digit.
- Dislocation of the metatarsophalangeal joint typically manifests as dorsal prominence of the base of the proximal phalanx.

DESCRIPTIVE CLASSIFICATION
- Location
- Angulation
- Displacement
- Comminution
- Intraarticular involvement
- Presence of fracture-dislocation

Treatment

Nonoperative treatment

Simple dislocations or nondisplaced fractures may be managed by gentle reduction with longitudinal traction and buddy taping for 4 weeks, with a rigid shoe orthosis to limit metatarsophalangeal joint motion as necessary.

Operative treatment

Intraarticular fractures of the metatarsal head or the base of the proximal phalanx may be treated by excision of a small fragment, by benign neglect of severely comminuted fractures, or by open reduction and internal fixation with Kirschner wires or screw fixation for fractures with a large intraarticular fragment.

Complications
- Posttraumatic osteoarthritis: may result from articular incongruity or chondral damage at the time of injury.
- Recurrent subluxation: uncommon; may be addressed by capsular imbrication, tendon transfer, cheilectomy, or osteotomy if symptomatic.

Sesamoid

Epidemiology
- Highest incidence is seen with repetitive hyperextension at the metatarsophalangeal joints, such as in ballet dancers and runners.
- The medial sesamoid is more frequently fractured than the lateral due to increased weight bearing on the medial side of the foot.

Anatomy

Bipartite sesamoids are common (10% to 30% incidence in the general population); they must not be mistaken for acute fractures.

- Bilateral in 85% of cases.
- Exhibit smooth, sclerotic, rounded borders.
- Do not show callus formation after 2 to 3 weeks of immobilization.

Mechanism of Injury
- Acute trauma: hyperextension of the first metatarsophalangeal joint with tensile loading of the flexor complex. The fracture line is usually transverse, except in Jahss type IIB dislocations and in markedly comminuted fractures.
- Stress-related or avulsions: found in dancers and runners with repetitive loading of the flexor complex.

Clinical Evaluation

- Patients typically present with pain well localized on the plantar aspect of the "ball" of the foot.
- Local tenderness is present over the fractured sesamoid, as well as accentuation of symptoms with passive extension or active flexion of the metatarsophalangeal joint, which stresses the flexor hallucis brevis tendon in which the sesamoids lie.

Radiographic Evaluation

- Anteroposterior, lateral, and oblique views of the forefoot are usually sufficient to demonstrate transverse fractures of the sesamoids.
- Occasionally, a tangential view of the sesamoids is necessary to visualize a small osteochondral or avulsion fracture.
- Technetium-99m bone scanning or magnetic resonance imaging may be used to identify stress fractures that are not apparent by plain radiography.

DESCRIPTIVE CLASSIFICATION

- Transverse versus longitudinal
- Displacement
- Location: medial versus lateral

Treatment

- Nonoperative management should initially be attempted with soft padding combined with a short-leg walking cast for 4 weeks. This is followed by a bunion last shoe with a metatarsal pad for 4 to 8 weeks.
- Sesamoidectomy is reserved for cases of failed conservative treatment; the flexor hallucis brevis must be repaired. The patient is maintained postoperatively in a short-leg walking cast for 3 to 4 weeks.

Complications

Sesamoid excision may result in problems of hallux valgus (medial sesamoid excision) or transfer pain to the remaining sesamoid due to overload.

Phalanges and Interphalangeal Joints

Epidemiology

Most of these fractures arise as a result of the use of improper footwear.

Anatomy

- The first and fifth digits are in especially vulnerable positions, because they form the medial and lateral borders of the distal foot.

Mechanism of Injury

- Fractures of the phalanges and interphalangeal joints most commonly occur as a result of "stub" injuries, in which axial load transmission occurs through the distal tip of the distal phalanx and proximally though the digit.
- Direct trauma to the dorsal aspect of the phalanges may occur when a heavy object is dropped onto the foot.
- Rarely, athletes or dancers may present with stress fractures at the base of the proximal phalanx of the great toe.

Clinical Evaluation

- Patients typically present with pain, swelling, and variable deformity of the affected digit.
- Tenderness can typically be elicited over the site of injury.

Radiographic Evaluation

- Anteroposterior, lateral, and oblique views of the foot should be obtained.
- If possible, isolation of the digit of interest for the lateral radiograph may aid in visualization of the injury. Alternatively, the use of small dental radiographs placed between the toes has been described.

- Technetium-99m bone scanning or magnetic resonance imaging may aid in the diagnosis of stress fracture when the injury is not apparent on plain radiographs.

DESCRIPTIVE CLASSIFICATION

- Location: proximal, middle, or distal phalanx
- Angulation
- Displacement
- Comminution
- Intraarticular involvement
- Presence of fracture-dislocation

Treatment

Nonoperative treatment

- Distal phalangeal fractures of all digits are managed with splinting, buddy taping, and/or rigid soled shoe orthosis.
- Proximal interphalangeal and distal interphalangeal joint function in the lesser toes is not essential for normal function; therefore, fractures involving the interphalangeal joints may be treated with splinting.
- Diaphyseal fractures of the proximal and middle phalanges of the lesser toes may be treated with simple splinting or buddy taping.
- A rigid soled shoe orthosis may limit the stress placed on the fracture site, thus decreasing symptoms of pain.
- Immobilization may be discontinued after 3 to 4 weeks when the symptoms subside.

Operative treatment

- Proximal phalanx and interphalangeal joint injuries of the great toe should be treated more aggressively than in the lesser toes; anatomic reduction may be achieved with Kirschner wires or lag screws if necessary.
- Capsular or collateral ligament damage should be repaired at the time of surgery.
- Postoperative immobilization in the form of a compressive dressing and a rigid soled shoe orthosis should be continued for 2 to 3 weeks.

Complications

- Nonunion: uncommon; nonunited displaced fragments may be addressed by simple excision with reattachment of any involved capsule or collateral ligament.
- Posttraumatic osteoarthritis: may complicate fractures with intraarticular injury with resultant incongruity. May be disabling if it involves the great toe.

V. PEDIATRIC FRACTURES AND DISLOCATIONS

40. PEDIATRIC ORTHOPEDIC SURGERY: GENERAL PRINCIPLES

OVERVIEW

- The development and growth of the skeletal system from gestation to skeletal maturity results in interrelated fibrous, tendinous, cartilaginous, and osseous changes that result in patterns of susceptibility and reparative response that distinguish the pediatric patient from the adult.
- As a rule, the younger the patient is, the greater the remodeling potential; thus, absolute anatomic reduction in a child is less important than in a comparable injury in an adult.

EPIDEMIOLOGY

- The overall mortality rate of children has fallen from 1 in 250 per year in 1900 to 1 in 4,000 per year in 1986; this is attributed to improved public education, preventive devices, and medical care.
- Except for the first year of life, the leading cause of death in children aged 1 to 14 years is accidents.
- Skeletal trauma accounts for 10% to 15% of all childhood injuries, with approximately 15% of these representing physeal injuries.
- The overall ratio of boys to girls who suffer a single isolated fracture is 2.7:1. The peak incidence of fractures in boys occurs at age 16, with an incidence of 450 per 10,000 per year; the peak incidence in girls occurs at age 12, with an incidence of 250 per 10,000 per year.

ANATOMY

- Pediatric bone has a higher water content and lower mineral content per unit volume than adult bone. Therefore, pediatric bone has a lower modulus of elasticity (less brittle) and a higher ultimate strain-to-failure ratio than adult bone.
- The physis (growth plate) is a unique cartilaginous structure that varies in thickness depending on age and location. It is frequently weaker than bone in torsion, shear, and bending, predisposing the child to injury through this delicate area.
- The periosteum in a child is a thick fibrous structure (up to several millimeters) that encompasses the entire bone except for the articular ends. The periosteum thickens and is continuous with the physis at the perichondral ring, offering additional resistance to shear force.
- As a general rule, ligaments in children are functionally stronger than are bones. Thus, a high proportion of injuries that produce sprains in adults result in fractures in children.
- The blood supply to the growing bone includes a rich metaphyseal circulation with fine capillary loops ending at the physis (in the neonate, small vessels may traverse the physis, ending in the epiphysis). This differs from adult bone.

MECHANISM OF INJURY

- Because of structural differences, pediatric fractures tend to occur at lower energies than adult fractures do. Most are a result of compression, torsion, or bending moments.
- Compression fractures are found most commonly at the metaphyseal-diaphyseal junction and are referred to as "buckle fractures" or "torus fractures." Torus fractures rarely result in physeal injury but may result in acute angular deformity. Because torus fractures are impacted, they are stable and rarely require manipulative reduction. If manipulated, they usually regain the original fracture deformity as swelling subsides.
- Torsional injuries result in two distinct patterns of fracture, depending on the maturity of the physis.
  - In the very young child with a thick periosteum, the diaphyseal bone fails before the physis, resulting in a long spiral fracture.
  - In the older child, similar torsional injury results in a physeal fracture.

- Bending moments in the young child cause "greenstick fractures" in which the bone is plastically deformed. In the older child, bending moments result in transverse or short oblique fractures. Occasionally, a small butterfly fragment may be seen; however, as pediatric bone fails more easily in compression, only a buckle of the cortex may be found.

CLINICAL EVALUATION

- Pediatric trauma patients should undergo a full trauma evaluation with attention to airway, breathing, circulation, and disability. This should ideally be performed under the direction of a general surgical trauma team or a pediatric emergency specialist (see Chapter 1).
- Children are typically not good historians; therefore, keen diagnostic skills are required for even the simplest problems. Parents may not be present at the time of injury and cannot always provide an accurate history. Evaluating the entire extremity is important because young children cannot always localize the injury.
- As a general rule, children will tolerate more pain and hardship than adults, especially if they understand what you are about to do and trust you. Thus, explaining everything to children, listening to their suggestions whenever possible, and stopping when they ask you to do so are important.
- Evaluation of the neurovascular status, both pre- and postmanipulation, is mandatory.
- Periodic evaluation for compartment syndrome should be performed, particularly in a nonverbal patient who is extremely irritable and who presents with a crush-type mechanism of injury. A high index of suspicion should be followed by compartment pressure monitoring.
- Intracompartmental blood loss from long-bone fractures of the lower extremities can be a serious problem for the young child.
- Child abuse must be suspected under the following scenarios:
  - Spiral fractures of the long bones;
  - A history (mechanism of injury) that is inconsistent with the fracture pattern;
  - An unwitnessed injury that results in fracture;
  - Multiple fractures in various stages of healing;
  - Skin stigmata suggestive of abuse: multiple bruises in various stages of resolution, cigarette burns, and so on.
- The physician's obligation is to ensure that the child is in a safe environment. If any questions remain regarding abuse, the child should be admitted to the hospital and social services should be notified.

RADIOGRAPHIC EVALUATION

- Radiographs should include appropriate views of the involved bone and the joint proximal and distal to the suspected area of injury. If one is uncertain as to the location of a suspected injury, the entire extremity may be placed on the radiographic plate.
- Comparison views of the opposite extremity may aid in appreciating subtle deformities or in localizing a minimally displaced fracture.
- "Soft signs," such as the posterior fat pad sign in the elbow, should be closely evaluated.
- A skeletal survey in children or a "babygram" in infants may help in searching for other fractures in cases of suspected child abuse or multiple trauma.
- Computed tomographies and tomograms may be useful for evaluating complicated intraarticular fractures in the older child.
- Magnetic resonance imaging can be invaluable in the preoperative evaluation of a complicated fracture or soft-tissue injury; it may also help evaluate a fracture that is not clearly identifiable on plain films.
- Arthrograms are essential in the evaluation of intraarticular fractures intraoperatively because radiolucent cartilaginous structures will not be apparent on fluoroscopic or plain radiographic evaluation.
- Bone scans may be used in the evaluation of osteomyelitis or tumor.

SALTER-HARRIS/OGDEN CLASSIFICATION (FIG. 40.1)

Pediatric physeal fractures have traditionally been described by the five-part Salter-Harris classification. More recently, the Ogden classification has extended the Salter-Harris classification to include periphyseal fractures, which do not radiographically appear to involve the physis but which may interfere with the physeal blood supply and may result in growth disturbance.

Salter-Harris Types I to V

Type I: Transphyseal fracture involving the hypertrophic and calcified zones; prognosis is usually excellent, although complete or partial growth arrest may occur in displaced fractures.

Type II: Transphyseal fracture that exits the metaphysis; the metaphyseal fragment is known as the Thurston-Holland fragment; the periosteal hinge is intact on the side with the metaphyseal fragment; prognosis is excellent, although complete or partial growth arrest may occur in displaced fractures.

Type III: Transphyseal fracture that exits the epiphysis, causing intraarticular disruption; anatomic reduction and fixation without violating the physis are essential; prognosis is guarded because partial growth arrest and resultant angular deformity are common problems.

Type IV: Fracture that traverses the epiphysis and the physis, exiting the metaphysis; anatomic reduction and fixation without violating the physis are essential; prognosis is guarded, because partial growth arrest and resultant angular deformity are common.

Type V: Crush injury to the physis; diagnosis is generally made retrospectively; prognosis is poor because growth arrest and partial physeal closure commonly result.

Ogden Types VI to IX

Type VI: Injury to the perichondral ring at the periphery of the physis; usually it is the result of an open injury; close follow-up may allow early identification of a peripheral physeal bar that is amenable to excision; prognosis is guarded because peripheral physeal bridges are common.

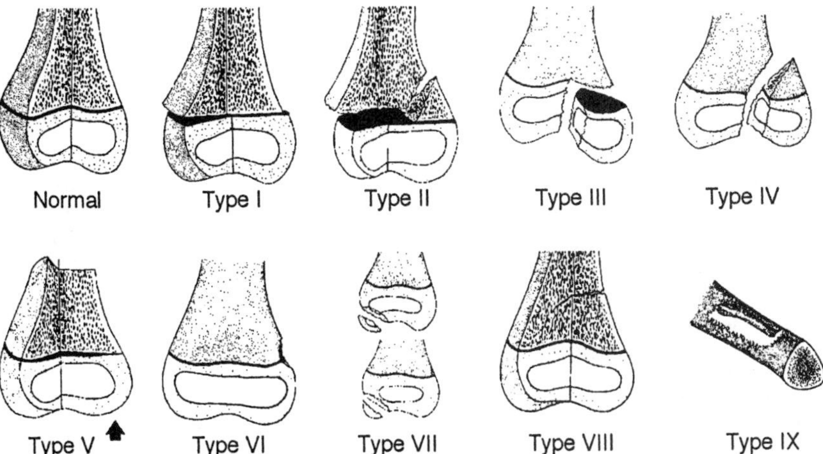

FIG. 40.1. Salter-Harris (types I–V) and Ogden (types VI–IX) classifications of physeal injuries in children. (From Ogden JA. *Pocket guide to pediatric fractures.* Baltimore: Williams & Wilkins, 1987:25–42, with permission.)

Type VII: Fracture involving the epiphysis only; includes osteochondral fractures and epiphyseal avulsions; prognosis is variable and is dependent on the location of the fracture and the amount of displacement.

Type VIII: Metaphyseal fracture; primary circulation to the remodeling region of the cartilage cell columns is disrupted; hypervascularity may cause angular overgrowth.

Type IX: Diaphyseal fracture; interruption of the mechanism for appositional growth (the periosteum); prognosis is generally good if reduction is maintained; cross-union between the tibia and fibula and between the radius and ulna may occur if intermingling of the respective periosteum occurs.

TREATMENT

- Fracture management in the child differs from that in an adult due to the presence of a thick periosteum in the case of a diaphyseal fracture or of an open physis in metaphyseal fractures.
  - The tough periosteum can be an aid to reduction as the periosteum on the concave side of the deformity is usually intact; it can be made to serve as a hinge, preventing overreduction. Longitudinal traction will not reliably unlock the fragments when the periosteum is intact. Controlled re-creation and exaggeration of the fracture deformity are effective means of disengaging the fragments to obtain reduction.
  - A periosteal flap entrapped in the fracture site or button-holing of a sharp fracture end through the periosteum can prevent an adequate reduction.
- Unlike in the adult, considerable physical deformity of the fracture may be permitted because the remodeling potential of the child is great.
  - In general, the closer the fracture is to the joint (physis), the better the deformity is tolerated (e.g., 45 to 60 degrees of angulation in a proximal humeral fracture in a young child is permissible, whereas a midshaft fracture of the radius or tibia should be brought to within 10 degrees of normal alignment).
  - Rotational deformity does not spontaneously correct or remodel to an acceptable extent even in the young child and should be avoided.
- Severely comminuted fractures or shortened fractures may require skin or skeletal traction. Traction pins should be placed proximal to the nearest distal physis (e.g., distal femur); care should be taken not to place them through the physis.
- Fracture reduction should be performed under conscious sedation, followed by immobilization in either a splint or bivalved cast. Univalving, particularly with a synthetic cast, does not provide adequate cast flexibility to accommodate extremity swelling.
- In children, casts or splints should encompass the joint proximal and distal to the site of injury because post-immobilization stiffness is not a common problem for children. Only in rare fractures (e.g., stable torus fractures of the distal radius) should short-arm or short-leg casts be applied. In as few as 2 days after cast application, children will run on short-leg casts or climb monkey bars in short-arm casts.
- All fractures should be elevated at heart level, iced, and frequently monitored by responsible individuals, with attention to extremity warmth, color, capillary refill, and sensation. Children in which pronounced swelling is an issue or in which the reliability of the guardian is in question should be admitted to the hospital for observation.
- Nerves, particularly at the elbow, or ankle tendons frequently become entrapped in the fracture site, preventing reduction.
- Fractures in which a reduction cannot be achieved or maintained should be splinted, and the child should be prepared with general anesthesia, in which complete relaxation may be achieved.
- Intraarticular fractures (Salter-Harris types III or IV) require anatomic reduction (<1 to 2 mm of displacement) to restore articular congruity and to minimize physeal bar formation.
- Indications for open reduction include the following:
  - Open fractures;
  - Displaced intraarticular fractures (Salter-Harris types III or IV);

Fractures with vascular injury;
Fractures with an associated compartment syndrome;
Unstable fractures that require abnormal positioning to maintain closed reduction.

COMPLICATIONS

Complications unique to pediatric fractures include the following:

- Growth arrest: may occur with physeal injuries in Salter-Harris fractures. May result in limb length inequalities that necessitate the use of orthotics, prosthetics, or operative procedures, including epiphysiodesis or limb lengthening.
- Progressive angular or rotational deformities may result from physeal injuries or malunion. If these result in significant functional disabilities or cosmetic deformities, they may require operative intervention, such as osteotomy, for correction.
- Osteonecrosis: may result from disruption of the tenuous vascular supply in skeletally immature patients in whom vascular development is not complete (e.g., osteonecrosis of the femoral head in cases of slipped capital femoral epiphysis).

41. PEDIATRIC SHOULDER

PROXIMAL HUMERUS FRACTURES

Epidemiology

- Account for <5% of fractures in children.
- Incidence ranges from 1.2 to 4.4 fractures per 10,000 children per year.
- Most common in adolescents due to increased sports participation with a peak at 15 years of age.
- Neonates may sustain birth trauma to the proximal humeral physis, representing 1.9% to 6.7% of physeal injuries.

Anatomy

- Eighty percent of humeral growth occurs at the proximal physis, giving this region great remodeling potential.
- The three centers of ossification in the proximal humerus are as follows:
  Humeral head: ossifies at 6 months;
  Greater tuberosity: ossifies at 3 years;
  Lesser tuberosity: ossifies at 5 years.
  All coalesce between the ages of 6 to 7 years.
- The joint capsule extends to the metaphysis, rendering some fractures of the metaphysis intraarticular.
- The primary vascular supply is via the anterolateral ascending branch of the anterior humeral circumflex artery with a small portion of the greater tuberosity and inferior humeral head supplied by branches from the posterior circumflex artery.
- The physis closes between the ages of 14 to 17 years in girls and 16 to 18 in boys.
- The physeal apex is posteromedial; it is associated with a strong, thick periosteum.
- Type I physeal fractures occur through the hypertrophic zone adjacent to the zone of provisional calcification. The layer of embryonal cartilage is preserved, leading to normal growth.

Mechanism of Injury

- Indirect mechanisms include a fall backward onto an outstretched hand with the elbow extended and the wrist dorsiflexed. Birth injuries may occur as the arm is hyperextended or rotated when the infant is being delivered. Shoulder dystocia is strongly associated with macrosomia from maternal diabetes.
- Direct mechanisms include direct trauma to the posterolateral aspect of the shoulder.
- The proximal fragment is held by the rotator cuff muscles in neutral or in slight abduction and external rotation.
- The distal fragment pierces the periosteum anterolateral to the biceps tendon. It is held in adduction by the pectoralis major and is pulled proximally by the deltoid.
- The thick posterior periosteum remains intact.

Clinical Evaluation

- Newborns present with pseudoparalysis with the arm held in extension. A history of birth trauma may be elucidated. A fever is variably present. Infection, clavicle fracture, and brachial plexus injury must be ruled out.
- Older children present with pain, dysfunction, swelling, and ecchymosis; the humeral shaft fragment may be palpable anteriorly. The shoulder is tender to palpation with a painful range of motion that may reveal crepitus.
- A careful neurovascular examination, including the axillary, musculocutaneous, radial, ulnar, and median nerves, is required.

Radiographic Evaluation

- Anteroposterior, lateral (in the plane of the scapula; "Y" view), and axillary views should be obtained, with comparison views of the opposite side as necessary.
- An ultrasound may be necessary in the newborn because the epiphysis is not yet ossified.

SALTER-HARRIS CLASSIFICATION (FIG. 41.1)

Type I: Separation through the physis; usually a birth injury.
Type II: Most occur in adolescents (>12 years); the metaphyseal fragment is always posteromedial.
Type III: Intraarticular fracture; uncommon; associated with dislocations.
Type IV: Rare; intraarticular transmetaphyseal fracture; associated with open fractures.

NEER-HOROWITZ CLASSIFICATION

Grade I: Less than 5 mm displacement
Grade II: displacement less than one-third the width of the shaft
Grade III: displacement one-third to two-thirds the width of the shaft
Grade IV: displacement more than two-thirds the width of the shaft, including total displacement

Treatment

Treatment depends on the age of the patient and on the fracture pattern encountered.

Newborns

- Most fractures are Salter-Harris type I. The prognosis is excellent.
- Ultrasound can be used to guide reduction.
- Closed reduction is the treatment of choice; it is achieved by applying gentle traction, 90 degrees of flexion and then 90 degrees of abduction and external rotation.
- In a stable fracture, the arm is immobilized against the chest for 5 to 10 days.
- In an unstable fracture, the arm is held abducted and externally rotated for 3 to 4 days to allow early callus formation.

Ages 1 to 4 Years

- These are typically Salter-Harris type I or, less frequently, type II fractures.
- Treatment is by closed reduction.

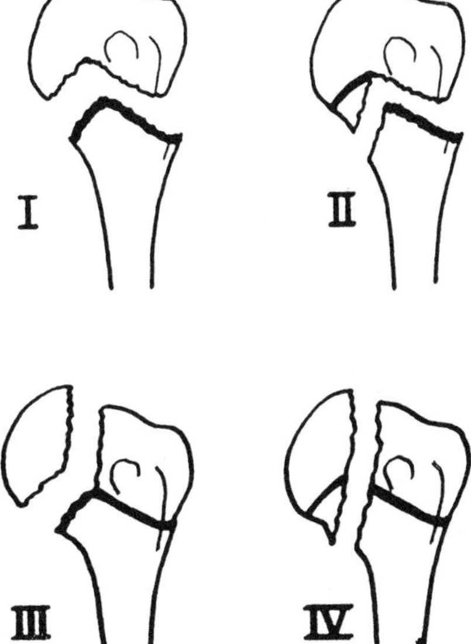

FIG. 41.1. The Salter-Harris classification as applied to fractures of the proximal humerus involving the physis. Type II injuries are by far the most common in children older than 5 years of age. Type I injuries are more common in children younger than 5 years of age. Type III injuries are rare, and type IV injuries have not been reported. (From Rockwood CA Jr, Wilkins KE, Beaty JH, eds. *Rockwood and Green's fractures in children*, 4th ed. Vol. 3. Philadelphia: Lippincott-Raven, 1996:934, with permission.)

- The arm is held in a sling for 10 days, followed by progressive activity.
- Extensive remodeling is possible.

Ages 5 to 12 Years
- The metaphyseal fracture (type II) is the most common in this age group because this area is undergoing the most rapid remodeling and is therefore structurally vulnerable.
- Treatment is by closed reduction.
- In a stable fracture, a sling and swathe is used.
- In an unstable fracture, the arm is placed in a shoulder spica cast with the arm in the salute position for 2 to 3 weeks, after which the patient may be changed to a sling with progressive activity.

Ages 12 Years to Maturity
- These are either Salter-Harris type II or, less frequently, type I fractures.
- Treatment is by closed reduction.
- At this age, less remodeling potential exists than in younger children.
- In a stable fracture, a sling and swathe is used for 2 to 3 weeks followed by progressive range-of-motion exercises.
- An unstable fracture is immobilized in a shoulder spica cast with the arm in the salute position for 2 to 3 weeks, after which the patient may be changed to a sling with progressive activity.

Acceptable Deformity
- Ages 1 to 4 years: 70 degrees of angulation with any displacement.
- Ages 5 to 12 years: 40 to 45 degrees of angulation and displacement one-half the width of the shaft.
- Ages 12 to maturity: 15 to 20 degrees of angulation and displacement of <30%.

Open Treatment
- Indications for open reduction and internal fixation include the following:
  - Open fractures;
  - Fractures with associated neurovascular compromise;
  - Salter-Harris type III and IV fractures;
  - Irreducible fractures with soft-tissue interposition (biceps tendon).
- Fixation is most often achieved with percutaneous smooth Kirschner wires or Steinmann pins.

Prognosis
- Neer-Horowitz grade I and II fractures heal well because of the remodeling potential of the proximal humeral physis.
- Neer-Horowitz grade III and IV fractures may be left with up to 3 mm of shortening or residual angulation. This is well tolerated by the patient and is often clinically insignificant.
- As a rule, the younger the patient, the higher the potential for remodeling and the greater the acceptable initial deformity.

Complications
- Humerus varus: rare; usually affects patients less than 1 year of age, but may complicate fractures in patients as old as 5 years of age. May result in a marked decrease of the neck-shaft angle to 90 degrees with marked humeral shortening and mild to moderate loss of glenohumeral abduction. Remodeling potential is great in this age group, however, so observation alone may result in improvement. Proximal humeral osteotomy may be performed in cases of extreme functional limitation.
- Limb length inequality: rarely significant; tends to occur more commonly in surgically treated patients as opposed to those treated nonoperatively.
- Loss of motion: uncommon; tends to occur more commonly in surgically treated patients. Older patients tend to have more postfracture difficulties with shoulder stiffness than do younger patients.

- Inferior glenohumeral subluxation: may be a complication in patients with Salter-Harris type II fractures of the proximal humerus secondary to a loss of deltoid and rotator cuff tone. May be addressed by a period of immobilization, followed by rotator cuff strengthening exercises.
- Osteonecrosis: may occur with associated disruption of the anterolateral ascending branch of the anterior circumflex artery, especially in fractures or dislocations that are not acutely reduced.
- Nerve injury: most commonly occurs as an axillary nerve injury in fracture-dislocations. Lesions that do not show signs of recovery in 4 months should be explored.
- Growth arrest: may occur in cases in which the physis is crushed or significantly displaced or in those in which a physeal bar forms. May require excision of the physeal bar.

CLAVICLE FRACTURES

Epidemiology

- The most frequent fracture in children.
- Occurs in 0.5% of normal deliveries and 1.6% of breech deliveries.
- Incidence of 13% in macrosomic infants (>4,000 g).
- Eighty percent of cases in the shaft, most frequently just lateral to the insertion of the subclavius muscle, which protects the underlying neurovascular structures. Ten percent to 15% involve the lateral aspect, with the remainder representing medial fractures.

Anatomy

- The clavicle is the first bone to ossify; this occurs by intramembranous ossification.
- The secondary centers develop via endochondral ossification as follows:
  - The medial epiphysis, where 80% of growth occurs, ossifies between the ages 12 to 19 years and fuses by ages 22 to 25 years.
  - The lateral epiphysis does not ossify until it fuses at the age of 19 years.
- Clavicular range of motion includes rotation about its long axis of approximately 50 degrees, accompanied by elevation of 30 degrees with full shoulder abduction and 35 degrees of anterior-posterior angulation with shoulder protraction and retraction.
- The periosteal sleeve always remains in the anatomic position. Therefore, remodeling is ensured.

Mechanism of Injury

- Indirect: fall onto an outstretched hand.
- Direct: most common mechanism, resulting from direct trauma to the clavicle or acromion; carries the highest incidence of injury to the underlying neurovascular and pulmonary structures.
- Birth injury: occurs during delivery of the shoulders through a narrow pelvis with direct pressure from the symphysis pubis or from obstetric pressure directly applied to the clavicle during delivery.
- Medial clavicle fractures or dislocations: usually represent Salter-Harris type I or II fractures. True sternoclavicular joint dislocations are rare. The inferomedial periosteal sleeve remains intact and provides a scaffold for remodeling. As 80% of the growth occurs at the medial physis, great potential for remodeling exists.
- Lateral clavicle fractures: occur as a result of direct trauma to the acromion. The coracoclavicular ligaments always remain intact and are attached to the inferior periosteal tube. The acromioclavicular ligament is always intact and is attached to the distal fragment.

Clinical Evaluation

- Birth fractures of the clavicle are usually obvious, with an asymmetric palpable mass overlying the fractured clavicle. An asymmetric Moro reflex is usually present. Nonobvious injuries may be misdiagnosed as congenital muscular torticollis.
- Children with clavicle fractures typically present with a painful palpable mass along the clavicle. Tenderness is usually discrete over the site of injury but may be diffuse in cases of plastic bowing. Tenting of the skin, crepitance, and ecchymosis may occur.

- Neurovascular status must be evaluated carefully because injuries to the brachial plexus and upper extremity vasculature may result.
- Pulmonary status must be assessed, especially if direct trauma is the mechanism of injury. Medial clavicular fractures may be associated with tracheal compression, especially with severe posterior displacement.
- Differential diagnoses include the following:
  - Cleidocranial dysostosis: defect in intramembranous ossification, most commonly affecting the clavicle; characterized by absence of the distal end of the clavicle, a central defect, or complete absence of the clavicle. Treatment is symptomatic only.
  - Congenital pseudarthrosis: most commonly occurs at the junction of the middle and distal thirds of the right clavicle, with smooth pointed bone ends. Pseudarthrosis of the left clavicle is found only in patients with dextrocardia. Patients present with no antecedent history of trauma, only a palpable bump. Treatment is supportive only, with bone grafting and intramedullary fixation reserved for symptomatic cases.

Radiographic Evaluation

- Ultrasound evaluation may be used in the diagnosis of clavicular fracture in neonates. Due to the S shape of the clavicle, an anteroposterior view is usually sufficient for diagnostic purposes; however, special views have been described in cases in which a fracture is suspected but not well visualized on a standard anteroposterior view:
  - Cephalic tilt view (cephalic tilt of 35 to 40 degrees) minimizes overlapping structures.
  - Apical oblique view (injured side rotated 45 degrees toward tube with cephalic tilt of 20 degrees) is best for visualizing nondisplaced middle third fractures.
- Patients with difficulty breathing should have an anteroposterior radiograph of the chest to evaluate a possible pneumothorax or associated rib fractures.
- Computed tomography or tomograms may be useful in the evaluation of medial clavicular fractures or suspected dislocation because most represent Salter-Harris types I or II fractures rather than true dislocations.

DESCRIPTIVE CLASSIFICATION

- Location
- Open versus closed
- Displacement
- Angulation
- Fracture type: segmental, comminuted, greenstick, etc.

ALLMAN CLASSIFICATION

Type I: middle third
Type II: distal to the coracoclavicular ligaments
Type III: proximal third

Treatment

Newborn to the Age of 2 Years

- Complete fracture under the age of 2 years is unusual; it may be caused by birth injuries or excessive force.
- Clavicle fracture in a newborn will unite in approximately 1 week. Reduction is not indicated. Care with lifting and/or a soft bandage may be used.
- Infants may be treated with a simple sling or figure-of-eight bandage applied for 2 to 3 weeks or until the patient is comfortable.

Ages 2 to 12 Years

Figure-of-eight bandage or sling for 2 to 4 weeks, at which time union is complete.

Ages 12 Years to Maturity

- Higher incidence of complete fracture.
- Figure-of-eight bandage or sling for 3 to 4 weeks.
- If grossly displaced with tenting of the skin, reduction done under general anesthesia with towel clip.

Open Treatment

- Operative treatment is indicated in open fractures and in those with neurovascular compromise.
- Comminuted fragments that tent the skin may be manipulated, and the dermis should be released from the bone ends with a towel clip.
- Bony prominences from the callus will usually remodel; exostectomy may be performed at a later date if necessary, although from a cosmetic standpoint, the surgical scar is often more noticeable than the prominence.

Complications

- Neurovascular compromise: rare in children because of the thick periosteum that protects the underlying structures, although brachial plexus and vascular injury (subclavian vessels) may occur with severe displacement.
- Malunion: rare due to high remodeling potential; well tolerated when present, with cosmetic issues of the bony prominence being the only long-term issue.
- Nonunion: rare (1% to 3%); probably associated with a congenital pseudarthrosis; never occurs at <12 years of age.
- Pulmonary injury: rare injuries to the apical pulmonary parenchyma with pneumothorax may occur, especially with severe direct trauma in an anterosuperior to posteroinferior direction.

ACROMIOCLAVICULAR JOINT INJURIES

Epidemiology

- Rare in children under age 16.
- True incidence unknown because many actually represent pseudodislocation of the acromioclavicular joint.

Anatomy

- The acromioclavicular joint is a diarthrodial joint; in mature individuals an intra-articular disk is present.
- The distal clavicle is surrounded by a thick periosteal sleeve that extends to the acromioclavicular joint.

Mechanism of Injury

- Athletic injuries and falls comprise most acromioclavicular injuries with direct trauma to the acromion.
- Unlike acromioclavicular injuries in adults, in children, the coracoclavicular (conoid and trapezoid) ligaments remain intact. Because of the tight approximation of the coracoclavicular ligaments to the periosteum of the distal clavicle, true dislocation of the acromioclavicular joint is rare.
- The defect is a longitudinal split in the superior portion of the periosteal sleeve though which the clavicle is delivered, much like a banana being peeled from its skin.

Clinical Evaluation

- The patient should be examined in the standing or sitting position to allow the upper extremity to be in the dependent position, thus stressing the acromioclavicular joint and emphasizing any deformity.
- A thorough shoulder examination, including assessment of neurovascular status and possible associated upper extremity injuries, should be performed. Inspection may reveal an apparent step-off deformity of the injured acromioclavicular joint, with possible tenting of the skin overlying the distal clavicle. Range of motion may be limited by pain. Tenderness may be elicited over the acromioclavicular joint.

Radiographic Evaluation

- A standard trauma series of the shoulder (anteroposterior, scapular-Y, and axillary views) is usually sufficient for the recognition of acromioclavicular injury, although closer evaluation requires targeted views of the acromioclavicular joint, which requires one-third to one-half the radiation to avoid overpenetration.
- Ligamentous injury may be assessed via stress radiographs, in which weights (5 to 10 pounds) are strapped to the wrists and an anteroposterior radiograph is taken of both shoulders for comparison.

ROCKWOOD CLASSIFICATION (FIG. 41.2)

Type I: Mild sprain of the acromioclavicular ligaments without periosteal tube disruption. Distal clavicle stable to examination, and radiographs show no abnormalities.

Type II: Partial disruption of the periosteal tube with mild distal clavicle instability. Slight widening of the acromioclavicular space is appreciated on radiographs.

Type III: Longitudinal split of the periosteal tube with gross instability of the distal clavicle to examination. Superior displacement of 25% to 100% is present on radiographs as compared with the normal contralateral shoulder.

Type IV: Posterior displacement of the distal clavicle through a periosteal sleeve disruption with button-holing through the trapezius. Anteroposterior radiographs demonstrate superior displacement similar to type II injuries, but axillary radiographs demonstrate posterior displacement.

Type V: Type III injury with >100% displacement. The distal clavicle may be subcutaneous to palpation, and disruption of deltoid or trapezial attachments may occur.

Type VI: Infracoracoid displacement of the distal clavicle as a result of a superior to inferior force vector.

Treatment

- Types I to III: nonoperative treatment with sling immobilization, ice, and early range-of-motion exercises as pain subsides. Remodeling is expected. Complete healing generally takes place in 4 to 6 weeks.
- Types IV to VI: operative, with reduction of the clavicle and repair of the periosteal sleeve. Internal fixation may be needed.

Complications

- Neurovascular injury: rarely associated with posteroinferior displacement. The intact periosteal sleeve is thick; it usually provides protection to neurovascular structures underlying the distal clavicle.
- Open lesion: severe displacement of the distal clavicle, such as with type V acromioclavicular dislocation, may result in tenting of the skin, with possible laceration necessitating irrigation and local debridement.

SCAPULA FRACTURES

- The scapula is relatively protected from trauma by the thoracic cavity and the rib cage anteriorly and by the encasing musculature posteriorly.
- Scapular fractures are often associated with other life-threatening injuries that take priority over the scapular fracture, such as intrathoracic and neck injuries.

Epidemiology

These constitute only 1% of all fractures and 5% of shoulder fractures in the general population and are even less common in children.

Anatomy

- The scapula forms from intramembranous ossification. The body and spine are ossified at birth.
- The center of the coracoid is ossified at 1 year of age. The base of the coracoid and the upper one-fourth of the glenoid ossifies by 10 years. A third center at the tip of the coracoid ossifies at a variable time. All three structures fuse by ages 15 to 16.

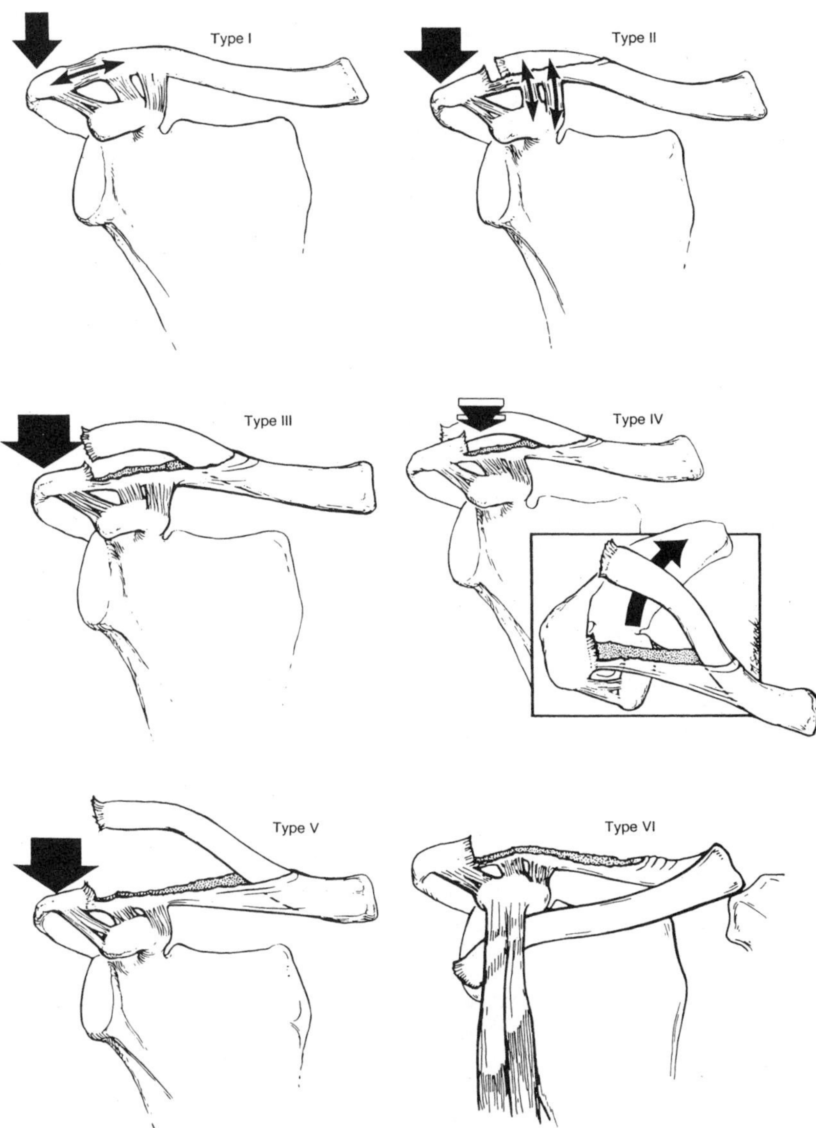

FIG. 41.2. Rockwood classification of clavicular-acromioclavicular joint injuries in children. (From Rockwood CA Jr, Wilkins KE, Beaty JH, eds. *Rockwood and Green's fractures in children*, 4th ed. Vol. 3. Philadelphia: Lippincott-Raven, 1996:974, with permission.)

- The acromion fuses by age 22 via two to five centers, which begin to form at puberty.
- Centers for the vertebral border and inferior angle and the center for the lower three-fourths of the glenoid appear at puberty and fuse by age 22.
- The suprascapular nerve traverses the suprascapular notch on the superior aspect of the scapula, medial to the base of the coracoid process, thus rendering it vulnerable to fractures in this region.

Mechanism of Injury

- In children, the most common scapular fractures represent avulsion fractures associated with glenohumeral joint injuries. Other fractures are usually the result of high energy trauma.
- As isolated scapula fractures are extremely uncommon, particularly in children, child abuse should be suspected unless a clear and consistent mechanism of injury exists.
- The presence of a scapular fracture should raise suspicion of associated injuries because 35% to 98% of scapular fractures occur in the presence of comorbid injuries, including the following:
  - Ipsilateral upper torso injuries—fractured ribs, clavicle, sternum, shoulder trauma.
  - Pneumothorax—seen in 11% to 55% of scapular fractures.
  - Pulmonary contusion—present in 11% to 54% of scapular fractures.
  - Injuries to neurovascular structures—brachial plexus injuries, vascular avulsions.
  - Spinal column injuries—20% lower cervical spine, 76% thoracic spine, 4% lumbar spine.
  - Others—concomitant skull fractures, blunt abdominal trauma, pelvic fracture, and lower extremity injuries are all seen with higher incidences in the presence of a scapular fracture.

Clinical Evaluation

- Full trauma evaluation with attention to airway, breathing, circulation, and disability should be performed, if indicated.
- Patient typically presents with the upper extremity supported by the contralateral hand in an adducted and immobile position, with painful range of shoulder motion, especially with abduction.
- A careful examination for associated injures should be pursued, with a comprehensive assessment of neurovascular status and an evaluation of breath sounds.

Radiographic Evaluation

- Initial radiographs should include a trauma series of the shoulder, consisting of a true anteroposterior view, an axillary view, and a scapular-Y view (true scapular lateral); these generally are able to demonstrate most glenoid, neck, body, and acromion fractures.
  - The axillary may be used to delineate further acromial and glenoid rim fractures.
  - An acromial fracture should not be confused with an *os acromiale*, which is a rounded unfused apophysis at the epiphyseal level and which is present in approximately 3% of the population. When present, it is bilateral in 60% of cases.
  - *Glenoid hypoplasia*, or *scapular neck dysplasia*, is an unusual abnormality that may resemble glenoid impaction and may be associated with humeral head or acromial abnormalities. It has a benign course and is usually noted incidentally.
- A 45-degree cephalic tilt (Stryker notch) radiograph helps to identify coracoid fractures.
- Tomography or computed tomography may be useful for further characterizing intra-articular glenoid fractures.
- Due to the high incidence of associated injuries, especially to thoracic structures, a chest radiograph is an essential part of the evaluation.

CLASSIFICATION BY LOCATION

Body and Neck Fractures

I. Isolated versus associated disruption of the clavicle axis.
II. Displaced versus nondisplaced.
- A high incidence of concomitant injury is found. Ipsilateral rib fractures with pneumothorax and pulmonary contusion occur in 50% of cases. Associated C-spine, clavicle, and brachial plexus injuries are also common. Computed tomography may be used to demonstrate associated glenoid fractures.

- Suprascapular nerve injury must be suspected if the fracture involves the suprascapular notch. Conservative treatment is recommended.

Glenoid Fractures

I: anterior avulsion fracture
II: transverse with inferior free fragment
III: upper third, including the coracoid
IV: horizontal fracture extending through body
V: combined II and III
VI: extensively comminuted

- These are associated with scapular neck fractures and shoulder dislocations.
- Treatment is nonoperative in most cases. Open reduction and internal fixation (ORIF) is indicated if a large anterior or posterior rim fragment is associated with glenohumeral instability.

Coracoid Fractures

Isolated versus associated disruption of the acromioclavicular joint.

- These are avulsion-type injuries, usually occurring through the common physis of the base of the coracoid and the upper one-fourth of the glenoid.
- The coracoacromial ligament remains intact, but the acromioclavicular ligaments may be stretched.

Acromial Fractures

I: nondisplaced
  IA: avulsion
  IB: direct trauma
II: displaced without subacromial narrowing
III: displaced with subacromial narrowing

- These are very rare and are usually the result of a direct blow.
- The os acromiale, which is an unfused ossification center, should not be mistaken for a fracture.
- Conservative treatment is recommended unless severe displacement of the acromioclavicular joint is found.

Treatment

- Scapular body fractures in children are treated nonoperatively, with the surrounding musculature maintaining reasonable proximity of the fracture fragments. Operative treatment is indicated for fractures that fail to unite, which may benefit from partial body excision.
- Scapular neck fractures that are nondisplaced and that are not associated with clavicle fractures may be treated expectantly. Significantly displaced fractures may be treated in a thoracobrachial cast. Associated clavicular disruption, either by fracture or by ligamentous instability, may be treated with open reduction and internal fixation of the clavicle alone or may include open reduction and internal fixation of the scapular fracture though a separate incision.
- Coracoid fractures that are nondisplaced may be treated with sling immobilization. Displaced fractures are usually accompanied by acromioclavicular dislocation or lateral clavicular injury and should be treated with open reduction and internal fixation.
- Acromial fractures that are nondisplaced may be treated with sling immobilization. Displaced acromial fractures with associated subacromial impingement should be reduced and stabilized with screw or plate fixation.
- Glenoid fractures in children, if not associated with glenohumeral instability, are rarely symptomatic when healed and can generally be treated nonoperatively if nondisplaced.

  Type I. Fractures involving greater than one-fourth of the glenoid fossa that result in instability may be amenable to open reduction and lag screw fixation.

Type II. Inferior subluxation of the humeral head may result, necessitating open reduction, especially when associated with an articular step-off greater than 5 mm. An anterior approach usually provides adequate exposure.

Type III. Reduction may be difficult; fracture occurs through the junction between the ossification centers of the glenoid and is often accompanied by a fractured acromion or clavicle or an acromioclavicular separation. Open reduction and internal fixation followed by early range of motion are indicated.

Types IV, V, and VI. These are difficult to reduce with little bone stock for adequate fixation in pediatric patients. A posterior approach is generally used for open reduction and internal fixation with Kirschner wire, plate, suture, or screw fixation.

Complications

- Posttraumatic osteoarthritis: may result from a failure to restore articular congruity adequately.
- Associated injuries: account for most serious complications due to the high energy nature of these injuries.
- Malunion: fractures of the body generally unite with nonoperative treatment; when malunion occurs, it is generally well tolerated but may result in painful scapulothoracic crepitus.
- Nonunion: extremely rare, but when present and symptomatic, may require open reduction and plate fixation for adequate relief.
- Suprascapular nerve injury: may occur in association with body, neck, or coracoid fractures that involve the suprascapular notch. The high association with coracoid fractures prompted Neer to favor early exploration of the suprascapular nerve.

GLENOHUMERAL DISLOCATIONS

Epidemiology

- Rare in children; Rowe reported that only 1.6% of shoulder dislocations occurred in patients <10 years of age, whereas 10% occurred in patients 10 to 20 years of age.
- Ninety percent are anterior dislocations.

Anatomy

- The glenohumeral articulation, with its large convex humeral head and correspondingly flat glenoid, is ideally suited to accommodate a wide range of motion. The articular surface and radius of curvature of the humeral head are about three times those of the glenoid fossa.
- Numerous static and dynamic stabilizers of the shoulder exist; these are covered in detail in Chapter 15.
- The humeral attachment of the glenohumeral joint capsule is along the anatomic neck of the humerus except medially, where the attachment is more distal along the shaft. The proximal humeral physis is therefore extraarticular, except along its medial aspect.
- As in most pediatric joint injuries, the capsular attachment to the epiphysis renders failure through the physis much more common than true capsuloligamentous injury; therefore, fracture through the physis is more common than a shoulder dislocation in a skeletally immature patient.
- In neonates, an apparent dislocation may actually represent a physeal injury.

Mechanism of Injury

- In neonates, pseudodislocation may occur with traumatic epiphyseal separation of the proximal humerus. This is much more common than a true shoulder dislocation, which may occur in neonates with underlying birth trauma to the brachial plexus or central nervous system.
- Anterior glenohumeral dislocation may occur as a result of either direct or indirect trauma.

  Direct. Anteriorly directed impact to the posterior shoulder may produce an anterior dislocation.

Indirect. Trauma to the upper extremity with the shoulder in abduction, extension, and external rotation is the most common mechanism for anterior shoulder dislocation.

- Posterior glenohumeral dislocation may occur as a result of trauma, either direct or indirect, as follows:

  Direct trauma: results from force application to the anterior shoulder, forcing the humeral head posteriorly.

  Indirect trauma: most common mechanism.

  1. The shoulder is typically in the position of adduction, flexion, and internal rotation at the time of injury.
  2. Electric shock or convulsive mechanisms may produce posterior dislocation due to the overwhelming of the external rotators of the shoulder (infraspinatus and teres minor muscles) by the internal rotators (latissimus dorsi, pectoralis major, and subscapularis muscles).
- Recurrent instability related to congenital or acquired laxity or to volitional mechanisms may result in an anterior dislocation with minimal trauma.

Clinical Evaluation

Patient presentation varies according to the type encountered.

Anterior Dislocation

- Determining the nature of the trauma, the chronicity of the dislocation, patterns of recurrence with inciting events, and the presence of instability in the contralateral shoulder helps.
- The patient typically presents with the affected shoulder held in slight abduction and external rotation. The acutely dislocated shoulder is painful, with muscular spasm in an attempt to stabilize the joint.
- Examination typically reveals squaring of the shoulder due to a relative prominence of the acromion, a relative hollow beneath the acromion posteriorly, and a palpable mass anteriorly.
- A careful neurovascular examination with attention to axillary nerve integrity is important. Deltoid muscle testing is usually not possible, but sensation over the deltoid may be assessed. Deltoid atony may be present and should not be confused with axillary nerve injury. Musculocutaneous nerve integrity can be assessed by the presence of sensation on the anterolateral forearm.
- Patients may present after spontaneous reduction or reduction in the field. If the patient is not in acute pain, examination may reveal a positive *apprehension test*, in which passive placement of the shoulder in the provocative position (abduction, extension, and external rotation) reproduces the patient's sense of instability and pain. Posteriorly directed counterpressure over the anterior shoulder may mitigate the sensation of instability.

Posterior Dislocation

- Clinically, a posterior glenohumeral dislocation does not present with striking deformity; moreover, the injured upper extremity is typically held in the traditional sling position of shoulder internal rotation and adduction.
- A careful neurovascular examination is important to rule out axillary nerve injury, although it is much less common than with anterior glenohumeral dislocations.
- On examination, limited external rotation (often <0 degrees) and limited anterior forward elevation (often <90 degrees) may be appreciated.
- A palpable mass posterior to the shoulder, flattening of the anterior shoulder, and a coracoid prominence may be observed.

Atraumatic Dislocation

- Patients present with a history of recurrent dislocations with spontaneous reduction.
- Often the patient will report a history of minimal trauma or volitional dislocation, frequently without pain.
- Multidirectional instability may be present bilaterally, as may characteristics of multiple joint laxity, including hyperextensibility of the elbows, knees, and metacarpophalangeal joints. Skin striae may be present.

Superior and Inferior (Luxatio Erecta) Dislocation

- This injury is extremely rare in children, although cases have been reported.
- It may be associated with hereditary conditions, such as Ehlers-Danlos syndrome.

Radiographic Evaluation

- Trauma series of the affected shoulder. Anteroposterior, scapular-Y, and axillary views should be obtained.
  - *Hill-Sachs lesion.* This is a posterolateral head defect caused by an impression fracture on the glenoid rim.
  - *Atraumatic dislocations.* Radiographs may demonstrate congenital aplasia or absence of the glenoid on radiographic evaluation.
- Special views taken should include the following:
  - Velpeau axillary: compliance is frequently an issue with an irritable injured child in pain. If a standard axillary cannot be obtained, the patient may be left in a sling and can be leaned obliquely backward 45 degrees over the cassette. The beam is directed caudally, orthogonal to the cassette, resulting in an axillary view with magnification.
  - West Point axillary: taken with patient prone with the beam directed cephalad to the axilla 25 degrees from the horizontal and 25 degrees medially; provides tangential view of the anteroinferior glenoid rim.
  - Hill-Sachs view: anteroposterior radiograph taken with shoulder in maximal internal rotation to visualize a posterolateral defect.
  - Stryker notch view: patient supine with ipsilateral palm on crown of head and elbow pointing straight up. X-ray beam is directed 10 degrees cephalad, aimed at the coracoid; able to visualize 90% of posterolateral humeral head defects.
- *Computed tomography.* This may be useful in defining humeral head or glenoid impression fractures, loose bodies, and anterior labral bony injuries (bony Bankart lesion).
- *Single or double contrast arthrography.* These may be used in cases in which the diagnosis may be unclear; they may demonstrate pseudosubluxation, or traumatic epiphyseal separation of the proximal humerus, in a neonate with an apparent glenohumeral dislocation.
- *Magnetic resonance imaging.* This technique may be used to identify rotator cuff, capsular, and glenoid labral (Bankart lesion) pathology.

DESCRIPTIVE CLASSIFICATION

Degree of stability: dislocation versus subluxation

Chronology: Congenital
Acute versus chronic
Locked (fixed)
Recurrent

Acquired: generally from repeated minor injuries (swimming, gymnastics, weights); labrum often intact; capsular laxity; increased glenohumeral joint volume; subluxation is common

Force:

- Atraumatic: usually due to congenital laxity; no injury; often asymptomatic; self-reducing
- Traumatic: etiology usually due to one major injury; anterior/inferior labrum may be detached (Bankart lesion); unidirectional; generally requires assistance for reduction

Patient contribution: voluntary versus involuntary

Direction: Subcoracoid
Subglenoid
Intrathoracic

Treatment

- Closed reduction should be performed after adequate clinical evaluation and administration of analgesics and/or sedation. Described techniques include the following:

Traction-countertraction. In the supine position a sheet is placed in the axilla of the affected shoulder with traction applied to counter axial traction placed on the affected upper extremity. Steady continuous traction eventually results in fatigue of the shoulder musculature in spasm, allowing reduction of the humeral head.

Stimson technique. The patient is placed prone on the stretcher with the affected upper extremity hanging free. Gentle manual traction or 5 pounds of weight is applied to the wrist, with reduction effected over 15 to 20 minutes.

Steel maneuver. With the patient supine, the examiner supports the elbow in one hand while supporting the forearm and wrist with the other. The upper extremity is abducted to 90 degrees and is slowly externally rotated. Thumb pressure is applied by the physician to push the humeral head into place, followed by adduction and internal rotation of the shoulder as the extremity is placed across the chest.

- After reduction, acute anterior dislocations are treated with sling immobilization for 4 weeks, following which an aggressive program of rehabilitation for rotator cuff strengthening is instituted. Posterior dislocations are treated for 4 weeks in a commercial splint or shoulder spica cast with the shoulder in neutral rotation, followed by physical therapy.
- Recurrent dislocation or associated glenoid rim avulsion fractures ("bony" Bankart lesion) may necessitate operative management, including reduction and internal fixation of the anterior glenoid margin, repair of a Bankart lesion (anterior labral tear), capsular shift, or capsulorraphy. Postoperatively, the child is placed in sling immobilization for 4 to 6 weeks with gradual increases in range-of-motion and strengthening exercises.
- Atraumatic dislocations rarely require reduction maneuvers as spontaneous reduction is the rule. Only after an aggressive supervised rehabilitation program for rotator cuff and deltoid strengthening has been completed should surgical intervention be considered. Vigorous rehabilitation may obviate the need for operative intervention in up to 85% of cases (Rockwood).
- Psychiatric evaluation may be necessary for the management of voluntary dislocators.

Complications

- Recurrence. A recurrence of 50% to 90% has been found, with rates of recurrence decreasing with increasing age. This may necessitate operative intervention, which has a >90% success rate in preventing future redislocation.
- Stiffness. Procedures aimed at tightening static and dynamic constraints (subscapularis tendon shortening, capsular shift, etc.) may produce "overtightening," resulting in a loss of range of motion and possible subluxation in the opposing direction with subsequent accelerated glenohumeral arthritis.
- Neurologic injury. Neurapraxic injury may occur to nerves in proximity to the glenohumeral articulation, especially the axillary nerve and less commonly the musculocutaneous nerve. These typically resolve with time; a lack of neurologic recovery by 3 months may warrant surgical exploration.
- Vascular injury. Traction injury to the axillary artery has been reported in conjunction with nerve injury to the brachial plexus.

42. PEDIATRIC ELBOW

EPIDEMIOLOGY

- These fractures represent 8% to 9% of all fractures in children.
- Some 86% of all elbow fractures occur at the distal humerus; 80% of those are supracondylar.
- Most fractures occur in patients 5 to 10 years of age; they are more common in males.
- A seasonal distribution for elbow fractures in children is found, with the most occurring during the summer months and the fewest during the winter months.

Anatomy

- The elbow consists of three joints: the ulnohumeral, radiocapitellar, and proximal radioulnar.
- The vascular supply to the elbow is a broad anastomotic network that forms the intra- and extraosseous supplies.
  - The capitellum is supplied by a posterior branch that enters the lateral crista.
  - The trochlea is supplied by a medial branch that enters along the nonarticular medial crista and by a lateral branch that crosses the physis.
  - No anastomotic connection exists between these two vessels.
- The articulating surface of the capitellum and trochlea projects distally and anteriorly at an angle of approximately 45 degrees. The centers of the arcs of rotation of the articular surfaces of each condyle lie on the same horizontal axis; thus, malalignment in the relationships of the condyles to one other changes their arcs of rotation, limiting flexion and extension.
- The carrying angle is influenced by the obliquity of the distal humeral physis; this averages 6 degrees in females and 5 degrees in males, and it is important in the assessment of angular growth disturbances.
- In addition to anterior distal humeral angulation, horizontal rotation of the humeral condyles is found in relation to the diaphysis, with the lateral condyle rotated 5 degrees medially. This medial rotation is often significantly increased with displaced supracondylar fractures.
- The elbow accounts for only 20% of the longitudinal growth of the upper extremity.
- Ossification: The mnemonic CRMTOL is used (Figs. 42.1 and 42.2):
  - **C**apitellum—6 months to 2 years of age; includes the lateral crista of the trochlea;
  - **R**adial head—4 years;
  - **M**edial epicondyle—6 to 7 years;
  - **T**rochlea—8 years;
  - **O**lecranon—8 to 10 years; often multiple centers, which ultimately fuse;
  - **L**ateral epicondyle—12 years.

MECHANISM OF INJURY

- *Indirect.* This occurs most commonly a result of a fall onto an outstretched upper extremity.
- *Direct.* Direct trauma to the elbow may occur from falls onto a flexed elbow or due to an object striking the elbow (e.g., baseball bat, automobile).

CLINICAL EVALUATION

- Patients typically present with varying degrees of gross deformity, usually accompanied by pain, swelling, tenderness, irritability, and refusal to use the injured extremity.
- The ipsilateral shoulder, humeral shaft, forearm, wrist, and hand should be examined for associated injuries.
- A careful neurovascular examination, with documentation of the integrity of the median, radial, and ulnar nerves and distal pulses and capillary refill, should be performed. Massive swelling in the antecubital fossa should alert the examiner to evaluate for compartment syndrome of the forearm. Flexion of the elbow in the presence

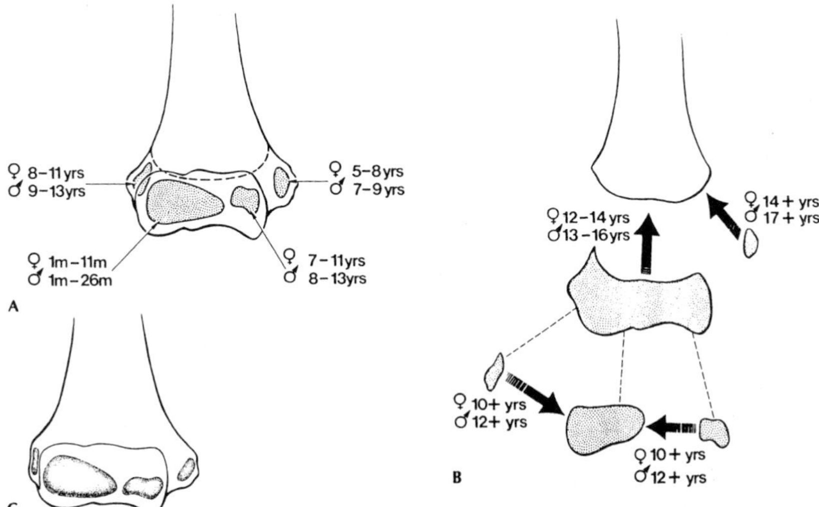

FIG. 42.1. Ossification and fusion of the secondary centers of the distal humerus. **A.** The average ages of the onset of ossification of the various ossification centers are shown for both males and females. **B.** The ages at which these centers fuse with each other are shown for both males and females. **C.** The contribution of each secondary center to the overall architecture of the distal humerus is represented by the *stippled areas.* (From Rockwood CA, Wilkins KE, Beaty JH. *Fractures and dislocations in children.* Philadelphia: Lippincott-Raven, 1999:662, with permission.)

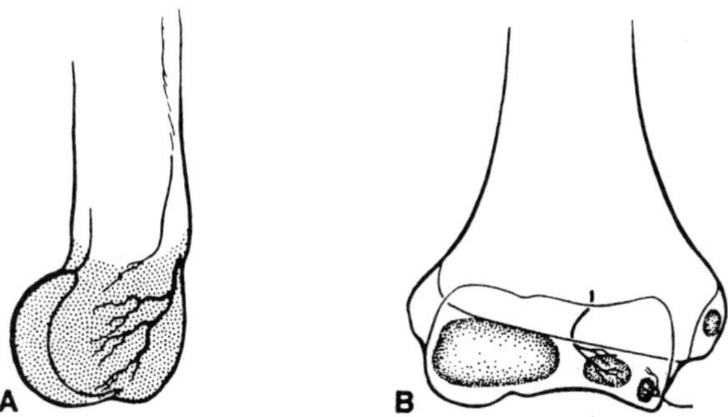

FIG. 42.2. Intraosseous blood supply of the distal humerus. **A.** The vessels supplying the lateral condyla epiphysis enter on the posterior aspect and course for a considerable distance before reaching the ossific nucleus. **B.** Two definite vessels supply the ossification center of the medial crista of the trochlea. The lateral one enters by crossing the physis. The medial one enters by way of the nonarticular edge of the medial crista. (From Rockwood CA, Wilkins KE, Beaty JH. *Fractures and dislocations in children.* Philadelphia: Lippincott-Raven, 1999:663, with permission.)

of antecubital swelling may cause neurovascular embarrassment; redocumentation of neurovascular integrity is thus essential after any manipulation or treatment.
- All aspects of the elbow should be examined for possible open lesions; clinical suspicion may be followed with intraarticular injection of saline into the elbow to evaluate possible intraarticular communication of a laceration.

RADIOGRAPHIC EVALUATION

- Standard anteroposterior and lateral views of the elbow should be obtained. On the anteroposterior radiographs, the following angular relationships may be determined:
  - Baumann angle: angulation of the lateral condylar physeal line with respect to the perpendicular of the long axis of the humerus; normal = 15 to 20 degrees and equal to the opposite side.
  - Humeral-ulnar angle: angle subtended by the intersection of the diaphyseal bisectors of the humerus and ulna.
  - Metaphyseal-diaphyseal angle: angle formed by a bisector of the humeral shaft with respect to a line delineated by the widest points of the distal humeral metaphysis (Fig. 42.3).
- On a true lateral radiograph of the elbow flexed to 90 degrees, the following landmarks may be observed:
  - *Teardrop.* This is the radiographic shadow formed by the posterior margin of the coronoid fossa anteriorly, the anterior margin of the olecranon fossa posteriorly, and the superior margin of the capitellar ossification center inferiorly (Fig. 42.4).
  - *Diaphyseal-condylar angle.* This projects 40 to 45 degrees anteriorly.
  - *Anterior humeral line.* When extended distally, this line should intersect the middle third of the capitellar ossification center.
  - *Coronoid line.* A proximally directed line along the anterior border of the coronoid process should be tangent to the anterior aspect of the lateral condyle.
- Special views should include the following:
  - *Jones view.* Extreme pain may limit an anteroposterior radiograph of the elbow in extension; in these cases, a radiograph may be taken with the elbow hyperflexed and the beam directed at the elbow through the overlying forearm with the arm flat on the cassette in neutral rotation.
  - *Internal and external rotation views.* These may be obtained in cases in which a fracture is suspected but is not clearly demonstrated on routine views. These may be particularly useful in the identification of coronoid process or radial head fractures.
- A view of the contralateral elbow should be obtained for comparison and identification of ossification centers. A *pseudofracture* of an ossification center may exist, in which apparent fragmentation of an ossification center may represent a developmental variant rather than a true fracture. This may be clarified on the basis of comparison views of the uninjured contralateral elbow.
- Fat pad signs are when three fat pads overlie major structures of the elbow as follows:
  - *Anterior (coronoid) fat pad.* A triangular lucency that is seen anterior to the distal humerus may represent displacement of the fat pad due to underlying effusion. The coronoid fossa is shallow; therefore, anterior displacement of the fat pad is sensitive to small effusions. However, an exuberant fat pad may be seen without associated trauma, diminishing the specificity of the anterior fat pad sign.
  - *Posterior (olecranon) fat pad.* The deep olecranon fossa normally completely contains the posterior fat pad. Thus, only moderate to large effusions will cause posterior displacement, resulting in a high specificity of the posterior fat pad sign for intraarticular pathology.
  - *Supinator fat pad.* This represents a layer of fat on the anterior aspect of the supinator muscle as it wraps around the proximal radius. Anterior displacement of this fat pad may represent a fracture of the radial neck; however, this sign has been demonstrated to be positive in only 50% of cases (Schunk).

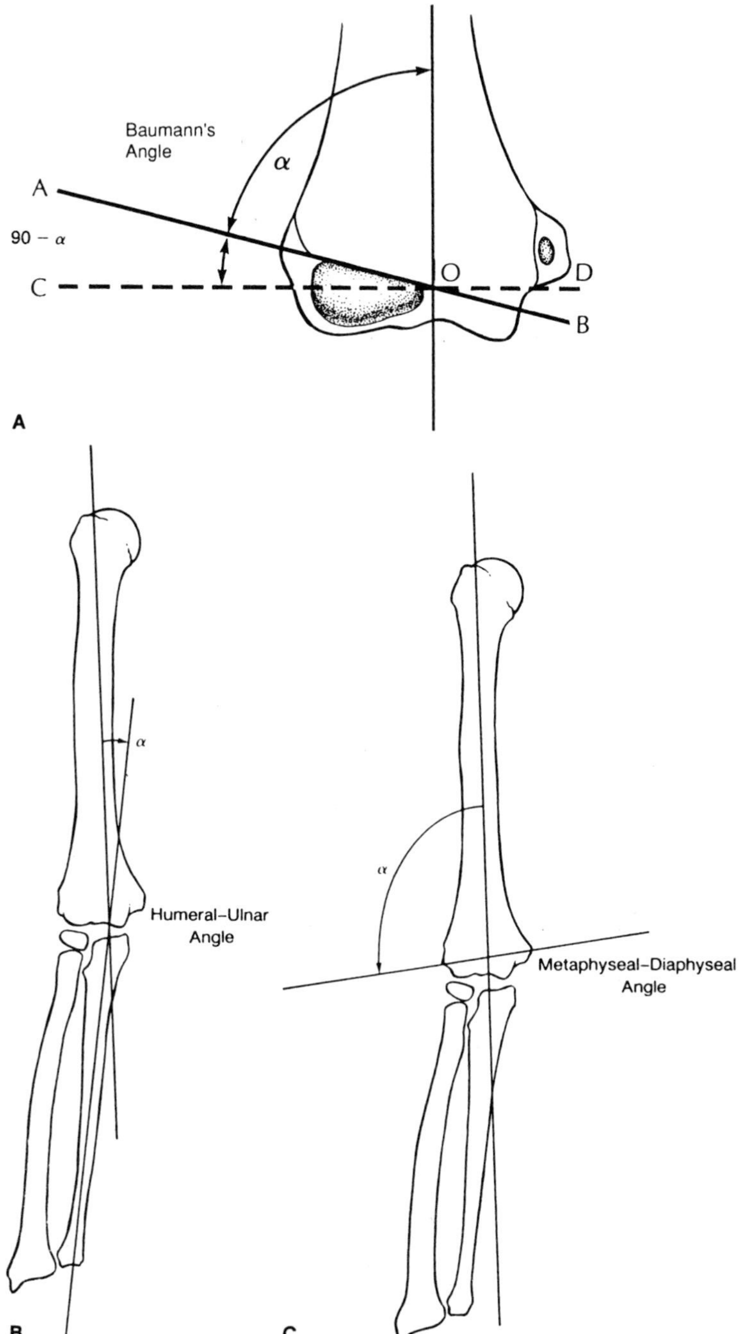

FIG. 42.3. Anteroposterior x-ray angles for the elbow. **A.** Baumann angle (α). **B.** The humeral-ulnar angle. **C.** The metaphyseal-diaphyseal angle. (From O'Brien WR, Eilert RE, Chang FM, et al. The metaphyseal-diaphyseal angle as a guide to treating supracondylar fractures of the humerus in children, 1999. Unpublished data.)

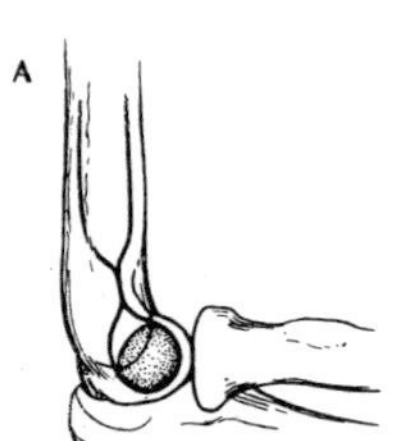

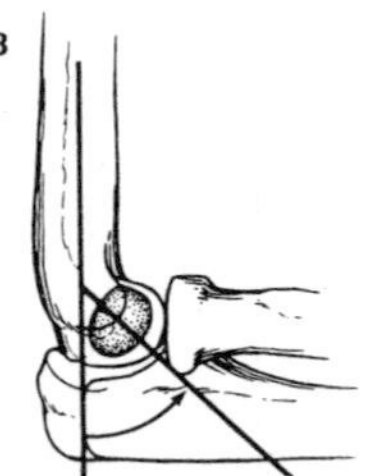

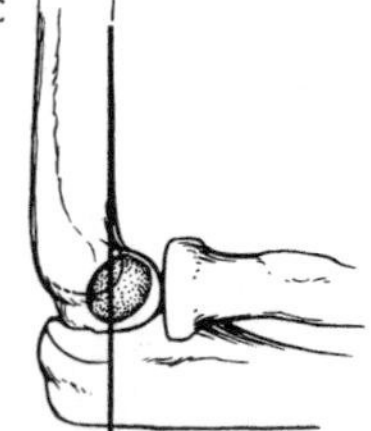

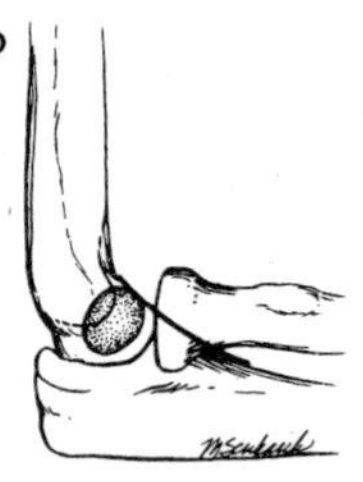

FIG. 42.4. Lateral x-ray lines of the distal humerus. **A.** The "teardrop" of the distal humerus. **B.** The angulation of the lateral condyle with the shaft of the humerus. **C.** The anterior humeral line. **D.** The coronoid line. (From Rockwood CA Jr, Wilkins KE, Beaty JH, eds. *Rockwood and Green's fractures in adults*, 4th ed. Vol. 3. Philadelphia: Lippincott-Raven, 1996:666, with permission.)

SUPRACONDYLAR HUMERUS FRACTURES

Epidemiology

- Sixty percent of all elbow fractures.
- Male/female ratio: 2:1.
- Peak incidence: 5 to 8 years of age, after which dislocations become more frequent.

Anatomy

- Remodeling of bone in the 5 to 8 year-old causes a decreased anteroposterior diameter in the supracondylar region, making this area susceptible to injury.
- Ligamentous laxity in this age range increases the likelihood of hyperextension injury.
- The anterior capsule is thickened and is stronger than the posterior capsule. In extension, the fibers of the anterior capsule are taut, serving as a fulcrum by which the olecranon becomes firmly engaged in the olecranon fossa. With extreme force, hyperextension may cause the olecranon process to impinge on the superior olecranon fossa and supracondylar region.
- The periosteal hinge remains intact on the side of the displacement.

Mechanism of Injury

- Extension type: hyperextension during a fall onto an outstretched hand with or without varus/valgus force; the triceps displaces proximally and medially.
- Flexion type: direct trauma or a fall onto the flexed elbow.

Clinical Evaluation

- Patients typically present with a swollen, tender elbow with painful range of motion.
- An S-shaped angulation at the elbow may be found. A complete (type III) fracture results in two points of angulation to give it an "S" shape.
- The "pucker" sign refers to anterior dimpling of the skin secondary to penetration of the proximal fragment into the brachialis muscle and should alert the examiner to the fact that reduction of the fracture with simple manipulation may be difficult.
- A careful neurovascular examination with documentation of the integrity of the median, radial, and ulnar nerves and their terminal branches should be performed. Capillary refill and distal pulses should be documented. The neurovascular examination should be repeated after splinting or manipulation.

CLASSIFICATION BY EXTENSION TYPE

Represents 98% of supracondylar humerus fractures in children.

Gartland Classification

Based on degree of displacement:

Type I: nondisplaced
Type II: displaced with intact posterior cortex; may be slightly angulated or rotated
Type III: complete displacement; posteromedial or posterolateral

CLASSIFICATION BY FLEXION TYPE

Comprises 2% of supracondylar humerus fractures in children.

Gartland Classification

- Type I: nondisplaced
- Type II: displaced with intact anterior cortex
- Type III: complete displacement; usually anterolateral

ORTHOPAEDIC TRAUMA ASSOCIATION CLASSIFICATION OF FRACTURES OF THE DISTAL HUMERUS

Type A: extraarticular fracture
- A1: apophyseal avulsion
- A2: metaphyseal simple
- A3: metaphyseal multifragmentary

Type B: partial articular
- B1: lateral sagittal
- B2: medial sagittal
- B3: frontal

Type C: complete articular
- C1: articular simple, metaphyseal simple
- C2: articular simple, metaphyseal multifragmentary
- C3: articular, metaphyseal multifragmentary

Treatment

Extension Type

- Type I: immobilization in a long arm cast at >90 degrees of flexion for 2 to 3 weeks.
- Type II: usually reducible by closed methods, followed by casting; may require pinning if unstable (crossed pins versus two lateral pins).

  Concepts involved in reduction are as follows:
  1. Correction of displacement in the coronal and horizontal planes before the sagittal plane.
  2. Hyperextension of the elbow with longitudinal traction to obtain apposition.
  3. Flexion of the elbow while applying a posterior force to the distal fragment.
  4. Stabilization with control of displacement in the coronal, sagittal, and horizontal planes.
  5. Immobilization with reduction held in >90 degrees of elbow flexion. The neurovascular examination should be repeated because extreme flexion of a swollen elbow may cause neurovascular compromise.
- Type III: attempt closed reduction and pinning; traction (olecranon skeletal traction) may be needed for comminuted fractures with marked soft-tissue swelling or damage.

  Open reduction and internal fixation may be necessary for rotationally unstable fractures, open fractures, and those with neurovascular injury; these should be pinned with two lateral pins and one medial pin.

  Immobilization in a long-arm cast (or posterior splint, if swelling is an issue) with the elbow flexed to 90 degrees and the forearm in neutral should be undertaken for 2 to 3 weeks postoperatively, at which time the cast may be discontinued and the pins may be removed. The patient should then be maintained in a sling with range-of-motion exercises and restricted activity for an additional 4 to 6 weeks.

Flexion Type

Type I: immobilization in a long-arm cast in near extension for 2 to 3 weeks.

Type II: closed reduction, followed by percutaneous pinning with two lateral pins or crossed pins.

Type III: reduction often difficult; most require open reduction and internal fixation with crossed pins.

Postoperative immobilization in a long-arm cast at 90 degrees should be undertaken for 2 to 3 weeks, followed by cast discontinuation and pin removal. Sling immobilization should then be instituted, accompanied by active range-of-motion exercises and restricted activity for 4 to 6 weeks.

Complications

- Neurologic injury (7%): may be due to traction injury during reduction due to tenting or entrapment at the fracture site. Also may occur as a result of Volkmann ischemic contracture, angular deformity, or incorporation into the callus or scar. Most are neurapraxias requiring no treatment.
  - Radial nerve, 45%;
  - Median nerve/anterior interosseous nerve, 32%;
  - Ulnar nerve, 23%: most common in flexion type supracondylar fractures. Early injury may be due to tenting over the medial spike of the proximal fragment, whereas late injury may represent progressive valgus deformity of the elbow.
- Vascular injury (0.5%): may represent direct injury to the brachial artery or may be secondary to antecubital swelling. This emphasizes the need for a careful neurovascular examination both on initial presentation and after manipulation or splinting, especially after elbow flexion is performed.
- Loss of motion (5%): more than 5-degree loss secondary to poor reduction or soft-tissue contracture.
- Myositis ossificans: rare; seen after vigorous manipulation.
- Angular deformity (varus more frequently than valgus): significant in 20% to 60% of patients.

LATERAL CONDYLAR PHYSEAL FRACTURES

Epidemiology

- These fractures represent 17% of all distal humerus fractures.
- They represent 54% percent of distal humeral physeal fractures.
- The peak age of occurrence is 6 years.
- Often, less satisfactory outcomes are seen here than in supracondylar fractures because of the following:
  - Diagnosis is less obvious and may be missed in subtle cases.
  - Loss of motion is more severe due to the intraarticular nature.
  - A higher incidence of growth disturbance occurs.

Anatomy

- The ossification center of the lateral condyle extends to the lateral crista of the trochlea.
- Lateral condylar physeal fractures are typically accompanied by a soft-tissue disruption between the origins of the extensor carpi radialis longus and the brachioradialis muscles; these origins remain attached to the free distal fragment, accounting for initial and late displacement of the fracture.
- Disruption of the lateral crista of the trochlea (Milch type II fractures) results in posterolateral subluxation of the proximal radius and ulna with consequent cubitus valgus; severe posterolateral translocation may lead to the erroneous diagnosis of primary elbow dislocation.

Mechanism of Injury

- "Pull-off" theory: avulsion injury by the common extensor origin due to a varus stress exerted on the extended elbow.
- "Push-off" theory: a fall onto an extended upper extremity resulting in axial load transmitted through the forearm, causing the radial head to impinge on the lateral condyle traumatically.

Clinical Evaluation

- Unlike the patient with a supracondylar fracture of the elbow, patients with lateral condylar fractures typically present with little gross distortion of the elbow, other than mild swelling due to a fracture hematoma, which is most prominent over the lateral aspect of the distal humerus.

- Crepitus associated with supination-pronation motions of the elbow may be elicited.
- Pain, swelling, tenderness to palpation, painful range of motion, and pain on resisted wrist extension may be observed.

Radiographic Evaluation

- Anteroposterior, lateral, and oblique views of the elbow should be obtained.
- Varus stress views may accentuate displacement of the fracture.
- In a young child in whom the lateral condyle is not ossified, distinguishing between a lateral condylar physeal fracture versus a complete distal humeral physeal fracture may be difficult; an arthrogram may be helpful. In such cases, the relationship of the lateral condyle to the proximal radius is critical:
  - Lateral condyle physeal fracture: disruption of the normal relationship with displacement of the proximal radius laterally due to loss of stability provided by the lateral crista of the distal humerus.
  - Fracture of the entire distal humeral physis: intact relationship of the lateral condyle to the proximal radius; often accompanied by posteromedial displacement of the proximal radius and ulna.
- Magnetic resonance imaging may help in appreciating the direction of the fracture line and the pattern of fracture.

MILCH CLASSIFICATION (FIG. 42.5)

Type I (less common): Fracture line courses lateral to the trochlea and into the capitulotrochlear groove, representing a Salter-Harris type IV fracture. The elbow is stable because the trochlea is intact.

Type II (more common): Fracture line extends into the apex of the trochlea, representing a Salter-Harris type II fracture. The elbow is unstable because the trochlea is disrupted.

JAKOB CLASSIFICATION

Stage I: nondisplaced fracture with an intact articular surface
Stage II: complete fracture with moderate displacement
Stage III: complete displacement and rotation with elbow instability

Treatment

Nonoperative Treatment

- Nondisplaced or minimally displaced fractures (stage I; <2 mm) may be treated with simple immobilization in a posterior splint or long-arm cast with the forearm in neutral position and the elbow flexed to 90 degrees. This is maintained for 3 to 4 weeks, after which range-of-motion exercises are instituted.

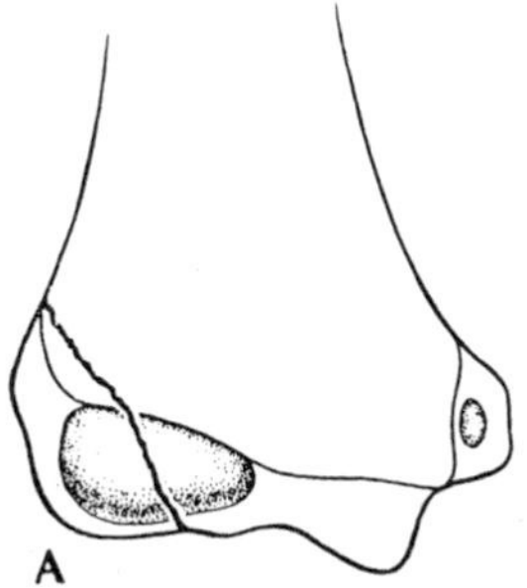

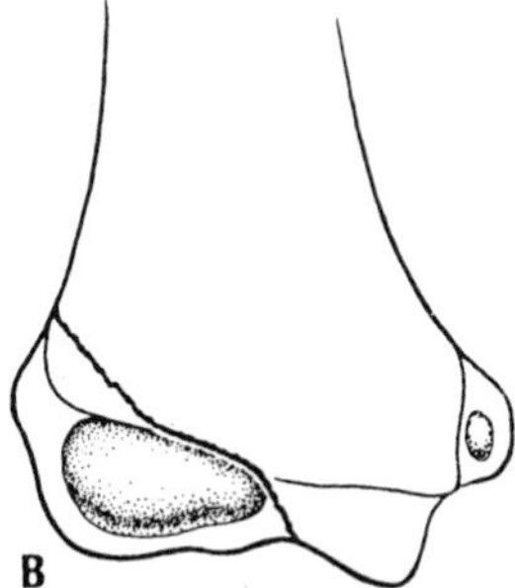

FIG. 42.5. Physeal fractures of the lateral condyle. **A.** Salter-Harris type IV physeal injury (Milch type I). **B.** Salter-Harris type II physeal injury (Milch type II). (From Rockwood CA Jr, Wilkins KE, Beaty JH, eds. *Rockwood and Green's fractures in children*, 4th ed. Vol. 3. Philadelphia: Lippincott-Raven, 1996:753, with permission.)

- Closed reduction of fractures (stage II or III) may be performed with the elbow extended and the forearm supinated. Further room for manipulation may be provided by exerting varus stress on the elbow. If the reduction is unable to be held (especially with Jakob stage III fractures), percutaneous pins may be placed. Closed reduction is unsuccessful in 50% of cases due to rotation.

Operative Treatment

- Open reduction is required for unstable Jakob stage II and stage III fractures (60% of cases).
  - The fragment may be secured with two crossed smooth Kirschner wires that diverge in the metaphysis.
  - The passage of smooth pins through the physis does not typically result in growth disturbance, as only 20% of growth occurs at the distal humeral physis.
  - Extreme care must be taken when dissecting near the posterior aspect of the lateral condylar fragment as the sole vascular supply is provided through soft tissues in this region.
  - Postoperatively, the elbow is maintained in a long-arm cast at 90 degrees with the forearm in neutral rotation. The cast is discontinued after 3 to 4 weeks with pin removal. Active range-of-motion exercises are then instituted.
- If treatment is delayed (>3 weeks), closed treatment should be strongly considered, regardless of displacement, due to the high incidence of osteonecrosis of the condylar fragment with late open reduction.

Complications

- Lateral condylar overgrowth with spur formation (30%): usually due to an ossified periosteal flap that is raised from the distal fragment at the time of injury or surgery. May represent a cosmetic problem (cubitus pseudovarus) as the elbow gains the appearance of varus due to a lateral prominence, but generally it is not a functional problem.
- Delayed union (>12 weeks) or nonunion: due to pull of extensors and poor metaphyseal circulation of the lateral condylar fragment; most common in patients treated nonoperatively. May result in cubitus valgus, necessitating ulnar nerve transposition for tardy ulnar nerve palsy. Treatment ranges from benign neglect to osteotomy and compressive fixation late (following healing with malunion) or at skeletal maturity.
- Angular deformity: cubitus valgus more frequently than varus due to lateral physeal arrest. Tardy ulnar nerve palsy may develop and necessitate transposition.
- Neurologic compromise: rare in the acute setting. Tardy ulnar nerve palsy may develop as a result of cubitus valgus as above.
- Osteonecrosis: usually iatrogenic, especially in cases in which surgical intervention was delayed. May result in a "fish-tail" deformity with a persistent gap between the lateral physeal ossification center and the medial ossification of the trochlea.
- Myositis ossificans: rare; may cause loss of elbow extension.

MEDIAL CONDYLAR PHYSEAL FRACTURES

Epidemiology

- Represents <1% of elbow fractures.
- Typical age range is between 8 to 12 years.

Anatomy

- Medial condylar fractures are Salter-Harris type IV fractures with an intraarticular component involving the trochlea and an extraarticular component involving the medial metaphysis and the medial epicondyle (common flexor origin).
- Only the medial crista is ossified by the secondary ossification centers of the medial condylar epiphysis.
- The vascular supply to the medial epicondyle and metaphysis is derived from the flexor muscle groups. Noting that the vascular supply to the lateral condylar physis traverses the surface of the medial condylar physis is important, as this renders it

vulnerable to medial physeal disruption with possible avascular complications and fish-tail deformity (sharp, angled, laterally directed wedge of bone due to a persistence of a gap between the lateral condylar physeal ossification center and the medial ossification center of the trochlea, resulting in an underdeveloped lateral trochlear crista with a functional "bony bar" of the distal humeral physis).

Mechanism of Injury
- *Direct.* Trauma to the point of the elbow, such as a fall onto a flexed elbow, results in the semilunar notch of the olecranon traumatically impinging upon the trochlea and splitting it, with the fracture line extending proximally to the metaphyseal region.
- *Indirect.* Fall onto an outstretched hand with valgus strain on the elbow results in an avulsion injury with the fracture line starting in metaphysis and propagating distally through the articular surface.
- *Rotation.* Once dissociated from the elbow, the powerful forearm flexor muscles produce a sagittal anterior rotation of the fragment.

Clinical Evaluation
- Patients typically present with pain, swelling, and tenderness to palpation over the medial aspect of the distal humerus. Range of motion is painful, especially with resisted flexion of the wrist.
- A careful neurovascular examination is important because ulnar nerve symptoms may be present.
- A common mistake is to diagnose a medial condylar physeal fracture erroneously as an isolated medial epicondylar fracture. This occurs based on tenderness and swelling medially in conjunction with radiographs demonstrating a medial epicondylar fracture due to the absence of a medial condylar ossification center in younger patients.
- Medial epicondylar fractures are often associated with elbow dislocations, usually posterolateral; elbow dislocations are extremely rare before ossification of the medial condylar epiphysis begins. With medial condylar physeal fractures, subluxation of the elbow is often observed posteromedially.

Radiographic Evaluation
- Anteroposterior, lateral, and oblique views of the elbow should be obtained.
- In young children in whom the medial condylar ossification center is not yet present, radiographs may demonstrate a fracture in the epicondylar region; in such cases an arthrogram may delineate the course of the fracture through the articular surface, indicating a medial condylar physeal fracture.
- Stress views may help distinguish epicondylar fractures (valgus laxity) from condylar fractures (both varus and valgus laxity).
- Magnetic resonance imaging may be helpful for appreciating the direction of the fracture line and the pattern of fracture.

MILCH CLASSIFICATION (FIG. 42.6)
Type I: Fracture line traverses through the apex of the trochlea; Salter-Harris type II; more common presentation.
Type II: Fracture line through capitulotrochlear groove; Salter-Harris type IV; infrequent presentation.

JAKOB CLASSIFICATION
Stage I: nondisplaced, articular surface intact
Stage II: fracture line complete with minimal displacement
Stage III: complete displacement with rotation of fragment due to pull of flexor mass

Treatment

Nonoperative
- Nondisplaced or minimally displaced fractures (stage I) may be treated with immobilization in a long-arm cast or posterior splint with the forearm in neutral rotation

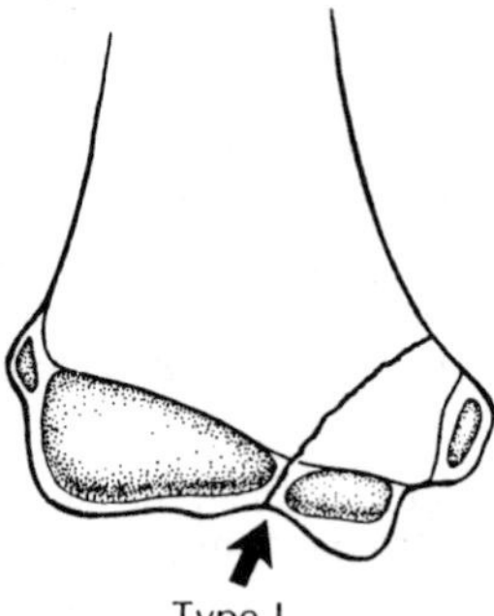

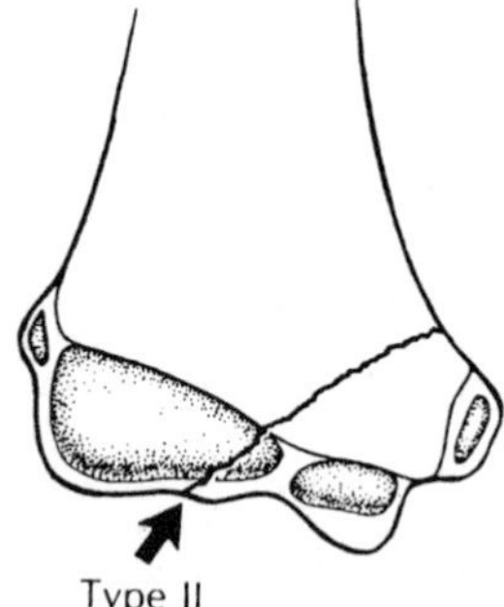

FIG. 42.6. Fracture patterns. **Left:** In the Milch type I injury, the fracture line terminates in the trochlea notch *(arrow)*. **Right:** In the Milch type II injury, the fracture line terminates in the capitulotrochlear groove *(arrow)*. (From Rockwood CA Jr, Wilkins KE, Beaty JH, eds. *Rockwood and Green's fractures in children*, 4th ed. Vol. 3. Philadelphia: Lippincott-Raven, 1996:786, with permission.)

and the elbow flexed to 90 degrees for 3 to 4 weeks, followed by range-of-motion and strengthening exercises.

- Closed reduction may be performed with the elbow extended and the forearm pronated to relieve tension on the flexor origin. This is followed by placement of a posterior splint or long-arm cast as above. Unstable reductions may require percutaneous pinning with two parallel metaphyseal pins.

Operative

- Irreducible or unstable stage II or III fractures of the medial condylar physis may require open reduction and internal fixation. Rotation of the condylar fragment may preclude successful closed treatment.
  - A medial approach may be used with identification and protection of the ulnar nerve.
  - The posterior surface of the condylar fragment and the medial aspect of the medial crista of the trochlea should be avoided in the dissection because these provide the vascular supply to the trochlea.
  - Smooth Kirschner wires in a parallel configuration extending to the metaphysis may be used for fixation. Cancellous screw fixation may be used in adolescents near skeletal maturity.
  - Postoperative immobilization consists of long-arm casting with the forearm in neutral rotation and the elbow flexed to 90 degrees for 3 to 4 weeks, at which time the pins and the cast may be discontinued and active range-of-motion exercises should be instituted.
- If treatment is delayed (>3 weeks), closed treatment should be strongly considered, regardless of displacement, due to the high incidence of osteonecrosis of the trochlea and lateral condylar fragment associated with extensive dissection with late open reduction.

Complications

- *Missed diagnosis.* Failures of treatment may represent misdiagnosis; the most common is medial epicondylar fracture due to the absence of ossification of the medial condylar ossification center. Late diagnosis of a medial condylar physeal fracture should be treated nonoperatively.
- *Nonunion.* This is uncommon, but it usually represents untreated displaced medial condylar physeal fractures secondary to the pull of flexors with rotation. These tend to demonstrate varus deformity. After ossification, the lateral edge of the fragment may be observed to extend to the capitulotrochlear groove.

- *Angular deformity.* Untreated or treated medial condylar physeal fractures may demonstrate angular deformity, usually varus, that is either secondary to angular displacement or is due to medial physeal arrest. Cubitus valgus may result from overgrowth of the medial condyle.
- *Osteonecrosis.* This may result after open reduction and internal fixation, especially when extensive dissection is undertaken. It may interrupt the vascular supply to the trochlea, especially the medial crista, as well as the lateral condyle.
- *Ulnar neuropathy.* This may occur early (related to trauma) or, more commonly, later (related to the development of angular deformities or scarring). Recalcitrant symptoms may be addressed with ulnar nerve transposition.

TRANSPHYSEAL FRACTURES

Epidemiology

Most of these fractures occur in patients younger than the age of 6 or 7 years. Originally this was thought to be an extremely rare injury; with advanced imaging (e.g., magnetic resonance imaging) its occurrence now seems fairly frequent, although the exact incidence is not known due to misdiagnoses.

Anatomy

- The epiphysis includes the medial epicondyle until the ages of 6 to 7 years in girls and 8 to 9 years in boys, at which time ossification occurs. Fractures before this age will include the medial epicondyle.
- The younger the child is, the greater the volume of the distal humerus that is occupied by the distal epiphysis; as the child matures, the physeal line progresses distally with a V-shaped cleft forming between the medial and lateral condylar physes. This cleft protects the distal humeral epiphysis from fracture in the mature child because fracture lines tend to exit through this cleft.
- The joint surface is not involved in this injury, and the relationship between the radius and capitellum is maintained.
- The anteroposterior diameter of the bone in this region is wider than in the supracondylar region, and consequently, not as much tilting or rotation occurs.
- The vascular supply to the medial crista of the trochlea courses directly through the physis; in cases of fracture, this may lead to avascular changes.
- As the physeal line assumes a more proximal location in younger patients, hyperextension injuries to the elbow tend to result in physeal separations instead of supracondylar fractures through bone.

Mechanism of Injury

- *Birth injuries.* Rotatory forces coupled with hyperextension injury to the elbow during delivery may result in traumatic distal humeral physeal separation.
- *Child abuse.* Bright demonstrated that the physis fails most often in shear rather than in pure bending or tension. Thus, in young infants or children, child abuse must be suspected because a high incidence of transphyseal fractures are associated with abuse.
- *Trauma.* These injuries may result from hyperextension injuries with posterior displacement coupled with a rotation moment.

Clinical Evaluation

- Young infants or newborns may present with pseudoparalysis of the affected extremity, minimal swelling, and "muffled crepitus," because the fracture involves softer cartilage rather than firm osseous tissue.
- Older children may present with pronounced swelling, refusal to use the affected extremity, and pain that precludes a useful clinical examination or palpation of bony landmarks. In general, because of the large, wide fracture surface, less tendency for tilting or rotation of the distal fragment is found, resulting in less gross deformity than that seen in supracondylar fractures. The bony relationship between the humeral epicondyles and the olecranon is maintained.
- A careful neurovascular examination should be performed because swelling in the cubital fossa may result in neurovascular compromise.

Radiographic Evaluation

- Anteroposterior, lateral, and oblique radiographs should be obtained.
- The proximal radius and ulna maintain normal anatomic relationships to each other but are displaced posteromedially with respect to the distal humerus. This is considered diagnostic of a transphyseal fracture.
- Comparison views of the contralateral elbow may be used to identify posteromedial displacement.
- In the child in whom the lateral condylar epiphysis is ossified, the diagnosis is much more obvious with an intact lateral condylar epiphysis to radial head relationship and posteromedial displacement of the distal humeral epiphysis with respect to the humeral shaft.
- Transphyseal fractures with large metaphyseal components may be mistaken for a low supracondylar fracture or a fracture of the lateral condylar physis. These may be differentiated by the presence of a smooth outline of the distal metaphysis in fractures involving the entire distal physis as compared with the irregular border of the distal aspect of the distal fragment seen in supracondylar fractures.
- Elbow dislocations in this age group are extremely rare, but they may be differentiated from transphyseal fractures by primarily posterolateral displacement and by a disrupted relationship between the lateral condylar epiphysis and the proximal radius.
- An arthrogram may useful for clarification of the fracture pattern and for differentiation from an intraarticular fracture.
- Magnetic resonance imaging may help to appreciate the direction of the fracture line and the pattern of fracture.
- Ultrasound may be useful for evaluating neonates and infants in whom ossification has not yet begun.

DELEE CLASSIFICATION

Based on ossification of the lateral condyle.

Group A: infant, before appearance of lateral condylar ossification center (birth to 7 months of age); diagnosis easily missed; Salter-Harris type I.

Group B: lateral condyle ossified (7 months to 3 years); Salter-Harris type I or II (fleck of metaphysis).

Group C: large metaphyseal fragment, usually exiting laterally (ages 3 to 7 years).

Treatment

Because many of these injuries in infants and toddlers represent child abuse injuries, for parents to delay seeking treatment is not uncommon.

Nonoperative Treatment

- Closed reduction with immobilization with the forearm pronated and the elbow in 100 to 120 degrees of flexion should be used, if recognized early (within 4 to 5 days of injury). This is maintained for 3 weeks, at which time the patient is allowed to resume active range of motion.
- Severe swelling of the elbow may necessitate Dunlop-type sidearm traction. Skeletal traction is typically not necessary.
- Cases in which treatment is delayed beyond 6 to 7 days of injury should not be manipulated regardless of displacement because the epiphyseal fragment is no longer mobile and other injuries may be precipitated; rather, splinting for comfort should be performed. Most will eventually completely remodel by maturity.

Operative Treatment

- DeLee Group C fracture patterns or unstable injuries may necessitate percutaneous pinning for fixation. An arthrogram is usually performed to determine the adequacy of reduction.
- Angulation of rotational deformities that cannot be reduced by closed methods may require open reduction and internal fixation with pinning for fixation.

- Postoperatively, the patient may be immobilized with the forearm in pronation and the elbow flexed to 100 to 120 degrees. The pins and cast are discontinued at 3 weeks, at which time active range of motion is permitted.

Complications

- Malunion: cubitus varus most common, although the incidence is lower than with supracondylar fractures of the humerus. This is due to the wider fracture surface of the transphyseal fracture that does not allow as much angulation as compared with supracondylar fractures.
- Neurovascular injury: extremely rare because fracture surfaces are covered with cartilage. Closed reduction and immobilization should be followed by repeat neurovascular assessment, as swelling in the antecubital fossa may result in neurovascular compromise.
- Nonunion: extremely rare as the vascular supply to this region is good.
- Osteonecrosis: observed mainly in the trochlea or lateral condyle with the development of a fish-tail deformity (see "Lateral Condylar Physeal Fractures" above); may be related to severe displacement of the distal fragment or iatrogenic injury, especially with late exploration.

MEDIAL EPICONDYLAR APOPHYSEAL FRACTURES

Epidemiology

- Comprise 12% of all elbow fractures.
- Associated with 14% of distal humerus fractures.
- Fifty percent linked to elbow dislocations.
- Peak age of 9 to 12 years.
- Male/female ratio of 4:1.

Anatomy

- The medial epicondyle is a traction apophysis for the medial collateral ligament and wrist flexors. It does not contribute to humeral length. The forces across this physis are tensile rather than compressive.
- Ossification begins between 4 to 6 years of age; it is the last ossification center to fuse with the metaphysis (15 years of age), and it does so independently of the other ossification centers.
- The fragment is usually displaced distally; it may be incarcerated in the joint 15% to 18% of the time.
- It is often associated with fractures of the proximal radius, olecranon, and coronoid.
- In younger children, a medial epicondylar apophyseal fracture may have an intra-articular component because the elbow capsule may attach as proximally as the physeal line of the epicondyle. In the older child, these fractures are generally extra-articular as the capsular attachment is more distal to the medial crista of the trochlea.

Mechanism of Injury

- *Direct.* Trauma to the posterior or posteromedial aspect of the medial epicondyle may result in fracture, although instances of this are rare and they tend to produce fragmentation of the medial epicondylar fragment.
- *Indirect.* Indirect mechanisms are as follows:
  - Secondary to elbow dislocation: ulnar collateral ligament provides avulsion force.
  - Avulsion injury by flexor muscles: valgus and extension force during a fall onto an outstretched hand.
- *Chronic.* These are related to overuse injuries from repetitive throwing, as are seen in skeletally immature baseball pitchers.

Clinical Evaluation

- Patients typically present with pain, tenderness, and swelling medially.
- Symptoms may be exacerbated by resisted wrist flexion.
- A careful neurovascular examination is essential, as the injury occurs in proximity to the ulnar nerve, which can be injured during the index trauma or from swelling about the elbow.

- Decreased range of motion is usually elicited, possibly secondary to pain; occasionally, a mechanical block to range of motion may exist due to incarceration of the epicondylar fragment within the elbow joint.
- Valgus instability can be appreciated on stress testing when the elbow is flexed to 15 degrees to eliminate the stabilizing effect of the olecranon.

Radiographic Evaluation

- Anteroposterior, lateral, and oblique radiographs of the elbow should be obtained.
- Because of the posteromedial location of the medial epicondylar apophysis, the ossification center may be difficult to visualize on the anteroposterior radiograph, especially if the radiograph is even slightly oblique.
- The medial epicondylar apophysis is frequently confused with a fracture due to the occasionally fragmented appearance of the ossification center and the superimposition on the distal medial metaphysis. Better visualization may be obtained by a slight oblique view of the lateral radiograph, which demonstrates the posteromedial location of the apophysis.
- A gravity stress test may be performed, demonstrating medial opening on stress radiographs.
- Complete absence of the apophysis on standard elbow views should prompt a search for the displaced fragment after obtaining comparison views of the contralateral normal elbow. Specifically, incarceration within the joint must be sought because the epicondylar fragment may be obscured by the distal humerus.
- Fat pad signs are unreliable, as epicondylar fractures are extraarticular in older children and because capsular rupture associated with elbow dislocation may compromise its ability to confine the hemarthrosis.
- Differentiating this fracture from a medial condylar physeal fracture is important; magnetic resonance imaging or an arthrogram may delineate the fracture pattern, especially in cases in which the medial condylar ossification center is not yet present.

DESCRIPTIVE CLASSIFICATION

- Acute
  - Nondisplaced
  - Minimally displaced
  - Significantly displaced (>5 mm) with fragment proximal to joint
  - Incarcerated fragment within the olecranon-trochlea articulation
  - Fracture through or fragmentation of the epicondylar apophysis; typically from direct trauma
- Chronic
  - Tension stress injuries ("Little League elbow")

Treatment

Nonoperative Treatment

- Most medial epicondylar fractures may be managed nonoperatively with immobilization. Studies demonstrate that, although 60% may establish only fibrous union, 96% have good or excellent functional results.
- Nonoperative treatment is indicated for nondisplaced or minimally displaced fractures and for significantly displaced fractures in older or low-demand patients.
- The patient is initially placed in a posterior splint with the elbow flexed to 90 degrees and the forearm in neutral to pronation.
- The splint is discontinued 3 to 4 days following injury, and early active range of motion is instituted. A sling is worn for comfort.
- Aggressive physical therapy is generally unnecessary unless the patient is not able to perform active range-of-motion exercises.

Operative Treatment

- An absolute indication for operative intervention is an irreducible, incarcerated fragment within the elbow joint. Relative indications for surgery include ulnar nerve dysfunction due to scar or callus formation, valgus instability in an athlete, or significantly displaced fractures in younger or high demand patients.

- Acute fractures of the medial epicondyle may be managed with a longitudinal incision just anterior to the medial epicondyle. Ulnar nerve identification is important, but extensive dissection or transposition are generally unnecessary. After reduction and provisional fixation with Kirschner wires, fixation may be achieved with the lag-screw technique. A washer may be used in cases of poor bone stock or fragmentation.
- Postoperatively, the patient should be maintained in a posterior splint or long-arm cast with the elbow flexed to 90 degrees and the forearm pronated. This may be converted to a removable posterior splint or sling at 7 to 10 days following the procedure, at which time active range-of-motion exercises should be instituted. Again, early range of motion is important; formal physical therapy is generally unnecessary if the patient is able to perform active exercises.

Complications

- *Unrecognized intraarticular incarceration.* An incarcerated fragment tends to adhere and to form a fibrous union to the coronoid process, resulting in significant loss of elbow range of motion. Although earlier recommendations were to manage this nonoperatively, recent recommendations have been to explore the joint with excision of the fragment.
- *Ulnar nerve dysfunction.* This is found in 10% to 16% of patients, although cases associated with fragment incarceration may have up to a 50% incidence of ulnar nerve dysfunction. Tardy ulnar neuritis may develop in cases involving reduction of the elbow or manipulation in which scar tissue may be exuberant. Surgical exploration and release may be warranted for symptomatic relief.
- *Nonunion.* This may occur in up to 60% of cases with significant displacement that are treated nonoperatively, although this rarely represents a functional problem.
- *Loss of extension.* Usually a 5% to 10% loss of extension is seen in up to 20% of cases, although this rarely represents a functional problem. This emphasizes the need for early active range-of-motion exercises.
- *Myositis ossificans.* This is rare, and its occurrence is related to repeated and vigorous manipulation of the fracture. This may result in a functional block to motion; it must be differentiated from ectopic calcification of the collateral ligaments related to microtrauma, which does not result in functional limitation.

LATERAL EPICONDYLAR APOPHYSEAL FRACTURES

Epidemiology

Extremely rare in children.

Anatomy

- The lateral epicondylar ossification center appears between 10 and 11 years of age; however, ossification is not complete until the second decade of life.
- The lateral epicondyle represents the origin of many of the wrist and forearm extensors; thus, avulsion injuries account for a proportion of the fractures and for displacement once the fracture has occurred.

Mechanism of Injury

- Direct trauma to the lateral epicondyle may result in fracture; these fractures may be comminuted.
- Indirect trauma may occur with forced volarflexion of an extended wrist, causing avulsion of the extensor origin, often with significant displacement as the fragment is pulled distally by the extensor musculature.

Clinical Evaluation

- Patients typically present with lateral swelling and painful range of motion of the elbow and wrist, with tenderness to palpation of the lateral epicondyle.
- Loss of extensor strength may be appreciated.

Radiographic Evaluation

- The diagnosis is typically made on the anteroposterior radiograph, although a lateral view should be obtained to rule out associated injuries.
- The lateral epicondylar physis represents a linear radiolucency on the lateral aspect of the distal humerus that is commonly mistaken for a fracture. Overlying soft-tissue swelling, cortical discontinuity, and clinical examination should assist the examiner in the diagnosis of a lateral epicondylar apophyseal injury.

DESCRIPTIVE CLASSIFICATION

- Avulsion
- Comminution
- Displacement

Treatment

Nonoperative Treatment

With the exception of an incarcerated fragment within the joint, almost all lateral epicondylar apophyseal fractures may be treated with immobilization of the elbow in the flexed supinated position until comfortable, usually by 2 to 3 weeks.

Operative Treatment

Incarcerated fragments within the elbow joint may be simply excised. Large fragments with associated tendinous origins may be reattached with a screw or Kirschner wire fixation, followed by postoperative immobilization for 2 to 3 weeks until comfortable.

Complications

- Nonunion: commonly occurs with an established fibrous union of the lateral epicondylar fragment, although this rarely represents a functional or symptomatic problem.
- Retained fragments: may result in limited range of motion, most commonly in the radiocapitellar articulation, although free fragments may migrate to the olecranon fossa and may limit terminal extension.

CAPITELLAR FRACTURES

Epidemiology

- Thirty-one percent of cases are associated with injuries to the proximal radius.
- These are rare in children, representing only 1 in 2,000 fractures about the elbow.
- No verified isolated fractures of the capitellum have ever been described in children younger than 12 years of age.

Anatomy

- The fracture fragment is composed mainly of pure articular surface from the capitellum and of essentially nonossified cartilage from the secondary ossification center of the lateral condyle.

Mechanism of Injury

- The mechanism of injury is indirect force due to axial load transmission from the hand through the radial head, causing the radial head to strike the capitellum.
- The presence of recurvatum or cubitus valgus predisposes the elbow to this fracture pattern.

Clinical Evaluation

- Patients typically present with minimal swelling and painful range of motion. Flexion is often limited by the fragment.
- Valgus stress tends to reproduce the pain over the lateral aspect of the elbow.
- Supination and pronation may accentuate the pain.

Radiographic Evaluation

- Anteroposterior and lateral views of the elbow should be obtained.
- Radiographs of the normal contralateral elbow may be obtained for comparison.
- If the fragment is large and if it encompasses ossified portions of the capitellum, it is most readily appreciated on the lateral radiograph.
- Oblique views of the elbow should be obtained if a radiographic abnormality is not appreciated on standard anteroposterior and lateral views because a small fragment may be obscured by the density of the overlying distal metaphysis on the anteroposterior view.
- Arthrography or magnetic resonance imaging may help in cases in which a fracture is not apparent but in which it is suspected to involve purely cartilaginous portions of the capitellum.

CLASSIFICATION

Type I: Hahn-Steinthal fragment—large osseous component of capitellum; sometimes involves the lateral crista of the trochlea.

Type II: Kocher-Lorenz fragment—articular cartilage with minimal subchondral bone attached; "uncapping of the condyle."

Type III: markedly comminuted.

Treatment

Nonoperative Treatment

- Nondisplaced or minimally displaced fractures may be treated with casting with the elbow in hyperflexion.
- Immobilization should be maintained for 2 to 4 weeks or until evidence of radiographic healing, at which time active exercises should be instituted.

Operative Treatment

- Adequate reduction of displaced fractures is difficult with closed manipulation. A modified closed reduction involving placement of a Steinmann pin into the fracture fragment with manipulation into the reduced position may be undertaken. Postoperative immobilization consists of casting with the elbow in hyperflexion.
- Excision of the fragment is indicated for fractures in which the fragment is small, comminuted, or old (>2 weeks), or in which it is not amenable to anatomic reduction without significant dissection of the elbow.
- Open reduction and internal fixation may be achieved by the use of two compression screws or with Herbert screws or Kirschner wires placed posterior to anterior. The heads of the screws must be countersunk to avoid intraarticular impingement.
- Postoperative immobilization should consist of casting with the elbow in hyperflexion for 2 to 4 weeks depending on stability, followed by serial radiographic evaluation.

Complications

- *Osteonecrosis of the capitellar fragment.* This is uncommon; synovial fluid can typically sustain the fragment until healing occurs.
- *Posttraumatic osteoarthritis.* This may occur with secondary incongruity from malunion or, more particularly, after a large fragment is excised.
- *Stiffness.* Loss of extension is most common, especially with healing of the fragment in a flexed position. This is typically not significant because it usually represents the terminal few degrees of extension.

T-CONDYLAR FRACTURES

Epidemiology

- Rare, especially in young children; however, this may represent misdiagnosis because purely cartilaginous fractures are not seen on routine radiographs.
- Peak incidence is in patients 11 years of age.

Anatomy

- Due to the muscular origin of the flexor and extensor muscles of the forearm, fragment displacement is related not only to the inciting trauma but also to that from the tendinous attachments. Displacement therefore includes rotational deformities in both the sagittal and coronal planes.
- Fractures in the young child may have a relatively intact distal humeral articular surface despite osseous displacement of the overlying condylar fragments; this is due to the elasticity of the cartilage in the skeletally immature patient.

Mechanism of Injury

- Flexion: most represent wedge-type fractures as the anterior margin of the semilunar notch is driven into the trochlea by a fall onto the posterior aspect of the elbow in >90 degrees of flexion. The condylar fragments are usually anteriorly displaced with respect to the humeral shaft.
- Extension: an uncommon mechanism by which a fall onto an outstretched upper extremity results in a wedge-type fracture as the coronoid process of the ulna is driven into the trochlea. The condylar fragments are typically posteriorly displaced with respect to the humeral shaft.

Clinical Evaluation

- The diagnosis is most often confused with extension-type supracondylar fractures as the patient typically presents with the elbow extended, accompanied by pain, limited range of motion, variable gross deformity, and massive swelling about the elbow.
- The ipsilateral shoulder, humeral shaft, forearm, wrist, and hand should be examined for associated injuries.
- A careful neurovascular examination, with documentation of the integrity of the median, radial, and ulnar nerves and of the distal pulses and capillary refill, is essential. Massive swelling in the antecubital fossa should alert the examiner to evaluate for compartment syndrome of the forearm.
- Flexion of the elbow in the presence of antecubital swelling may cause neurovascular embarrassment; redocumentation of neurovascular integrity is thus essential after any manipulation or treatment.
- All aspects of the elbow should be examined for possible open lesions; clinical suspicion should be followed by an intraarticular injection of saline into the elbow to evaluate possible intraarticular communication of a laceration.

Radiographic Evaluation

- Standard anteroposterior and lateral views of the injured elbow should be obtained.
- Comparison views of the normal, contralateral elbow are often helpful. Oblique views may further aid in fracture definition.
- In younger patients, the vertical intercondylar component may involve only cartilaginous elements of the distal humerus; the fracture may thus appear to be purely supracondylar in nature, although differentiation between the two fracture patterns is important due to the potential for articular disruption and incongruity with T-type fractures. An arthrogram should be obtained in cases in which intraarticular extension is suspected.
- Computed tomography and magnetic resonance imaging are of limited value and are not typically used in the acute diagnosis of T-type fractures. In younger patients, these modalities often require heavy sedation or anesthesia outside of the operating room, making an arthrogram preferred as it allows for evaluation of the articular involvement and for treatment in the operating room setting.

WILKINS AND BEATY CLASSIFICATION

Type I: nondisplaced or minimally displaced
Type II: displaced, with no metaphyseal comminution
Type III: displaced, with metaphyseal comminution

Treatment

Nonoperative Treatment

- Reserved only for truly nondisplaced type I fractures. The thick periosteum may provide sufficient intrinsic stability so that the elbow may be immobilized in flexion with a posterior splint. Mobilization initiated 1 to 4 weeks following injury.
- Skeletal olecranon traction with elbow flexed to 90 degrees used for patients with extreme swelling and soft-tissue compromise or for delayed cases with extensive skin injury that precludes immediate operative intervention. If used as definitive treatment, skeletal traction is usually continued for 2 to 3 weeks, at which time sufficient stability exists for the patient to be converted to a hinged cast brace for an additional 2 to 3 weeks. Following this, protected active motion may be initiated.

Operative Treatment

- Closed reduction and percutaneous pinning have been used with increasing frequency recently for minimally displaced type I injuries, in keeping with the current philosophy that the articular damage, which cannot be appreciated on standard radiography, may be worse than the apparent osseous involvement.
  - Rotational displacement is corrected using a percutaneous joystick in the fracture fragment and placement of multiple oblique Kirschner wires for definitive fixation.
  - The elbow is then protected in a posterior splint with the removal of pins at 3 to 4 weeks postoperatively.
- Open reduction and internal fixation are undertaken for type II and III fractures using either a posterior triceps splitting approach or the triceps-sparing approach described by Bryan and Morrey. Olecranon osteotomy is generally not necessary for exposure and should be avoided.
  - The articular surface is anatomically reduced first and is provisionally fixed with Kirschner wires. This is followed by metaphyseal reconstruction with definitive fixation using a combination of Kirschner wires, compression screws, and plates.
  - Semitubular plates are usually inadequate; pelvic reconstruction plates or specifically designed pediatric J-type plates have been used with success, often with two plates placed at a 90 degree offset from one another.
  - Postoperatively, the elbow is placed in the flexed position for 5 to 7 days, at which time active range of motion is initiated and a removable cast brace is provided.

Complications

- *Loss of range of motion.* T-type condylar fractures are invariably associated with residual stiffness, especially to elbow extension, due to the significant soft-tissue injury and articular disruption. This can be minimized by ensuring anatomic reduction of the articular surface, using arthrographic visualization if necessary, and guaranteeing stable internal fixation to minimize soft-tissue scarring.
- *Neurovascular injury.* This is rare, but it is related to often significant antecubital soft-tissue swelling. Nerve injury to the median, radial, or ulnar nerves may occur due to initial fracture displacement or to intraoperative traction, although these typically represent neurapraxias that resolve without intervention.
- *Growth arrest.* Partial or total growth arrest may occur in the distal humeral physis, although these are rarely of clinical significance because T-type fractures tend to occur in older children. Similarly, the degree of remodeling is limited, and anatomic reduction should be sought at the time of initial treatment.
- *Osteonecrosis of the trochlea.* This may occur, especially in association with comminuted fracture patterns in which the vascular supply to the trochlea may be disrupted.

RADIAL HEAD AND NECK FRACTURES

Epidemiology

- Ninety percent involve either the physis or neck; the head is rarely involved.
- These represent 5% to 8.5% of elbow fractures.
- The peak age of incidence is from 9 to 10 years.

- Common associated fractures include the olecranon, the coronoid, and the medial epicondyle.

Anatomy

- Ossification of the proximal radial epiphysis begins between 4 to 6 years of age as a small flat nucleus. It may be spherical, or it may present as a bipartite structure; these are anatomic variants, which may be appreciated by their smooth rounded borders without cortical discontinuity.
- Normal angulation of the radial head with respect to the neck is between 0 to 15 degrees laterally and from 10 degrees anterior to 5 degrees posterior angulation.
- Much of the radial neck is extracapsular; therefore, fractures in this region may not result in a significant effusion or a positive anterior fat pad sign.
- No ligaments attach directly to the radial head or neck; the radial collateral ligament attaches to the orbicular ligament, which originates from the radial aspect of the ulna.

Mechanism of Injury

Acute

- Indirect: most common; usually due to a fall onto an outstretched hand with axial load transmission through the proximal radius from trauma against the capitellum.
- Direct: uncommon due to overlying soft-tissue mass.

Chronic

Repetitive stress injuries, most commonly due to overhead throwing activities, may occur. Although most Little League elbow injuries represent tension injuries to the medial epicondyle, compressive injuries from valgus stress may result in an osteochondritic-type pathology of the radial head or in angular deformity of the radial neck.

Clinical Evaluation

- Patients typically present with lateral swelling of the elbow and pain exacerbated by range of motion, especially supination and pronation.
- Crepitus may be elicited on supination and pronation.

Radiographic Evaluation

- Anteroposterior and lateral views of the elbow should be obtained. Oblique views may aid in further definition of the fracture line.
- Special views are as follows:
  - *Perpendicular views.* With an acutely painful flexed elbow, anteroposterior evaluation of the elbow may be obtained by taking one radiograph perpendicular to the humeral shaft and a second orthogonal view perpendicular to the proximal radius.
  - *Radiocapitellar (Greenspan) view.* An oblique lateral radiograph is obtained with the beam directed 40 degrees in a proximal direction, resulting in a projection of the radial head anterior to the coronoid process of the anterior ulna.
- A positive supinator fat pad sign may be present, indicating injury to the proximal radius.
- In cases in which a fracture through nonossified regions of the radial head is suspected, an arthrogram may be performed to determine displacement.
- Magnetic resonance imaging may help in appreciating the direction of the fracture line and the pattern of fracture.

O'BRIEN CLASSIFICATION

Based on degree of angulation.

Type I: 0 to 30 degrees
Type II: 30 to 60 degrees
Type III: >60 degrees

WILKINS CLASSIFICATION (FIG. 42.7)

- Based on mechanism of injury
- Valgus injuries: fall onto outstretched hand (compression); angular deformity of head usually seen as follows:
  - Type A: Salter-Harris type I or II physeal injury
  - Type B: Salter-Harris type III or IV intraarticular injury
  - Type C: fracture line completely within metaphysis
- Fracture associated with elbow dislocation:
  - Reduction injury
  - Dislocation injury

Treatment

Nonoperative Treatment

- Simple immobilization is indicated for type I fractures in which <30 degrees of angulation occurs. They can be immobilized with the use of a collar and cuff, a posterior splint, or a long-arm cast for 7 to 10 days, followed by early range of motion.
- Type II fractures in which 30 to 60 degrees of angulation are found should be managed with manipulative closed reduction.
  - This may be accomplished by distal traction with the elbow in extension and the forearm in supination; varus stress is applied to overcome the ulnar deviation of the distal fragment and to open up the lateral aspect of the joint, allowing for disengagement of the fragments for manipulation.
  - After reduction the elbow should be immobilized in a long-arm cast in pronation with 90 degrees of flexion. This should be maintained for 10 to 14 days, following which range-of-motion exercises should be instituted.

Operative Treatment

- Type II fractures (30 to 60 degrees of angulation) that are unstable after closed reduction may require the use of percutaneous Kirschner wire fixation. A Steinmann pin for manipulation is placed in the fracture fragment under image intensification, followed by oblique Kirschner wire placement after reduction is achieved. The patient is then placed in a long-arm cast in pronation with 90 degrees elbow flexion for 3 weeks. At this time the pins and cast are discontinued, and active range of motion is initiated.
- Indications for open reduction and internal fixation include fractures that are irreducible by closed means, type III fractures (>60 degrees of angulation), fractures with >4 mm translocation, and medial displacement fractures (these are notoriously difficult to reduce by closed methods).

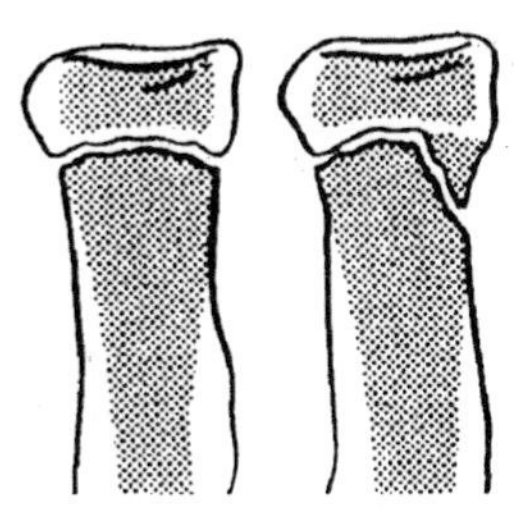

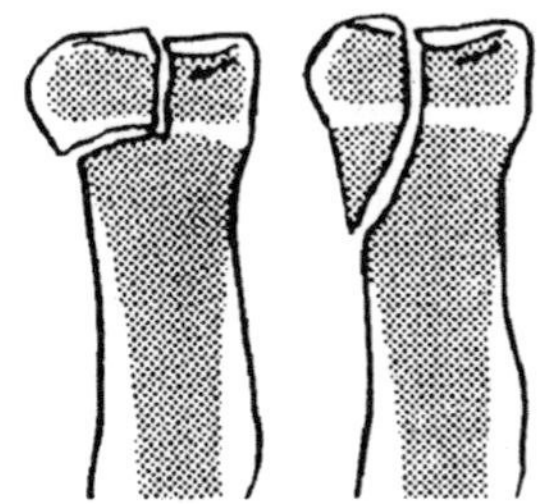

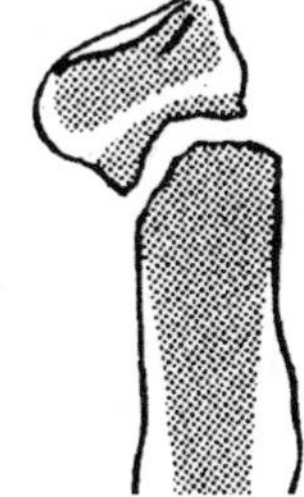

FIG. 42.7. Wilkins classification of radial head and neck fractures. (From Morrey BF. *The elbow and its disorders*, 2nd ed. Philadelphia: W.B. Saunders, 1993:260 with permission.)

- Open reduction with oblique Kirschner wire fixation is recommended; transcapitellar pins are contraindicated due to a high rate of breakage and of articular destruction from even slight postoperative motion.
- The results of open treatment do not differ significantly from those of closed treatment; thus, closed treatment should be performed when possible.
- Radial head excision gives poor results in children due to the high incidence of overgrowth.

Prognosis

- Fifteen percent to 23% of cases have poor results regardless of treatment.
- Indicators of a favorable prognosis include the following:
  - <10 years of age;
  - Isolated injury;
  - Minimal soft-tissue injury;
  - Good reduction;
  - <30 degrees of initial angulation;
  - <3 mm initial displacement;
  - Closed treatment;
  - Immediate treatment.

Complications

- Decreased range of motion is seen (in order of decreasing frequency) in pronation, supination, extension, and flexion. This is due to loss of joint congruity and fibrous adhesions. Additionally, enlargement of the radial head after the fracture may contribute to loss of motion.
- Radial head overgrowth is found in 20% to 40% of cases. In these instances, the patient experiences posttraumatic overgrowth of the radial head due to increased vascularity from the injury that stimulates epiphyseal growth.
- Premature physeal closure rarely results in shortening by >5 mm, although it may accentuate cubitus valgus.
- Avascular necrosis of the radial head occurs in 10% to 20% of cases and is related to the amount of displacement; 70% of cases of avascular necrosis are associated with open reduction.
- Neurologic complications occur usually as posterior interosseous nerve neurapraxia; during the surgical exposure, pronating the forearm causes the posterior interosseous nerve to move ulnarly and out of the surgical field.
- Radioulnar synostosis is the most serious complication, which usually occurs after open reduction with extensive dissection. However, it has been reported with closed manipulations and may require exostectomy to improve function.
- Myositis ossificans may complicate up to 32% of cases, most of which involve the supinator.

RADIAL HEAD SUBLUXATION

Epidemiology

- Referred to as "nursemaid's elbow" or "pulled elbow."
- Comprises 28% of all elbow injuries in children.
- Male/female ratio of 1:2.
- Occurs between the ages of 6 months to 6 years; peaks between the ages of 2 to 3.
- Recurrence rate of 5% to 30%.

Anatomy

- Primary stability of the proximal radioulnar joint is conferred by the annular ligament, which closely apposes the radial head within the radial notch of the proximal ulna.
- The annular ligament becomes taut in supination of the forearm because of the shape of the radial head.
- The substance of the annular ligament is reinforced by the radial collateral ligament at the elbow joint.
- After age 5, the distal attachment of the annular ligament to the neck of the radius strengthens significantly to prevent tearing or subsequent displacement.

Mechanism of Injury

Longitudinal traction force on extended elbow, although controversy remains as to whether the lesion is produced in forearm supination or pronation (that the forearm must be in pronation for the injury to occur is more widely accepted).

Clinical Evaluation

- Patients typically present with an appropriate history of sudden longitudinal traction applied to the extended upper extremity (e.g., a child "jerked" back from crossing the street), often with an audible snap. The initial pain subsides rapidly, and the patient allows the upper extremity to hang in the dependent position with refusal to use the ipsilateral hand (pseudoparalysis) and with the elbow slightly flexed.
- Effusion is rare, although tenderness can usually be elicited over the anterior and lateral aspects of the elbow.
- A neurovascular examination should be performed, although the presence of neurovascular compromise should alert the physician to consider other diagnostic possibilities because neurovascular injury is not associated with simple radial head subluxation.

Radiographic Evaluation

- Standard anteroposterior and lateral views of the elbow should be obtained.
- Radiographic abnormalities are not typically comprehended, although some authors have suggested that on the anteroposterior radiograph, >3 mm lateral displacement of the radial head with respect to the capitellum is indicative of radial head subluxation. However, disruption of the radiocapitellar axis is subtle, and it is often obscured by even slight rotation; thus, even with a high index of suspicion, appreciation of this sign is present in only 25% of cases.
- Ultrasound is not routinely used in the evaluation of radial head subluxation; however, it may demonstrate an increase in the echo-negative area between the radial head and the capitellum (radiocapitellar distance is typically about 7.2 mm; a difference of >3 mm between the normal and injured elbow is suggestive of radial head subluxation).

CLASSIFICATION

- A classification scheme for radial head subluxation does not exist because the diagnosis is qualitative.
- Ruling out other diagnostic possibilities, such as early septic arthritis or proximal radial fractures, which may present in a similar fashion, is of utmost importance.

Treatment

- Closed reduction is as follows:
  - The forearm is supinated with thumb pressure on the radial head.
  - The elbow is then brought into maximum flexion with the forearm still in supination.
- A palpable "click" may be felt upon reduction.
- The child typically experiences a brief moment of pain with the reduction maneuver, followed by the absence of pain and the normal use of the upper extremity 5 to 10 minutes later.
- Postreduction films are generally unnecessary. A child that remains irritable may require further workup for other pathology or a repeat attempt at reduction. If the subluxation injury occurred 12 to 24 hours before evaluation, a reactive synovitis that may account for elbow tenderness and a reluctance to move the joint may be present.
- Sling immobilization is generally unnecessary if the child is able to use the upper extremity without complaint.

Complications

- *Chronically unreduced subluxation.* Unrecognized subluxation of the radial head generally reduces spontaneously with the relief of painful symptoms. In these cases,

the subluxation is realized retrospectively. True unreduced subluxation may result in changes in radial head architecture with time, causing painful symptoms that may require radial head resection for adequate relief and function.
- *Recurrence.* This occurs in 5% to 39% of cases but generally ceases after 4 to 5 years of age when the annular ligament strengthens, especially at its distal attachment to the radius.
- *Irreducible subluxation.* This rarely occurs; it is due to interposition of the annular ligament. Open reduction may be necessary with transection and repair of the annular ligament to obtain stable reduction.

ELBOW DISLOCATIONS

Epidemiology
- Represents 3% to 6% of all elbow injuries.
- Peak age of occurrence at 13 to 14 years, after the physes are closed.
- High incidence of associated fractures, including those to the medial epicondyle, coronoid, and radial head and neck.

Anatomy
- "Modified hinge" joint (ginglymotrochoid) with high degree of intrinsic stability due to joint congruity, opposing tension of triceps and flexors, and ligamentous constraints. Of these, the anterior bundle of the medial collateral ligament is the most important.
- Three separate articulations as follows:
  - Ulnohumeral (hinge);
  - Radiohumeral (rotation);
  - Proximal radioulnar (rotation).
- Stability provided as follows:
  - Anterior/posterior: trochlea/olecranon fossa (extension); coronoid fossa, radiocapitellar joint, biceps/triceps/brachialis (flexion).
  - Valgus: medial collateral ligament complex—the anterior bundle is the primary stabilizer in flexion and extension; anterior capsule and radiocapitellar joint (extension).
  - Varus: ulnohumeral articulation, lateral ulnar collateral ligament (static); anconeus muscle (dynamic).
- Range of motion of 0 to 150 degrees flexion, 85 degrees supination, and 80 degrees pronation; functional requirements of 30 to 130 degrees flexion, 50 degrees supination, and 50 degrees pronation.
- The olecranon provides bony stability in extension; the coronoid, in flexion.

Mechanism of Injury
- Most commonly due to a fall onto an outstretched hand or elbow, resulting in a levering force that unlocks the olecranon from the trochlea and combines with translation of the articular surfaces to produce the dislocation.
- Posterior dislocation: combination of elbow hyperextension, valgus stress, arm abduction, and forearm supination with resultant soft-tissue injuries to the capsule, collateral ligaments (especially medial), and musculature.
- Anterior dislocation: direct force striking the posterior aspect of the flexed elbow.

Clinical Evaluation
- Patients typically present guarding the injured upper extremity with variable gross instability and massive swelling.
- A careful neurovascular examination is crucial; it must be performed *immediately* before radiographs or manipulation. At significant risk of injury are the median, ulnar, radial, and anterior interosseous nerves and the brachial artery.
- Serial neurovascular examinations should be performed in cases in which massive antecubital swelling exists or in which the patient is believed to be at risk for compartment syndrome.
- After manipulation or reduction, repeat neurovascular examinations should be performed to monitor neurovascular status.

- Angiography may be necessary to identify vascular compromise. One must note that the radial pulse may be present with brachial artery compromise as a result of collateral circulation.

Radiographic Evaluation
- Standard anteroposterior and lateral radiographs of the elbow should be obtained.
- Radiographs should be scrutinized for associated fractures about the elbow, most commonly disruption of the apophysis of the medial epicondyle, and for fractures involving the coronoid process and radial neck.

CHRONOLOGIC CLASSIFICATION

Acute, chronic (unreduced), recurrent

DESCRIPTIVE CLASSIFICATION

Based on the relationship of the radius/ulna to the distal humerus.
- Posterior
  - Posterolateral: >90% dislocations
  - Posteromedial
- Anterior: represents only 1% of pediatric elbow dislocations
- Divergent: rare
- Medial and lateral: not described in the pediatric population
- Fracture dislocation: most associated osseous injuries involve the coronoid process of the olecranon, the radial neck, or the medial epicondylar apophysis of the distal humerus. Rarely, shear fractures of the capitellum or trochlea occur.

Treatment

Posterior Dislocation

Nonoperative treatment
- *Acute posterior elbow dislocations.* These should be managed initially with closed reduction under sedation and analgesia. Alternatively, general or regional anesthesia may be used.
- *Young children.* With the patient prone and the affected forearm hanging off the edge of the table, anteriorly directed pressure is applied to the olecranon tip, effecting reduction.
- *Older children.* With the patient supine, reduction should be performed with the forearm supinated and the elbow flexed while providing distal traction. Reduction with the elbow hyperextended is associated with median nerve entrapment and increased soft-tissue trauma.
- *Neurovascular status.* This should be reassessed, followed by evaluation of stable range of motion.
- *Radiographs.* Postreduction radiographs are essential.
- *Postreduction management.* This should consist of a posterior splint at 90 degrees with loose circumferential wraps and elevation. Attention should be paid to antecubital and forearm swelling.
- *Range of motion.* Early, gentle, active range of motion 5 to 7 days following reduction is associated with better long-term results. Forced passive range of motion should be avoided as redislocation may occur. Prolonged immobilization is associated with unsatisfactory results and with greater flexion contractures.
- *Instability.* A hinged elbow brace through a stable arc of motion may be indicated in cases of instability without associated fractures.
- *Recovery.* Full recovery of motion and strength requires 3 to 6 months.

Operative treatment
- This treatment is indicated for cases of soft-tissue and/or bony entrapment in which closed reduction is not possible.
- A large displaced coronoid fragment requires open reduction and internal fixation to prevent recurrent instability. Medial epicondylar apophyseal disruptions with entrapped fragments must be addressed.

- Lateral ligamentous reconstruction is usually unnecessary in cases of recurrent instability and dislocation.
- An external fixator for grossly unstable dislocations (with disruption of the medial collateral ligament) may be required as a salvage procedure.

Anterior Dislocation

- Acute anterior dislocation of the elbow may be managed initially with closed reduction under sedation/analgesia.
- Initial distal traction is applied to the flexed forearm to relax the forearm musculature and is followed by dorsally directed pressure on the volar forearm, coupled with posteriorly directed pressure on the distal humerus.
- Triceps function should be assessed after reduction as stripping of the triceps tendon from its olecranon insertion may occur.
- Associated olecranon fractures usually require open reduction and internal fixation.

Divergent Dislocation

This rare injury has two types as follows:

Anterior-posterior type (ulna posteriorly, radial head anteriorly): more common; reduction achieved in the same manner as a posterior dislocation concomitant with posteriorly directed pressure over the anterior radial head prominence.

Mediolateral (transverse) type (distal humerus wedged between the radius laterally and the ulna medially): extremely rare; reduction by direct distal traction on the extended elbow with pressure on the proximal radius and ulna to converge them.

Complications

- *Loss of motion (extension).* This is associated with prolonged immobilization and initially unstable injuries. Some authors recommend posterior splint immobilization for 3 to 4 weeks, although recent trends have been to begin early (1 week) supervised range of motion. Patients typically will experience a loss of the terminal 1 to 15 degrees of extension, which is usually not functionally significant.
- *Neurologic compromise.* Neurologic deficits occur in 10% of cases. Most complications occur with entrapment of the median nerve. Ulnar nerve injuries are most commonly associated with disruptions of the medial epicondylar apophysis. Radial nerve injuries occur rarely.

  Spontaneous recovery is usually expected; a decline in nerve function (especially after manipulation) or severe pain in nerve distribution should be explored and decompressed.

  Exploration is recommended if no recovery is seen after 3 months after an electromyogram and serial clinical examinations are conducted.
- *Vascular injury.* The brachial artery is most commonly disrupted during injury.

  Prompt recognition of vascular injury is essential; closed reduction should reestablish perfusion.

  If, after reduction, perfusion is not reestablished, an angiography is indicated to identify the lesion; arterial reconstruction with a reverse saphenous vein graft should be performed when indicated.
- *Compartment syndrome (Volkmann contracture).* This may result from massive swelling due to soft-tissue injury. Postreduction care must include aggressive elevation and avoidance of hyperflexion of the elbow. Serial neurovascular examinations and compartment pressure monitoring may be necessary. Forearm fasciotomy is used when indicated.
- *Instability/redislocation.* This is rare (<1%) after isolated traumatic posterior elbow dislocation; an increased incidence is found in the presence of associated coronoid process and radial head fracture (plus elbow dislocation = *terrible triad of the elbow*). It may necessitate hinged external fixation, capsuloligamentous reconstruction, internal fixation, or prosthetic replacement of the radial head.
- *Ectopic calcification.* Calcification of the capsule and/or collateral ligaments seldom contributes to the loss of motion and therefore does not usually require treatment.

- *Heterotopic bone/myositis ossificans.* This occurs in 3% of pure dislocations and in 18% when associated with fractures; it is most commonly caused by vigorous attempts at reduction.
  - Anteriorly, it forms between the brachialis muscle and the capsule; posteriorly, it may form medially or laterally between the triceps and the capsule.
  - The risk increases with a greater degree of soft-tissue trauma or the presence of associated fractures.
  - It may result in significant loss of function.
  - Forcible manipulation or passive stretching increases soft-tissue trauma and should be avoided.
  - Indocin or local radiation therapy is recommended for prophylaxis postoperatively and in the presence of significant soft-tissue injury and/or associated fractures. Radiation therapy is contraindicated in the presence of open physes.
- *Osteochondral fractures.* Anterior shear fractures of the capitellum or trochlea may occur with anterior dislocations of the elbow. The presence of an unrecognized osteochondral fragment in the joint may be the cause of an unsatisfactory result in what initially appeared to be an uncomplicated elbow dislocation.
- *Radioulnar synostosis.* The incidence increases with associated radial neck fracture.
- *Cubitus recurvatum.* With significant disrution of the anterior capsule, hyperextension of the elbow may occur later, although this is rarely of any functional or symptomatic significance.

43. PEDIATRIC FOREARM

EPIDEMIOLOGY

- This fracture is very common, comprising 45% of all pediatric fractures, with a 3:1 male predominance.
- Eighty percent occur in children >5 years of age.
- Peak incidence corresponds to the peak velocity of growth when the bone is weakest due to a dissociation between bone growth and mineralization.
- Fifteen percent of cases have an ipsilateral supracondylar fracture.
- Sixty-two percent of pediatric forearm fractures occur in the distal metaphyses of the radius or ulna; 20% in the shafts; 14% in the distal physes; and <4% in the proximal third.

ANATOMY

- The radial and ulnar shafts ossify during the eighth week of gestation.
- The distal radial epiphysis appears at the age of 1 year (often from two centers); the distal ulnar epiphysis appears at age 6; the radial head appears at ages 5 to 7; the olecranon appears at ages 9 to 10. These all close between the ages of 16 and 18.
- With advancing skeletal age, the tendency is for fractures to occur in an increasingly distal location due to the distal recession of the transition between the more vulnerable wider metaphysis and the more narrow and stronger diaphysis.
- Osteology is as follows:
  - The radius is a curved bone, cylindrical in the proximal third, triangular in the middle third, and flat distally with an apex lateral bow.
  - The ulna has a triangular shape throughout with an apex posterior bow in the proximal third.
  - The proximal radioulnar joint is most stable in supination where the broadest part of the radial head contacts the radial notch of the ulna and the interosseous membrane is most taut. The annular ligament is its major soft-tissue stabilizer.
  - The distal radioulnar joint is stabilized by the ulnar collateral ligament, the anterior and posterior radioulnar ligaments, and the pronator quadratus muscle.
  - The triangular fibrocartilage complex has an articular disk joined by volar and dorsal radiocarpal ligaments and by ulnar collateral ligament fibers. It attaches to the distal radius at its ulnar margin with its apex attached to the base of the ulna styloid. This firmly unites both bones.
  - The periosteum is very strong and thick in the child. It is generally disrupted on the convex side, whereas an intact hinge remains on the concave side. This is an important consideration when attempting closed reduction.
- Biomechanics of the forearm:
  - The posterior distal radioulnar ligament is taut in pronation, whereas the anterior ligament is taut in supination.
  - The radius effectively shortens with pronation and lengthens with supination.
  - The interosseous space is narrowest in pronation and widest in neutral to 30 degrees of supination. Further supination or pronation relaxes the membrane.
  - The average range of pronation/supination is 90 degrees/90 degrees (50 degrees/50 degrees for function).
  - Malreduction of 10 degrees in the middle third limits rotation by 20 to 30 degrees.
  - Bayonet apposition (overlapping) does not reduce forearm rotation.
- Deforming muscle forces include the following (Fig. 43.1):
  - Proximal third fractures:
    - Biceps and supinator: flexion and supination of proximal fragment.
    - Pronator teres and pronator quadratus: pronate distal fragment.
  - Middle third fractures:
    - Supinator, biceps, and pronator teres: proximal fragment in neutral.
    - Pronator quadratus: pronates distal fragment.
  - Distal third fractures:
    - Brachioradialis: dorsiflexes and radially deviates distal segment.

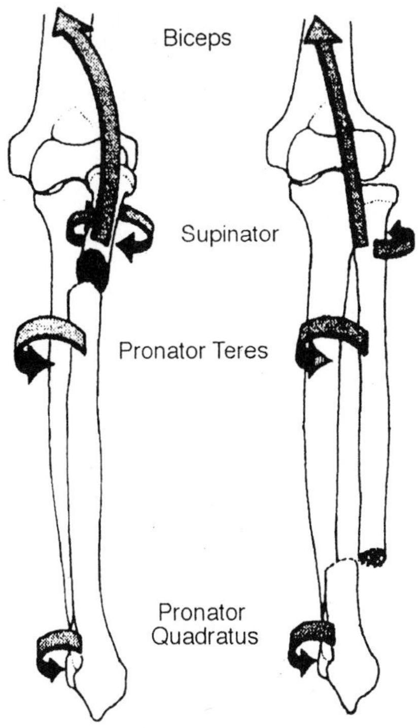

FIG. 43.1. Deforming muscle forces in both bone forearm fractures. (From Cruess RL. Importance of soft tissue evaluation in hand and wrist trauma: statistical evaluation. *Orthop Clin North Am* 1973;4:969, with permission.)

Pronator quadratus, wrist flexors and extensors, and thumb abductors: also cause fracture deformity.

MECHANISM OF INJURY

- Indirect: a fall onto an outstretched hand. Forearm rotation determines the direction of angulation:
  - Pronation: flexion injury (dorsal angulation).
  - Supination: extension injury (volar angulation).
- Direct: trauma to the radial shaft or ulnar shaft.

CLINICAL EVALUATION

- The patient typically presents with pain, swelling, variable gross deformity, and a refusal to use the injured upper extremity.
- A careful neurovascular examination is essential. Injuries to the wrist may be accompanied by symptoms of carpal tunnel compression.
- The ipsilateral hand, wrist, forearm, and arm should be palpated with examination of the ipsilateral elbow and shoulder to rule out associated fractures or dislocations.
- In cases of dramatic swelling of the forearm, compartment syndrome should be ruled out on the basis of serial neurovascular examinations with compartment pressure monitoring as indicated. Pain on passive extension of the digits is the most sensitive sign for recognition of a possible developing compartment syndrome; the presence of any of the "classic" signs of compartment syndrome (pain out of proportion to injury, pallor, paresthesias, pulselessness, paralysis) should be aggressively addressed with a possible forearm fasciotomy.
- Examination of skin integrity must be performed with removal of all bandages or splints placed in the field.

RADIOGRAPHIC EVALUATION

- Anteroposterior and lateral views of the forearm, wrist, and elbow should be obtained. The forearm should not be rotated to obtain these views; instead, the beam should be rotated to obtain a cross-table view.
- The bicipital tuberosity (Fig. 43.2) is the landmark for identifying the rotational position of the proximal fragment.
  90-degree supination: directed medially
  Neutral: directed posteriorly
  90-degree pronation: directed laterally
  Normal uninjured radius: bicipital tuberosity is 180 degrees to the radial styloid.

DESCRIPTIVE CLASSIFICATION

Location: proximal, middle, or distal third
Type: plastic deformation, incomplete ("greenstick"), compression ("torus" or "buckle"), or complete (Fig. 43.3)
Displacement
Angulation
Associated physeal injuries: Salter-Harris types I to V (see Chapter 40 for details)
- 75% occur in children from 10 to 16 years of age.
- Uncommon in children <5 years of age.
- Type II most common (50% to 60%).
- Type I most common in younger patients.
- Types III, IV, and V rare—generally seen with high energy trauma.

SPECIAL FRACTURES

Monteggia Fracture

- Proximal ulna fracture with associated dislocation of the radial head.
- Represents 0.4% of all forearm fractures in children.
- Peak incidence between 4 and 10 years of age.
- Ulnar fracture that is usually located at junction of proximal/middle thirds.

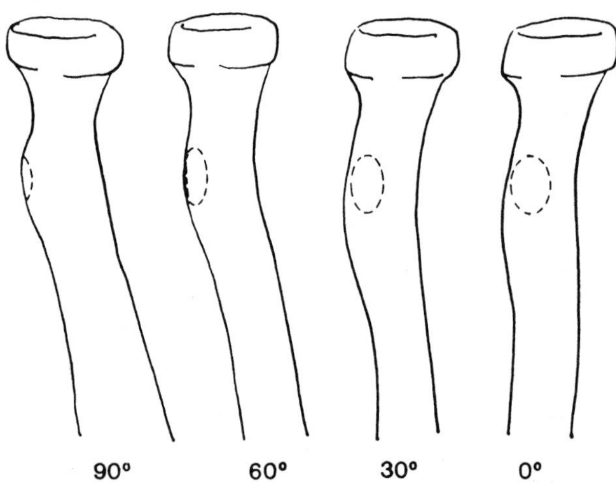

FIG. 43.2. The normal bicipital tuberosity from full supination (90 degrees) to mid-position (0 degrees). In children these characteristics are less clearly defined. (From Rockwood CA Jr, Wilkins KE, Beaty JH, eds. *Rockwood and Green's fractures in children*, 4th ed. Vol. 3. Philadelphia: Lippincott-Raven, 1996:515, with permission.)

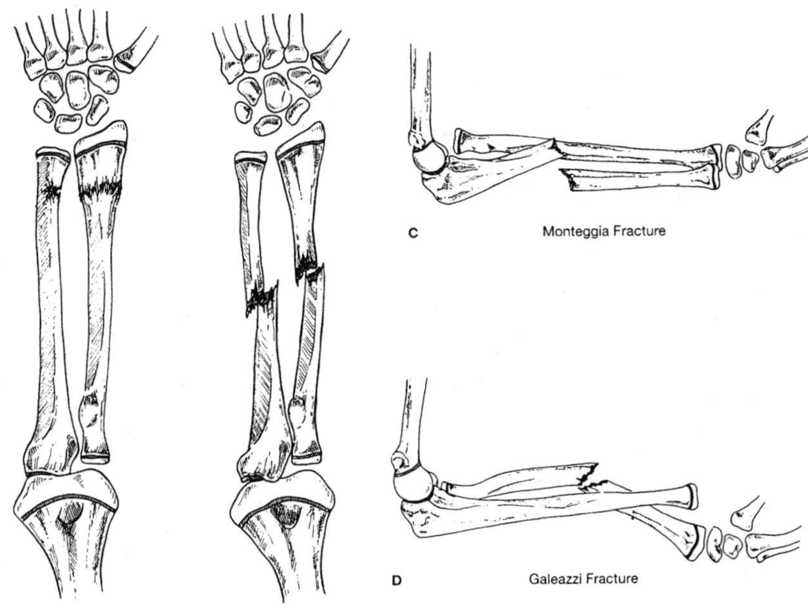

FIG. 43.3. A fall on the outstretched hand can produce any of these shaft fractures. **A.** Torus fracture; **B.** complete fracture; **C.** Monteggia fracture-dislocation; **D.** Galeazzi fracture-dislocation. (From Rockwood CA Jr, Wilkins KE, Beaty JH, eds. *Rockwood and Green's fractures in children*, 4th ed. Vol. 3. Philadelphia: Lippincott-Raven, 1996:518, with permission.)

- Bado classification of Monteggia fractures (Fig. 43.4):
  - Type I: Anterior dislocation of the radial head with fracture of the ulnar diaphysis at any level with anterior angulation.
  - Type II: Posterior/posterolateral dislocation of the radial head and fracture of the ulnar diaphysis with posterior angulation.
  - Type III: Lateral/anterolateral dislocation of the radial head with fracture of the ulnar metaphysis.
  - Type IV: Anterior dislocation of the radial head with fractures of both radius and ulna within proximal third at the same level.

Galeazzi Fracture

- Middle to distal third radius fracture with intact ulna and disruption of the distal radioulnar joint.
- Rare injury in children.
- Peak incidence between ages 9 and 12 years.

Combination Fractures

- Ipsilateral forearm fractures—make up 4% to 13% of elbow fractures.
- Forearm fracture with supracondylar humerus fracture (floating elbow).
- Distal radial epiphysis fracture with supracondylar humerus fracture (floating elbow).
- Elbow dislocation with forearm fracture.
- Olecranon physeal fracture with distal radial physeal fracture.
- Forearm fracture with lateral condylar humerus fracture.
- Distal forearm fracture with Monteggia type I or equivalent fracture.

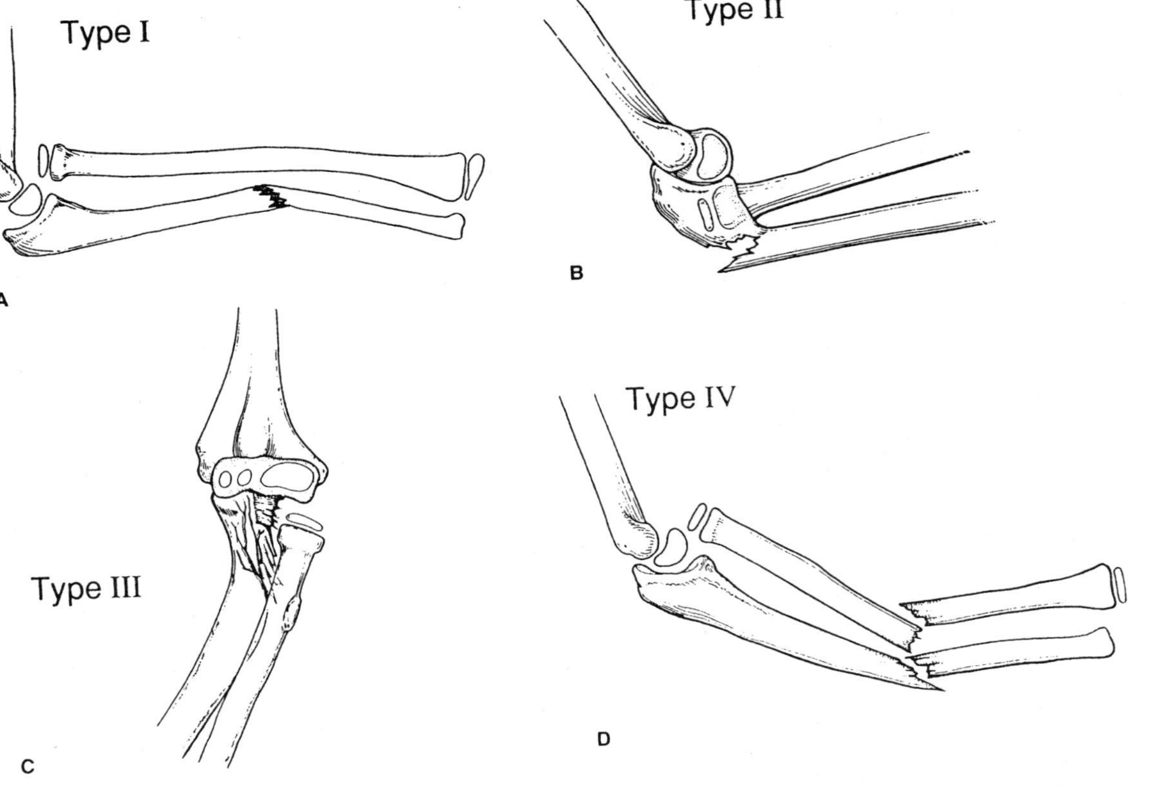

FIG. 43.4. Bado classification. **A.** Type I (anterior dislocation); **B.** type II (posterior dislocation); **C.** type III (lateral dislocation); **D.** type IV (anterior dislocation with radius shaft fracture). (From Rockwood CA Jr, Wilkins KE, Beaty JH, eds. *Rockwood and Green's fractures in children*, 4th ed. Vol. 3. Philadelphia: Lippincott-Raven, 1996:553, with

TREATMENT

Nonoperative Treatment

- Gross deformity should be corrected on presentation to limit injury to soft tissues. The extremity should be splinted for pain relief and for prevention of further injury if closed reduction will be delayed.
- The extent and type of fracture and the child's age are the factors that determine whether reduction can be carried out with sedation, local anesthesia, or general anesthesia.
- Finger traps may be applied with weights to aid in reduction.
- Closed reduction and application of a well-molded long-arm cast or splint should be performed for most fractures, unless the fracture is open, unstable, irreducible, or associated with compartment syndrome.
  - Exaggeration of the deformity (often >90 degrees) should be performed to disengage the fragments. The angulated distal fragment may then be apposed onto the end of the proximal fragment, with simultaneous correction of rotation.
  - Reduction should be maintained with pressure on the side of the intact periosteum (concave side).
- Because of deforming muscle forces, the level of the fracture determines the forearm rotation of immobilization:
  - Proximal third fractures—supination.
  - Middle third fractures—neutral.
  - Distal third fractures—pronation.
- The cast should be bivalved if forearm swelling is a concern, and the arm should be elevated.
- The cast should be maintained for 4 to 6 weeks until radiographic evidence of union is found. Conversion to a short-arm cast may be undertaken at 3 to 4 weeks if healing is adequate.
- Patients older than 10 years of age should be managed like adults; no deformity should be accepted.
  - Angular deformities: correction of 1 degree per month or 10 degrees per year due to epiphyseal growth. Exponential correction occurs over time; therefore, increased correction occurs for greater deformities.
  - Rotational deformities: do not appreciably correct; therefore, rotational alignment must be perfect.
  - Bayonet apposition: ≤1 cm acceptable; will remodel if the patient is <8 to 10 years old.
- Children younger than 4 years of age or with deformities <20 degrees usually remodel and require a long-arm cast for 4 to 6 weeks until the fracture site is nontender. Any plastic deformation that prevents reduction of a concomitant fracture, prevents full rotation in a child >4 years, or exceeds 20 degrees should be corrected.
  - General anesthesia is typically necessary because forces of 20 to 30 kg are usually required for correction.
  - The apex of the bow should be placed over a well-padded wedge, and a constant force should be applied for 2 to 3 minutes, followed by application of a well-molded long-arm cast.
  - The correction should be within 10 to 20 degrees of angulation.
- Nondisplaced or minimally displaced fractures, called greenstick fractures, may be immobilized in a well-molded long-arm cast. They should be slightly overcorrected to prevent the recurrence of the deformity.
  - Completing the fracture decreases the risk of recurrence of the deformity; however, reduction of the displaced fracture may be more difficult. Therefore, carefully cracking the intact cortex while preventing displacement may be beneficial. A well-molded long-arm cast should then be applied.
- In cases of complete displacement, the following should be done:
  - Patients <10 years of age have greater remodeling potential; an attempt at closed reduction and casting should be performed. If the fracture is irreducible, open reduction and internal fixation may be indicated.

Fractures in patients >10 years of age and proximal third fractures are very difficult to manage by closed means; open reduction and internal fixation generally should be performed.

- Physeal injuries should be handled as follows:
  Salter-Harris types I and II: gentle closed reduction followed by application of a long-arm cast or sugar tong splint with the forearm pronated; 50% apposition with no angular or rotational deformity is acceptable. Growth arrest occurs in 25% of patients on whom two or more manipulations are attempted.
  Salter-Harris type III: anatomic reduction necessary. Open reduction and internal fixation with smooth pins or screws parallel to the physis are recommended.
  Salter-Harris Types IV and V: rare injury. Open reduction and internal fixation if displaced; growth disturbance is likely.

Operative Treatment

- Surgical stabilization of pediatric forearm fractures is required in 1.5% to 31% of cases.
- Intramedullary fixation consists of percutaneous insertion of intramedullary rods or wires that are used for fracture stabilization. Typically, flexible rods or rods with an inherent curvature that permit anatomic restoration of the radial bow are employed.
  The radius is reduced first with insertion of the rod just proximal to the radial styloid after visualization of the two branches of the superficial radial nerve.
  The ulna is then reduced with insertion of the rod either antegrade through the olecranon or retrograde through the distal metaphysis while protecting the ulnar nerve.
  Postoperatively, a volar splint is placed for 4 weeks. The hardware is left in place for 6 to 9 months, at which time removal may take place if a solid callus is present across the fracture site and fracture lines have been obliterated.
- Plate fixation is used for severely comminuted fractures or for those associated with segmental bone loss. It is ideal for these because in these patterns rotational stability is questionable. Plate fixation is also used in cases of forearm fractures with skeletally mature patients.
- When ipsilateral supracondylar fractures are associated with forearm fractures, a "floating elbow" results. These may be managed by conventional pinning of the supracondylar fracture, followed by plaster immobilization of the forearm fracture.

COMPLICATIONS

- Malunion: common causes are inadequate follow-up, improper positioning in the cast, failure to perform cast changes when needed (redisplacement occurs in 7% to 13% of patients within the first 2 weeks), failure to correct inadequate reduction, and delay in diagnosis. Loss of pronation is more common in children than in adults. Over 60% have rotational losses of >20 degrees, yet more than 85% have satisfactory functional results.
- Refracture: incidence approaches 12%; therefore, refraining from active sports for 1 month after cast removal is recommended. Refracture may occur as late as 1 year after the initial injury.
- Nonunion: extremely rare in children; more likely after high energy trauma, open fractures, infection, or significant soft-tissue loss. Ulnar nonunion occurs more commonly than radial nonunion.
- Neurovascular injuries: direct injury unusual; however, anterior interosseous and median nerve injuries have been reported. Injury to the posterior interosseous nerve can be seen with Monteggia fractures (especially type III: lateral).
- Compartment syndrome: most commonly occurs after crush injuries or with ipsilateral supracondylar humerus fractures. The cardinal symptom is pain aggravated by passive stretching of the fingers. Management includes removal of constricting bandages and splitting casts (including the padding). Compartment pressures >30 mm Hg indicate compartment syndrome, at which time fasciotomies should be performed.

- Infection: usually a consequence of an open fracture. Contaminated fractures should undergo emergent irrigation and debridement with proper antibiotic coverage (including tetanus prophylaxis).
- Reflex sympathetic dystrophy: rare in children; continuous burning pain, hyperesthesia, sweating, discoloration, and swelling are the cardinal signs. Aggressive physical therapy, psychological counseling, transcutaneous nerve stimulation, and stellate ganglion blocks are the mainstays of treatment. It usually resolves 6 to 12 months after the injury.
- Overgrowth: rapid growth for the first 6 to 8 months after the injury. Overgrowth averages 6 to 7 mm, which is generally insignificant.

44. PEDIATRIC WRIST AND HAND

INJURIES TO THE CARPUS

Epidemiology

- These rarely occur, although carpal injuries may be under-appreciated due to difficulties in examining an injured child and the limited ability of plain radiographs to detail the immature skeleton.
- The adjacent physis of the distal radius is among the most commonly injured; this protects the carpus as load transmission is diffused by injury to the distal radial physis, thus partially accounting for the rarity of pediatric carpal injuries.

Anatomy

- The cartilaginous anlage of the wrist begins as a single mass; by the tenth week this transforms into eight distinct masses, each in the contour of its respective carpal bone in mature form.
- Appearance of ossification centers of the carpal bones ranges from 6 months of age for the capitate to 8 years for the pisiform (Fig. 44.1).
- The ossific nuclei of the carpal bones are uniquely protected by cartilaginous shells. As the child matures, a "critical bone-to-cartilage ratio" is reached in preadolescence after which carpal fractures are increasingly common.

Mechanism of Injury

- The most common mechanism of carpal injury in children is direct trauma to the wrist.
- Indirect injuries result from falls onto the outstretched hand, resulting in an axial compressive force with the wrist in hyperextension. In children, injury by this mechanism occurs from higher energy mechanisms, such as falling off a moving bicycle or a fall from a height.

CLINICAL EVALUATION

- The clinical presentation of individual carpal injuries is variable, but in general, the most consistent sign of carpal injury is well-localized tenderness. In the agitated child, however, appreciation of localized tenderness may be difficult because distal radial pain may be confused with carpal tenderness.
- A neurovascular examination with documentation of distal sensation in median, radial, and ulnar distributions; appreciation of movement of all digits; and assessment of distal capillary refill is important.
- Gross deformity, ranging from displacement of the carpus to the prominence of individual carpal bones, may be present.

Radiographic Evaluation

- Anteroposterior and lateral views of the wrist should be obtained.
- Comparison views of the uninjured, contralateral wrist may be helpful.

DESCRIPTIVE CLASSIFICATION

Based on the specific fracture.

Scaphoid (Fig. 44.2)

- The scaphoid is the most commonly fractured carpal bone.
- Peak incidence occurs at the age of 15 years; injuries in the first decade are extremely rare due to the abundant cartilaginous envelope.
- Unlike adults, the most common mechanism is direct trauma, with extraarticular fractures of the distal one-third appearing most often. The proximal pole fracture is rare; it typically is a result of scapholunate ligament avulsion.

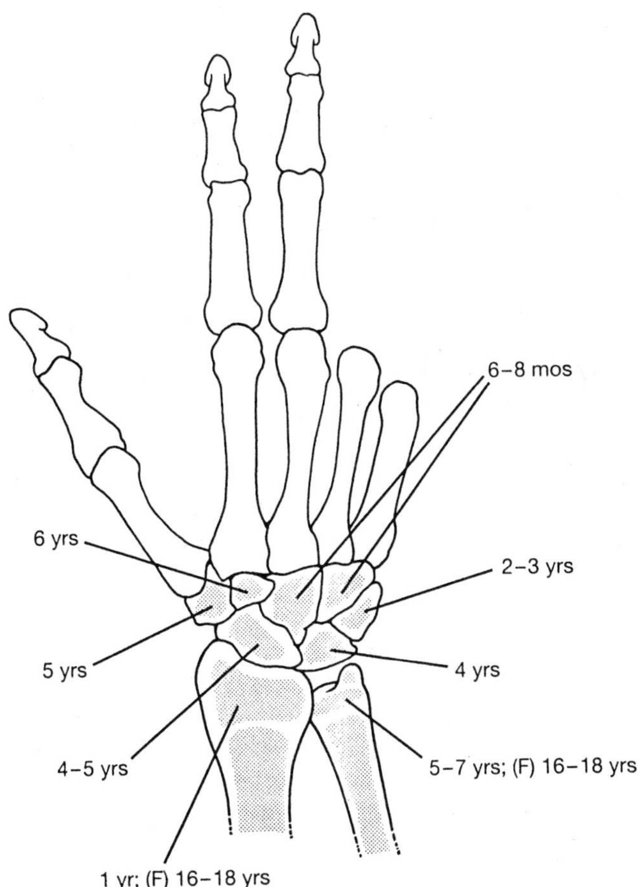

FIG. 44.1. The ages at the time of the appearance of the ossific nucleus of the carpal bones and distal radius and ulna are shown. The ossific nucleus of the pisiform (not shown) appears at about 6 to 8 years of age. (From Rockwood CA Jr, Wilkins KE, Beaty JH, eds. *Rockwood and Green's fractures in children*, 4th ed. Vol. 3. Philadelphia: Lippincott-Raven, 1996:406, with permission.)

Clinical Evaluation

Patients present with wrist pain and swelling and tenderness to deep palpation overlying the scaphoid and the anatomic snuffbox. The snuffbox is typically obscured by swelling.

Radiographic Evaluation

- The diagnosis can usually be made on the basis of anteroposterior and lateral views of the wrist.
- Oblique views and "scaphoid views," views of the scaphoid in radial and ulnar deviation of the wrist, may aid in the diagnosis or may assist in further fracture definition.
- Technetium-99m bone scan, magnetic resonance imaging, computed tomography, and ultrasound evaluation may be used to diagnose occult scaphoid fractures.

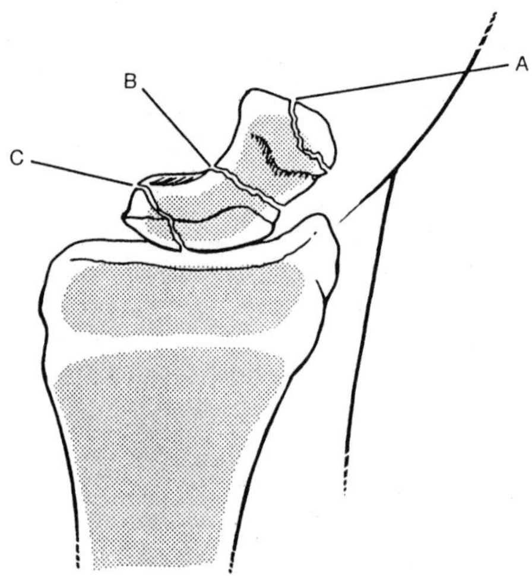

FIG. 44.2. The three types of scaphoid fractures: **A.** distal third, **B.** middle third, and **C.** proximal pole. (From Rockwood CA Jr, Wilkins KE, Beaty JH, eds. *Rockwood and Green's fractures in children*, 4th ed. Vol. 3. Philadelphia: Lippincott-Raven, 1996:407, with permission.)

CLASSIFICATION

Type A: fractures of the distal pole
  A.1: extraarticular distal pole fractures
  A.2: intraarticular distal pole fractures.
Type B: fractures of the middle third
Type C: fractures of the proximal pole

Treatment

- Initial treatment in the emergency setting should consist of a thumb spica splint or cast immobilization if swelling is not pronounced. In the pediatric population, a long-arm cast or splint is typically necessary for adequate immobilization. This should be maintained for 2 weeks at which time reevaluation may be undertaken.
- For stable nondisplaced fractures, a long-arm cast should be placed with the wrist in neutral deviation and flexion/extension and should be maintained for 6 to 8 weeks or until radiographic evidence of healing is found.
- Displaced fractures in the pediatric population may initially be addressed with closed reduction and percutaneous pinning if deemed necessary. Distal pole fractures can generally be reduced by traction and ulnar deviation.
- Residual displacement >1 mm, angulation >10 degrees, or scaphoid fractures in adolescents generally require open reduction and internal fixation. A headless compression screw or smooth Kirschner wires may be used for operative fixation; postoperative immobilization consists of a long-arm thumb spica cast for 6 weeks.

Complications

- Delayed union, nonunion, and malunion: rare in the pediatric population; may necessitate operative fixation with bone grafting to achieve union.
- Osteonecrosis: extremely rare in the pediatric population; occurs with fractures of the proximal pole in skeletally mature individuals.

Lunate

- Extremely rare injury occurring primarily from severe direct trauma (e.g., crush injury).
- Clinical evaluation reveals tenderness to palpation on the volar wrist overlying the distal radius and lunate and painful range of motion.

Radiographic Evaluation

- Anteroposterior and lateral views of the wrist are often inadequate for establishing the diagnosis of lunate fracture as osseous details are frequently obscured by overlapping densities.
- Oblique views may be helpful, but computed tomography or technetium-99m bone scanning best demonstrate the fracture.

Treatment

- Nondisplaced fractures or unrecognized fractures generally heal uneventfully and may be recognized only in retrospect. When diagnosed, they should be treated in a short-arm cast or splint for 2 to 4 weeks until radiographic and symptomatic healing occurs.
- Displaced or comminuted fractures must be treated surgically to allow adequate apposition for formation of vascular anastomoses. This may be achieved with open reduction and internal fixation, although the severity of the injury mechanism typically results in concomitant injuries to the wrist that may result in growth arrest.

Complications

Osteonecrosis: referred to as "lunatomalacia" in the pediatric population when it occurs in children less than 10 years of age. Symptoms are rarely dramatic, and radiography reveals mildly increased density of the lunate with no change in morphology. Immobilization of up to 1 year may be necessary for treatment but usually results in good functional and symptomatic recovery.

Triquetrum

- This is extremely rare, but the true incidence is unknown due to the late ossification of the triquetrum so that many potential injuries are unrecognized.
- The mechanism of fracture is typically direct trauma to the ulnar wrist or avulsion by dorsal ligamentous structures.
- Clinical evaluation reveals tenderness to palpation on the dorsoulnar aspect of the wrist and painful range of motion.
- In radiographic evaluation, transverse fractures of the body can generally be identified on anteroposterior views in older children and adolescents. Distraction views may be helpful in these cases.

Treatment

- Nondisplaced fractures of the body or dorsal chip fractures may be treated in a short-arm cast or ulnar gutter splint for 2 to 4 weeks when symptomatic improvement occurs.
- Displaced fractures may be amenable to open reduction and internal fixation.

Pisiform

- No specific discussions of pisiform fractures in the pediatric population exist in current literature.
- Direct trauma causing a comminuted fracture or a flexor carpi ulnaris avulsion may occur in late adolescence.
- Radiographic evaluation is typically unrevealing because ossification of the pisiform does not occur until the age of 8 years.
- Treatment is symptomatic only, with immobilization in an ulnar gutter splint until comfortable (usually 2–3 weeks).

Trapezium

- These are extremely rare in children and adults.
- The mechanism of injury is axial loading of the adducted thumb, which drives the base of the first metacarpal onto the articular surface of the trapezium with dorsal impaction. Avulsion fractures may occur with forceful deviation, traction, or rotation of the thumb. Direct trauma to the palmar arch may result in avulsion of the trapezial ridge by the transverse carpal ligament.
- Clinical evaluation reveals tenderness to palpation of the radial wrist, accompanied by painful range of motion at the first carpometacarpal joint with stress testing.

Radiographic Evaluation

- Fractures are difficult to identify due to the late ossification of the trapezium. In older children and adolescents, identifiable fractures may be appreciated on standard anteroposterior and lateral views.
- Superimposition of the first metacarpal base may be eliminated by obtaining a Robert view or a true anteroposterior view of the first carpometacarpal joint and trapezium.

Treatment

- Most fractures are amenable to thumb-spica splinting or casting to immobilize the first carpometacarpal joint for 3 to 5 weeks.
- Rarely, severely displaced fractures may require open reduction and internal fixation to restore articular congruity and to maintain carpometacarpal joint integrity.

Trapezoid

- Fractures of the trapezoid in children are extremely rare.
- Axial load transmitted through the second metacarpal may lead to dislocation (more often dorsal) with associated capsular ligament disruption. Direct trauma from blast or crush injuries may cause trapezoid fracture.
- Clinical evaluation demonstrates tenderness proximal to the base of the second metacarpal with painful range of motion of the second carpometacarpal joint.

Radiographic Evaluation

- Fractures are difficult to identify due to late ossification. In older children and adolescents, they may be identified on the anteroposterior radiograph based on a loss of the normal relationship between the second metacarpal base and the trapezoid.
- Comparison with the contralateral normal wrist may aid in the diagnosis.
- The trapezoid, or fracture fragments, may be superimposed over the trapezium or capitate, and the second metacarpal may be proximally displaced.

Treatment

- Most fractures may be treated with a splint or a short-arm cast for 3 to 5 weeks.
- Severely displaced fractures may require open reduction and internal fixation with Kirschner wires and attention to restoration of articular congruity.

Capitate

- This is uncommon as an isolated injury due to its relatively protected position.
- A fracture of the capitate is more commonly associated with a greater arc injury pattern (transscaphoid, transcapitate perilunate fracture-dislocation). A variation of this is the "naviculocapitate syndrome," in which the capitate and scaphoid are fractured without associated dislocation.
- The mechanism of injury is typically direct trauma or a crushing force that results in associated carpal or metacarpal fractures. Hyperdorsiflexion may result in impaction of the capitate waist against the lunate or the dorsal aspect of the radius.
- Clinical evaluation reveals point tenderness and variable painful dorsiflexion of the wrist as the capitate impinges on the dorsal rim of the radius.

Radiographic Evaluation

- The fracture can usually be identified on the anteroposterior radiograph; identification of the head of the capitate on lateral views is used to determine rotation or displacement.
- Distraction views may aid in fracture definition and in identification of associated greater arc injuries.
- Magnetic resonance imaging may assist in evaluating ligamentous disruption.

Treatment

- Simple splint or cast immobilization for 6 to 8 weeks may be performed for minimally displaced capitate fractures.

- Open reduction is indicated for fractures with extreme displacement or rotation to avoid osteonecrosis. Fixation may be achieved with Kirschner wires or compression screws.

Complications

- Midcarpal arthritis: due to capitate collapse as a result of displacement of the proximal pole.
- Osteonecrosis: rare; most often involves severe displacement of the proximal pole. May result in functional impairment; emphasizes need for accurate diagnosis and stable reduction.

Hamate

- No specific discussions concerning hamate fractures in the pediatric population are found in the literature.
- The mechanism of injury typically involves direct trauma to the volar aspect of the ulnar wrist, such as may occur with participation in racquet sports, softball, or golf.
- In clinical evaluation, patients typically present with pain and tenderness over the hamate. Ulnar and median neuropathy can also be seen, as well as rare injuries to the ulnar artery.

Radiographic Evaluation

- The diagnosis of hamate fracture can usually be made on the basis of the anteroposterior view of the wrist.
- Fracture of the hamate is best visualized on the carpal tunnel or 20-degree supination oblique view (oblique projection of the wrist in radial deviation and semisupination). A hamate fracture should not be confused with an os hamulus proprium, which represents a secondary ossification center.

Treatment

All hamate fractures should be initially treated with immobilization in a short-arm splint or cast unless compromise of neurovascular structures warrants exploration. Excision of fragments is generally not necessary in the pediatric population.

Complications

- Symptomatic nonunion: may be treated with excision of the nonunited fragment.
- Ulnar or median neuropathy: related to the proximity of the hamate to these nerves. May require surgical exploration and release.

INJURIES TO THE HAND

Epidemiology

- Hand fractures and dislocations are uncommon in very young children; the prevalence of these injuries rises sharply after they reach eight years of age due to a change in the ratio of cartilage to bone and because of participation in contact sports.
- The number of hand fractures in children is higher in males and peaks at 13 years of age, which coincides with the participation of boys in organized football.
- The annual incidence of pediatric hand fractures is 26.4 per 10,000 children, with the majority occurring about the metacarpophalangeal joint.

Anatomy (Fig. 44.3)

- As a rule, extensor tendons of the hand insert onto epiphyses.
- At the level of the metacarpophalangeal joints, the collateral ligaments originate from the metacarpal epiphysis and insert almost exclusively onto the epiphysis of the proximal phalanx; this accounts for the high frequency of Salter-Harris type II and III injuries in this region.
- The periosteum of the bones of the pediatric hand is usually well developed and accounts for intrinsic fracture stability in seemingly unstable injuries—this often serves as an aid to achieving or maintaining fracture reduction; conversely, the exuberant periosteum may become interposed in the fracture site, thus preventing effective closed reduction.

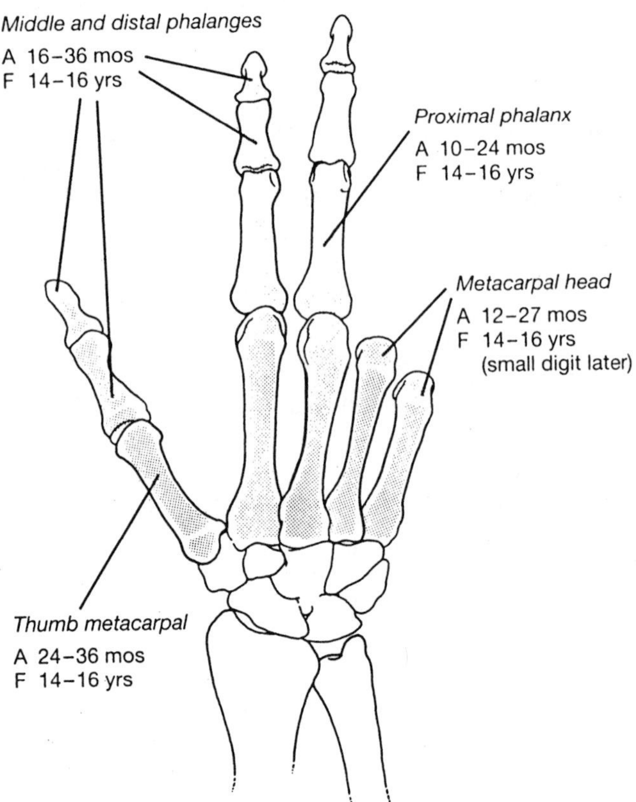

FIG. 44.3. Appearance (A) of secondary ossification centers and fusion (F) of secondary centers to the primary centers. (From Rockwood CA Jr, Wilkins KE, Beaty JH, eds. *Rockwood and Green's fractures in children*, 4th ed. Vol. 3. Philadelphia: Lippincott-Raven, 1996:325, with permission.)

Mechanism of Injury

- The mechanism of hand injuries varies considerably; in general, fracture patterns emerge based on the nature of the traumatic force:
  - Nonepiphyseal: torque, angular force, compressive load, direct trauma.
  - Epiphyseal: avulsion, shear, splitting.
  - Physeal: shear, angular force, compressive load.

Clinical Evaluation

- The child with a hand injury is typically uncooperative due to pain, unfamiliar surroundings, parent anxiety, and "white coat" fear. Simple observation of the child at play may provide useful information concerning the location and severity of injury. Game playing (e.g., "Simon says") with the child may be used for clinical evaluation.
- A careful history is essential because it may influence treatment and should include the following:
  - Age;
  - Dominant versus nondominant hand;
  - Refusal to use injured extremity;
  - Exact nature of injury—crush, direct trauma, twist, tear, laceration, etc.;
  - Exact time of injury (for open fractures);

Exposure to contamination—barnyard, brackish water, animal/human bite; Treatment provided—cleansing, antiseptic, bandage, tourniquet.

- In the physical examination, the entire hand should be exposed and examined for open injuries. Swelling should be noted, as well as the presence of gross deformity (rotational or angular).
- A careful neurovascular examination, with documentation of capillary refill and neurologic status (two-point discrimination), is critical. If the child is uncooperative and if nerve injury is suspected, the "wrinkle test" may be performed. This is accomplished by immersion of the affected digit in warm sterile water for 5 minutes; observe corrugation of the distal volar pad (absent in the denervated digit).
- Passive and active range of motion of each joint should be determined.
- Stress testing may be performed to determine collateral ligament and volar plate integrity.

Radiographic Evaluation

- Anteroposterior, lateral, and oblique radiographs of the affected digit or hand should be obtained. Injured digits should be viewed individually when possible to minimize overlap of other digits over the area of interest.
- Stress radiographs may be obtained in cases in which ligamentous injury is suspected.
- The examiner must be cognizant of the fact that cartilaginous injury may have occurred despite negative plain radiographs. Treatment must be guided by clinical and radiographic factors.

DESCRIPTIVE CLASSIFICATION

- Open versus closed injury (see below).
- Bone involved.
- Location within bone—proximal, middle, distal.
- Fracture pattern: comminuted, transverse, spiral, vertical split.
- Presence or absence of displacement.
- Presence or absence of deformity (rotation and/or angulation).
- Extra- versus intraarticular fracture.
- Physeal involvement (see Salter-Harris Classification in Chapter 40).
- Stable versus unstable.

Treatment

General Principles

- "Fight-bite" injuries: Any short curved laceration overlying a joint in the hand, particularly the metacarpal-phalangeal joint, must be suspected of having been caused by a tooth. These injuries must be assumed to be contaminated with oral flora and should be addressed with broad-spectrum antibiotics.
- The overwhelming majority of pediatric hand fractures are treated nonoperatively with closed reduction under conscious sedation or regional anesthesia (e.g., digital block). Hematoma blocks or fracture manipulation without anesthesia should be avoided in younger children.
- Finger traps may be used with older children or adolescents but are generally poorly tolerated in younger children.
- The likelihood of iatrogenic physeal injury substantially increases with repeated forceful manipulation, especially when involving late (>5 to 7 days following injury) manipulation of a periphyseal fracture.
- Immobilization may consist of short-arm splints (volar, dorsal, ulnar gutter, etc.) or long-arm splints in younger patients to enhance immobilization and to diminish chance of "escape." With conscientious follow-up and cast changes as indicated, immobilization is rarely necessary beyond 4 weeks.
- Operative indications include fractures in which stability is questionable, in which the patient may benefit from percutaneous Kirschner wire fixation; open fractures, which may require debridement, irrigation, and secondary wound closure; or fractures in which reduction is unattainable by closed means, which may signify interposed periosteum or soft tissue.

- Subungual hematomas should be evacuated with the use of a drill, cautery, or heated paper clip. DaCruz et al. reported a high incidence of late nail deformities associated with failure to decompress subungual hematomas.
- Nailbed injuries should be addressed with removal of the compromised nail, repair of the nailbed with 6-0 or 7-0 absorbable suture, and retention of the nail under the nailfold as a biologic dressing to protect the healing nailbed. Alternatively, commercially available stents are available for use as dressings.

Management of Specific Fracture Patterns

Metacarpals

Pediatric metacarpal fractures are classified as follows:

1. Type A: epiphyseal and physeal fractures
   - Fractures include the following:
     - Epiphyseal fractures;
     - Physeal fractures—Salter-Harris type II fractures of the fifth metacarpal most common;
     - Collateral ligament avulsion fractures;
     - Oblique, vertical, and horizontal head fractures;
     - Comminuted fractures;
     - Boxer fractures with an intraarticular component;
     - Fractures associated with bone loss.
   - Most require anatomic reduction (if possible) to reestablish joint congruity, thus minimizing posttraumatic arthrosis.
     - Stable reductions of fractures may be splinted in the "protected position," consisting of metacarpal-phalangeal flexion of >70 degrees to minimize joint stiffness.
     - Percutaneous pinning may be necessary to obtain stable reduction; if possible, the metaphyseal component (Thurston-Holland fragment) should be included in the fixation.
   - Early range of motion is essential.
2. Type B: metacarpal neck
   - Fractures of the fourth and fifth metacarpal necks are commonly seen as pediatric analogues to Boxer fractures in adults.
   - The degree of acceptable deformity varies according to which metacarpal is injured, especially in adolescents:
     - More than 15 degrees of angulation for the second and third metacarpals is unacceptable.
     - More than 40 to 45 degrees of angulation for the fourth and fifth metacarpals is unacceptable.
   - These fractures are typically addressed by closed reduction and splinting in the "protected position."
   - Unstable fractures require operative intervention with either percutaneous pins (may be intramedullary or transverse into the adjacent metacarpal) or plate fixation (adolescents).
3. Type C: metacarpal shaft
   - Most of these fractures may be reduced by closed means and splinted in the protected position.
   - Operative indications include unstable fractures, rotational deformity, and dorsal angulation of >10 degrees for second and third metacarpals or >20 degrees for fourth and fifth metacarpals, especially for older children and adolescents in whom significant remodeling is not expected.
   - Operative fixation may be achieved with closed reduction and percutaneous pinning (intramedullary or transverse into the adjacent metacarpal). Open reduction is rarely indicated; however, the child presenting with multiple, adjacent, displaced metacarpal fractures may require reduction by open means.
4. Type D: metacarpal base
   - The carpometacarpal joint is protected from frequent injury due to its proximal location in the hand and the stability afforded by the bony congruence and soft-tissue restraints.

- The fourth and fifth carpometacarpal joints are more mobile than are the second and third; thus, injury to these joints is uncommon, and it usually results from high energy mechanisms.
- Axial loading from punching mechanisms typically results in stable buckle fractures in the metaphyseal region.
- Closed reduction under regional or conscious sedation and splinting with a short-arm ulnar gutter splint, leaving the proximal interphalangeal joint mobile, may be performed for most of these fractures.
- Fracture-dislocations in this region may result from crush mechanisms or falls from heights; these may initially be addressed with attempted closed reduction, although transverse metacarpal pinning is usually necessary for stability. Open reduction may be necessary, especially in cases of multiple fracture-dislocations at the carpometacarpal level.

Thumb Metacarpal

- Fractures are uncommon and are typically related to direct trauma.
- Metaphyseal and physeal injury are the most common fracture patterns.
- Structures inserted on the thumb metacarpal constitute potential deforming forces:
  - Opponens pollicis: broad insertion over metacarpal shaft and base that displaces the distal fragment into relative adduction and flexion.
  - Abductor pollicis longus: multiple sites of insertion including the metacarpal base, resulting in an abduction moment or fracture-dislocation.
  - Flexor pollicis brevis: partially originates on the medial metacarpal base, resulting in flexion and apex dorsal angulation in metacarpal shaft fractures.
  - Adductor pollicis: may result in adduction of the distal fragment.
- Pediatric thumb metacarpal fractures are classified as follows:
  1. Thumb metacarpal head and shaft fractures
     These typically result from direct trauma.
     Closed reduction is usually adequate for the treatment of most fractures; post-reduction immobilization consists of a thumb spica splint or cast.
     Anatomic reduction is essential for intraarticular fractures; this may necessitate the use of percutaneous pinning with Kirschner wires.
  2. Thumb metacarpal base fractures are subclassified as follows:
     Type A: fractures distal to the physis
     - Often transverse or oblique in nature with apex-lateral angulation and an element of medial impaction.
     - Treated with closed reduction; extension is applied to the metacarpal head and direct pressure is placed on the apex of the fracture; it is then immobilized in a thumb spica splint or cast for 4 to 6 weeks.
     - Up to 30 degrees of residual angulation is acceptable in younger children.
     - Unstable fractures can possibly be treated with percutaneous Kirschner wire fixation, often with smooth pins to cross the physis. Trans-carpometacarpal pinning may be performed but is usually reserved for more proximal fracture patterns.

     Type B: Salter-Harris type II fracture, metaphyseal medial
     - The shaft fragment is typically angulated laterally and displaced proximally due to the pull of the abductor pollicis longus; adduction of the distal fragment is common due to the pull of the adductor pollicis.
     - Anatomic reduction is essential for avoiding growth disturbance.
     - Closed reduction followed by thumb spica splinting is initially indicated with close serial follow-up. With maintenance of reduction, immobilization is continued for 4 to 6 weeks.
     - Percutaneous pinning is indicated for unstable fractures with capture of the metaphyseal fragment if possible. Alternatively, trans-metacarpal pinning to the second metacarpal may be necessary. Open reduction is possibly required for anatomic restoration of the physis.

     Type C: Salter-Harris type II fracture, metaphyseal lateral
     - Similar to type B fractures but less common; typically due to more significant trauma, resulting in an apex medial angulation.

- Periosteal button-holing common; may prevent anatomic reduction.
- Open reduction frequently necessary for restoration of anatomic relationships.

Type D: intraarticular Salter-Harris type III or IV fractures
- Pediatric analogue to the adult Bennett fracture.
- Rare; deforming forces similar to type B fractures with the addition of lateral subluxation at the level of the carpometacarpal articulation due to the intraarticular component of the fracture.
- Results of nonoperative methods of treatment widely variable. Most consistent results obtained with open reduction and percutaneous pinning or with internal fixation in older children.
- Severe comminution or soft-tissue injuries initially addressed with oblique skeletal traction.
- External fixation used for cases of contaminated open fractures with potential bone loss.

Phalanges
- The physes are located at the proximal aspect of the phalanges.
- The collateral ligaments of the proximal and distal interphalangeal joints originate from the collateral recesses of the proximal bone and insert onto both the epiphysis and metaphysis of the distal bone and the volar plate.
- The volar plate originates from the metaphyseal region of the phalangeal neck and inserts onto the epiphysis of the more distal phalanx.
- The extensor tendons insert onto the dorsal aspect of the epiphysis of the middle and distal phalanges.
- The periosteum is typically well developed and exuberant, often resisting displacement and aiding reduction; occasionally, it interposes at the fracture site and prevents adequate reduction.

Proximal and Middle Phalanges
Pediatric fractures of the proximal and middle phalanges are subclassified as follows:

1. Type A: physeal
   - Forty-one percent of pediatric hand fractures involve the physis. The vast majority of these involve the proximal phalanx.
   - The collateral ligaments insert onto the epiphysis of the proximal phalanx; in addition to the relatively unprotected position of the physis at this level, this contributes to the high incidence of physeal injuries.
   - A pediatric "gamekeeper's" thumb is a Salter-Harris type III avulsion fracture in which the ulnar collateral ligament is attached to an epiphyseal fragment of the proximal aspect of the proximal phalanx.
   - Treatment is initially by closed reduction and splinting in the protected position.
   - Unstable fractures may require percutaneous pinning. Fractures with >25% articular involvement or >1.5-mm displacement require open reduction and internal fixation with Kirschner wires or screws.
2. Type B: shaft
   - Shaft fractures are not as common as those surrounding the joints.
   - Proximal phalangeal shaft fractures are typically associated with apex volar angulation and displacement; this is created by the forces caused by the distally inserting central slip and lateral bands coursing dorsal to the apex of rotation, as well as by the action of the intrinsics on the proximal fragment that pull it into flexion.
   - Oblique fractures may be associated with shortening and rotational displacement. This must be recognized and taken into consideration for treatment.
   - Closed reduction with immobilization in the protected position for 3 to 4 weeks is indicated for the majority of these fractures.
   - Residual angulation of >30 degrees in children who are <10 years of age and of >20 degrees in children who are >10 years of age requires operative intervention, consisting of closed reduction and percutaneous crossed pinning. Intramedullary pinning may allow rotational displacement.

3. Type C: neck
   - The fractures through the metaphyseal region of the phalanx are commonly associated with door-slamming injuries.
   - Rotational displacement and angulation of the distal fragment are common, as the collateral ligaments typically remain attached distal to the fracture site. This may allow interposition of the volar plate at the fracture site.
   - Closed reduction followed by splinting in the protected position for 3 to 4 weeks may be attempted initially, although closed reduction with percutaneous crossed pinning is usually required.
4. Type D: intraarticular (condylar)
   - These arise from a variety of mechanisms, ranging from shear or avulsion that result in simple fractures to combined axial and rotational forces that may result in comminuted intraarticular T- or Y-type patterns.
   - Open reduction and internal fixation are usually required for anatomic restoration of the articular surface. This is most often performed through a lateral or dorsal incision with operative fixation using Kirschner wires or miniscrews.

Distal Phalanx

- These injuries are frequently associated with soft-tissue or nail compromise and may require subungual hematoma evacuation, soft-tissue reconstructive procedures, or nailbed repair.
- Pediatric distal phalangeal fractures are subclassified as follows:
  1. Physeal

     Dorsal mallet injuries

     Type A: Salter-Harris I or II injuries
     Type B: Salter-Harris III or IV injuries
     Type C: Salter-Harris I or II associated with joint dislocation
     Type D: Salter-Harris fracture associated with extensor tendon avulsion

     - A mallet finger may result from a fracture of the dorsal lip with disruption of the extensor tendon. Alternatively, a mallet finger may result from a purely tendinous disruption; it therefore may not be radiographically apparent.
     - Treatment of type A and non- or minimally displaced type B injuries is with full-time extension splinting for 4 to 6 weeks.
     - Types C, D, and displaced type B injuries typically require operative management. Type B injuries are usually amenable to Kirschner wire fixation with smooth pins. Types C and D injuries generally require open reduction with internal fixation.

     Volar (reverse) mallet injuries

     - These are associated with flexor digitorum profundus rupture ("jersey finger," which is seen in football and rugby players and which most commonly involves the ring finger).
     - Treatment is primary repair using heavy suture, miniscrews, or Kirschner wires. Postoperative immobilization is continued for 3 weeks.
  2. Extraphyseal

     Type A: transverse diaphyseal
     Type B: longitudinal splitting
     Type C: comminuted

     - Mechanism of injury is almost always direct trauma.
     - Nailbed injuries must be recognized and addressed.
     - Treatment is typically with closed reduction and splinting for 3 to 4 weeks with attention to concomitant injuries. Unstable injuries may require percutaneous pinning, either longitudinally from the distal margin of the distal phalanx or across the distal interphalangeal joint (uncommon) for extremely unstable or comminuted fractures.

Complications

- *Impaired nail growth.* Failure to repair the nailbed adequately may result in germinal matrix disturbance that causes anomalous nail growth. This is frequently a cosmetic matter; however, it may be addressed with reconstructive procedures if pain, infection, or hygiene is an issue.

- *Extensor lag.* Despite adequate treatment, extensor lag of up to 10 degrees is common, although it is not typically of functional significance. This occurs most commonly at the level of the proximal interphalangeal joint secondary to tendon adherence. Exploration, release, and/or reconstruction may result in further cosmetic or functional disturbance.
- *Malunion.* Dorsal angulation can disturb intrinsic balance and can also result in prominence of the metacarpal heads in the palm that cause pain on gripping. Rotational or angulatory deformities, especially of the second and third metacarpals, may result in functional and cosmetic disturbances, emphasizing the need to maintain anatomic relationships as nearly as is possible.
- *Nonunion.* This is uncommon but may occur, especially with extensive soft-tissue injury and bone loss and with open fractures with gross contamination and infection. It may necessitate debridement, bone grafting, or flap coverage.
- *Infection and/or osteomyelitis.* Grossly contaminated wounds require meticulous management and appropriate antibiosis depending on the injury setting (e.g., barnyard contamination, brackish water, bite wounds), local wound care with debridements as necessary, and possible delayed closure.
- *Metacarpal-phalangeal joint extension contracture.* This may result if splinting is not performed in the protected position (i.e., metacarpal-phalangeal joints at >70 degrees), resulting in soft-tissue contracture.

45. PEDIATRIC HIP

FRACTURES

Epidemiology

Hip fractures are rare in children, occurring less than 1% as often as in adults.

Anatomy

- Ossification occurs as follows:
  - Proximal femur—week 7 *in utero*.
  - Proximal femoral epiphysis—between the ages of 4 to 8 months.
  - Trochanter—4 years of age.
- The proximal femoral epiphysis fuses by age 18 and the trochanteric apophysis between the ages of 16 to 18 years.
- The proximal femoral physis contributes significantly to metaphyseal growth of the femoral neck and less to primary appositional growth of the femoral head. Thus, disruptions in this region may lead to architectural changes that may affect the overall anatomic development of the proximal femur.
- The trochanteric apophysis contributes significantly to appositional growth of the greater trochanter and less to the metaphyseal growth of the femur.
- Blood is supplied to the hip by the lateral femoral circumflex artery and, more importantly, the medial femoral circumflex artery. Anastomoses at the anterosuperior portion of the intertrochanteric groove form the extracapsular ring. Ascending retinacular vessels go to the epiphysis. Vessels of the ligamentum teres contribute little before 8 years of age; they contribute approximately 20% in adulthood (Fig. 45.1).

Mechanism of Injury

- Direct: severe trauma, high energy injury, child abuse. Severe direct trauma (e.g., motor vehicle accidents) accounts for 75% to 80% of pediatric hip fractures.
- Pathologic: fracture through bone cyst, fibrous dysplasia, or tumor.
- Stress fractures: uncommon.

Clinical Evaluation

- The patient typically presents with a shortened and externally rotated lower extremity.
- Range of motion is painful with variable crepitus.
- Swelling, ecchymosis, and tenderness to palpation are generally present over the injured hip.
- A careful neurovascular examination should be performed.

Radiographic Evaluation

- Anteroposterior views of the pelvis and a cross-table lateral view of the affected hip should be obtained.
- Developmental coxa vara should not be confused with hip fracture, especially in patients <5 years of age. Comparison with the contralateral hip may aid in the distinction.
- Computed tomography may aid in the diagnosis of nondisplaced fractures or stress fractures.
- A radioisotope bone scan obtained 48 hours postinjury may demonstrate increased uptake at the occult fracture site.

DELBERT CLASSIFICATION OF PEDIATRIC HIP FRACTURES (FIG. 45.2)

Type I: transepiphyseal fracture

- This type comprises 8% of pediatric hip fractures.
- The incidence of osteonecrosis approaches 100%.
- The end of the spectrum is a slipped capital femoral epiphysis; consider hypothyroidism, hypogonadism, and renal disease.
- In newborns, differential diagnosis includes developmental dysplasia of the hip (DDH) and septic arthritis.

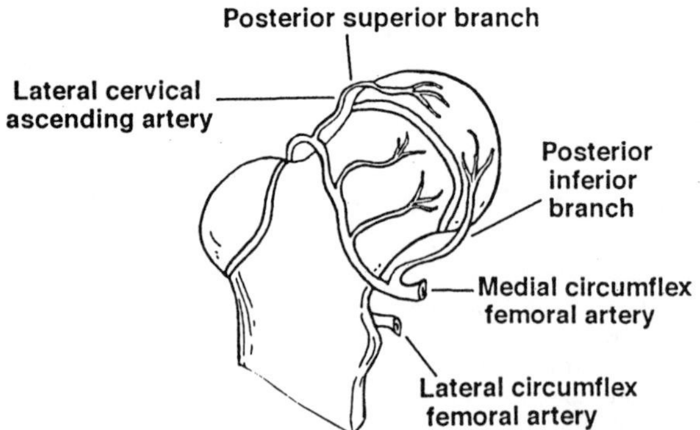

FIG. 45.1. Arterial supply of the proximal femur. The capital femoral epiphysis and physis are supplied by the medial circumflex artery through two retinacular vessel systems—the posterosuperior and posteroinferior. The lateral circumflex artery supplies the greater trochanter and its portion of the proximal femoral physis, as well as a small area of the anteromedial metaphysis. (From Rockwood CA Jr, Wilkins KE, Beaty JH, eds. *Rockwood and Green's fractures in children,* 4th ed. Vol. 3. Philadelphia: Lippincott-Raven, 1996:1149, with permission.)

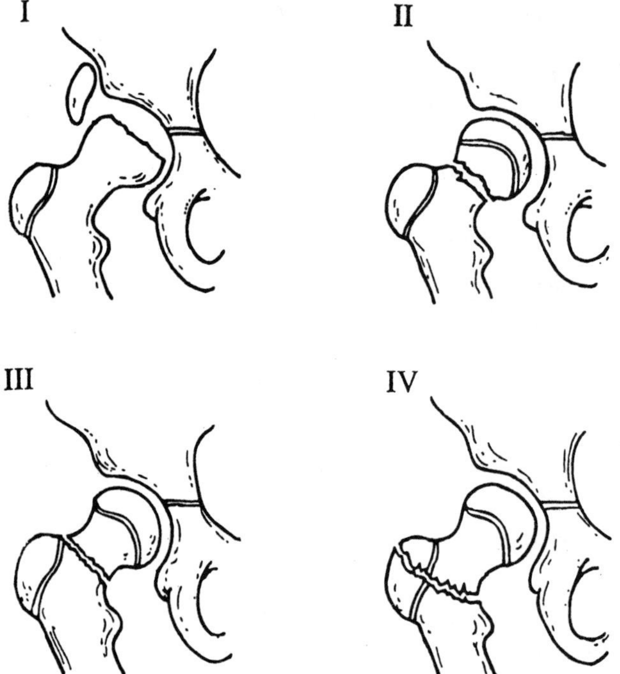

FIG. 45.2. Classification of hip fractures in children. Type I, Transepiphyseal, with or without dislocation from the acetabulum; type II, transcervical; type III, cervicotrochanteric; and type IV, trochanteric. (From Rockwood CA Jr, Wilkins KE, Beaty JH, eds. *Rockwood and Green's fractures in children,* 4th ed. Vol. 3. Philadelphia: Lippincott-Raven, 1996:1151, with permission.)

Type II: transcervical fracture

- This encompasses 45% of pediatric hip fractures (most common type).
- Eighty percent are displaced.
- Osteonecrosis occurs in up to 50% of cases.

Type III: cervicotrochanteric fracture

- This type includes 30% of pediatric hip fractures.
- It is more common in children than in adults.
- The rate of osteonecrosis is from 20% to 30%.

Type IV: intertrochanteric fracture

- This fracture comprises 10% to 15% of pediatric hip fractures.
- Fewer complications than in other hip fractures because vascular supply is more abundant.

Treatment

Type I: Closed reduction with pin fixation, using threaded pins in an older child and smooth pins in a young child. Open reduction and internal fixation may be necessary if irreducible by closed methods.

Type II: If nondisplaced, use of abduction spica cast versus *in situ* pinning; these fractures may go on to coxa vara or nonunion. With a displaced fracture, treat with closed reduction and pinning (open reduction used as necessary); transphyseal pinning should be avoided.

Type III: If nondisplaced, traction employed; then choose from spica versus immediate abduction spica versus *in situ* pinning. With a displaced fracture, treat with open reduction and internal fixation and avoidance of transphyseal pinning.

Type IV: 2 to 3 weeks of traction, then abduction spica for 6 to 12 weeks. Open reduction and internal fixation may be necessary for unstable fractures or if unable to achieve closed reduction with initial treatment.

Complications

- *Osteonecrosis.* Overall incidence is 40% after pediatric hip fracture; this is directly related to initial fracture displacement and fracture location. Ratliff described the following three types:
  - Type I: diffuse, complete head involvement, and collapse; poor prognosis (60%).
  - Type II: localized head involvement only; minimal collapse (22%).
  - Type III: femoral neck only involved; spares head (18%).
- *Premature physeal closure.* Incidence is no more than 60% and increases with pin penetration of the physis. This may result in femoral shortening, coxa vara, and a short femoral neck. The proximal femoral epiphysis contributes to only 15% of growth of the entire lower extremity. However, the presence of premature physeal closure in association with osteonecrosis may result in significant leg length discrepancies.
- *Coxa vara.* Incidence is 20%; it is usually secondary to inadequate reduction. Open reduction and internal fixation are associated with a reduced incidence of coxa vara.
- *Nonunion.* Incidence is 10% and is primarily due to inadequate reduction or inadequate internal fixation. This may require valgus osteotomy with or without a bone graft to achieve union.

DISLOCATION

Epidemiology

- More common than hip fractures.
- Bimodal distribution with incidence greater between 2 and 5 years, due to joint laxity and soft pliable cartilage, and between 11 and 15 years of age, as injuries associated with athletics and vehicular trauma become more common.
- Posterior dislocations 10 times more frequent than anterior dislocations.

Mechanism of Injury

- Younger patients (age of <5 years): may occur with relatively insignificant trauma, such as a fall from standing.

- Older patients (age >11 years): tend to occur with athletic participation and vehicular accidents (bicycles, automobiles, etc.). In this age group, a higher association with acetabular fractures is found.

Clinical Evaluation

- In cases of posterior hip dislocation, the patient typically presents with the affected hip flexed, adducted, and internally rotated. Anterior hip dislocation typically demonstrates extension, abduction, and external rotation of the affected hip.
- A careful neurovascular examination, with documentation of integrity of the sciatic nerve and its branches, is essential. This should be repeated after manipulation of the hip.
- Ipsilateral femoral fracture often occurs; it must be ruled out before forceful manipulation of the hip.

Radiographic Evaluation

- Anteroposterior views of the pelvis and a lateral view of the affected hip should be obtained.
- Pain, swelling, or obvious deformity in the femoral region is an indication for femoral radiographs to rule out an associated fracture.
- Fracture fragments from the femoral head or acetabulum are typically more readily appreciated on radiographs obtained after reduction of the hip dislocation as anatomic landmarks are better delineated.
- After reduction, computed tomography may be obtained to delineate associated femoral head or acetabular fracture and the presence of any interposing soft tissue.

DESCRIPTIVE CLASSIFICATION

- Direction: anterior versus posterior
- Fracture-dislocation: fractures to the femoral head or acetabulum
- Associated injuries: presence of ipsilateral femoral fracture, etc.

Treatment

Nonoperative Treatment

- Closed reduction under conscious sedation may be performed for patients presenting less than 12 hours after dislocation.
- Skeletal traction may be used for reduction of an old, overlooked, or neglected hip dislocation. Reduction should take place over a 3- to 6-day period, and traction should be continued for an additional 2 to 3 weeks to achieve stability.

Operative Treatment

- Dislocations more than 12 hours old may require reduction under general anesthesia. Open reduction with surgical removal of the interposing capsule, inverted limbus, or osteocartilaginous fragments may be necessary if the injury proves irreducible.
- Open reduction is also indicated in cases of sciatic nerve compromise in which surgical exploration is necessary.
- Hip dislocations associated with ipsilateral femoral shaft fractures should initially be addressed with reduction of the dislocation. If manipulative closed reduction is unsuccessful, skeletal traction may be applied to the trochanteric region to allow control of the proximal fragment. Internal or external fixation of the femoral shaft fracture may then be performed. Occasionally, operative fixation of the femoral shaft fracture is necessary to achieve stable reduction of the hip.
- Postoperatively, the patient should be placed in skeletal traction or a spica cast for 4 to 6 weeks to achieve hip stability.

Complications

- *Osteonecrosis (8% to 10%).* This has a decreased incidence with an age of <5 years and an increased incidence with severe displacement and delay in reduction.

- *Epiphyseal separation.* Traumatic physeal injury may occur at the time of dislocation and may result in osteonecrosis.
- *Recurrent dislocations.* In traumatic cases this may be due to absolute capsular tears or capsular attenuation. It is also associated with hyperlaxity or congenital syndromes (e.g., Down syndrome). It may be addressed with surgical "tightening" of the hip, consisting of capsular repair or plication and spica casting for 4 to 6 weeks postoperatively.
- *Degenerative joint disease.* This may result due to nonconcentric reductions that are secondary to trapped soft-tissue or bony fragments; it can also result from the initial trauma. Articular incongruity secondary to associated femoral head or acetabular fracture or entrapped osteochondral fragments may exacerbate the degenerative processes.

46. PEDIATRIC FEMORAL SHAFT

EPIDEMIOLOGY

- These fractures represent 1.6% of all fractures in the pediatric population.
- Males are more commonly affected at a ratio of 2.6:1.
- A bimodal distribution of incidence occurs; the first peak is from 2 to 4 years of age, and the second is in mid-adolescence.
- In children younger than walking age, 80% are caused by child abuse; this decreases to 30% in toddlers.
- In adolescence, >90% of femoral fractures are caused by motor vehicle accidents.

ANATOMY

- During childhood, remodeling in the femur triggers a change from primarily weaker woven bone to stronger lamellar bone.
- Up to age 16, a geometric increase in the shaft diameter and relative cortical thickness of the femur occurs, resulting in a markedly increased area moment of inertia and strength (Fig. 46.1). This partially explains the bimodal distribution of injury pattern, in which younger patients experience fractures under load conditions reached in normal play or minor trauma, whereas in adolescence high velocity trauma is required to reach the stresses necessary for fracture.

MECHANISM OF INJURY

- Direct trauma: motor vehicle accidents, pedestrian injuries, falls, and child abuse.
- Indirect trauma: rotational injuries.
- Pathologic fractures: osteogenesis imperfecta, nonossifying fibroma, bone cysts, tumors. Severe involvement from myelomeningocele or cerebral palsy may result in generalized osteopenia and a predisposition to fracture with minor trauma.

CLINICAL EVALUATION

- Patients with a history of high energy injury should undergo a full trauma evaluation dictated by that history.
- The presence of a femoral shaft fracture results in an inability to ambulate and in extreme pain, variable swelling, and variable gross deformity. The diagnosis is more difficult in patients with multiple trauma or head injuries or with nonambulatory, severely disabled children.
- A careful neurovascular examination is essential.
- Splints or bandages placed in the field must be removed, and a careful examination of the overlying soft tissues should be conducted to rule out the possibility of an open fracture.
- Hypotension from an isolated femoral shaft fracture is uncommon; the Waddell triad of head injury, intraabdominal or intrathoracic trauma, and femoral shaft fracture is strongly associated with vehicular trauma and is a more likely cause of volume loss. However, the presence of a severely swollen thigh may indicate high volume loss into muscle compartments surrounding the fracture.
- Compartment syndrome is rare; it occurs only with severe hemorrhage into thigh compartments.
- The ipsilateral hip and knee should be examined for associated injuries.

RADIOGRAPHIC EVALUATION

- Anteroposterior and lateral views of the femur should be obtained.
- Radiographs of the hip and knee should be taken to rule out associated injuries; intertrochanteric fractures, femoral neck fractures, hip dislocation, physeal injuries to the distal femur, ligamentous disruptions, meniscal tears, and tibial fractures have all been described in association with femoral shaft fractures.
- Magnetic resonance imaging and bone scans are generally unnecessary, but they may aid in the diagnosis of otherwise occult nondisplaced, buckle, or stress fractures.

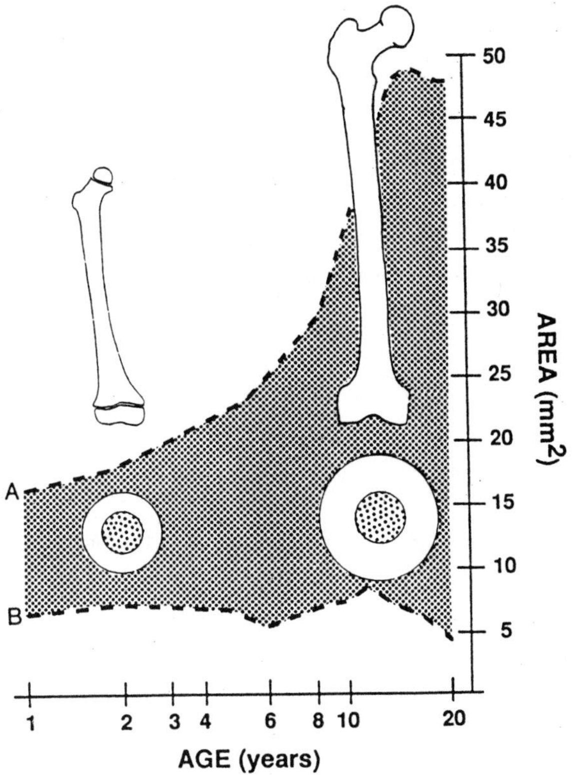

FIG. 46.1. Age-related changes in bone geometry. The shaded area represents cortical thickness by age group. This rapid increase in cortical thickness may contribute to the diminishing incidence of femoral fractures during late childhood. (From Netter FH. *The Ciba collection of medical illustrations*. Vol. 8. *Musculoskeletal system*. Part I. *Anatomy, physiology, and metabolic disorders*. Summit, NJ: Ciba-Geigy, 1987, with permission.)

DESCRIPTIVE CLASSIFICATION

- Open versus closed
- Level of fracture: proximal, middle, distal third
- Fracture pattern: transverse, spiral, oblique, butterfly fragment
- Comminution
- Displacement
- Angulation

ANATOMIC CLASSIFICATION

- Subtrochanteric
- Shaft
- Supracondylar

TREATMENT

Treatment depends on the age of the patient and the fracture pattern encountered.

Newborn to 2 Years of Age
Early spica cast.

From 2 to 10 Years of Age
- Less than 2 cm overriding: early spica cast.
- More than 2 cm overriding: traction (preferably distal femoral pin proximal to the physis), followed by a spica cast.
- External fixation: considered for multiple injuries or open fracture.

From 10 to 15 Years of Age
- Distal femoral traction, followed by intramedullary fixation for definitive care.
- External fixation considered for multiple injuries or open fracture.

Reduction Criteria
- Length
  - Two to 10 years of age: up to 2 cm overriding acceptable.
  - Age >10 years: up to 1 cm overriding acceptable.
- Angulation
  - Sagittal plane: up to 30 degrees is acceptable.
  - Frontal plane: up to 10 degrees is acceptable.
  - Varies with pattern, age, and location of fracture along femur.
- Rotation
  - Up to 10 degrees acceptable; external rotation is better tolerated than internal rotation.

Operative Indications
The following indicate the need for operative fixation:

- Multiple trauma, including head trauma
- Open fracture
- Vascular injury
- Pathologic fracture
- Uncooperative patient

Operative Options
- Intramedullary nailing
  - Flexible nails (Enders): applied from above the distal femoral physis.
  - Reamed locked intramedullary nails: place antegrade through the piriformis fossa. The distal physis should not be traversed. Not recommended for patients younger than 12 years of age (proximal femoral physis open) because proximal femoral growth abnormalities and osteonecrosis of the femoral head due to disruption of the vascular supply are possible complications.
  - Use: most effective in the isolated fracture or in the hemodynamically stable, multiply injured patient.
- External fixation
  - Lateral, unilateral frame: spares the quadriceps mechanism.
  - Multiple trauma: useful; especially in those who are hemodynamically unstable or have open fractures and in burn patients.
- Plate fixation
  - May be accomplished using a 4.5-mm compression plate and interfragmentary compression of comminuted fragments; less desirable because of the long incision necessary, significant periosteal stripping, scarring, plate removal, and infection.

COMPLICATIONS
- *Malunion.* Remodeling will not correct rotational defects; the older patient will not remodel as well as the younger patient. Anteroposterior remodeling in the femur occurs much more rapidly and completely in the femur than with varus/valgus angular deformity. For this reason, greater degrees of sagittal angulation are acceptable.

- *Nonunion.* This is rare; even with segmental fractures, children often have sufficient osteogenic potential to fill moderate deficiencies. Children from 5 to 10 years of age with established nonunion may require bone grafting and plate fixation; the trend in older (>12 years) children involves bone grafting and locked intramedullary nailing.
- *Muscle weakness.* Many patients demonstrate weakness, typically in the hip abductors, quadriceps, or hamstrings, and up to a 30% decrease in strength and 1-cm thigh atrophy when compared with the contralateral uninjured lower extremity; however, this is seldom clinically significant.
- *Leg length discrepancy.* This may be secondary to shortening or overgrowth. It represents the most common complication of femoral shaft fracture.
  - ***Overgrowth.*** An overgrowth of 1.5 to 2.0 cm is common in the ages from 2 to 10 years. It is most common during the initial 2 years following the fracture, especially with fractures of the distal third of the femur and those associated with greater degrees of trauma.
  - ***Shortening.*** Up to 2.0 cm (age dependent) of initial shortening is acceptable due to the potential for overgrowth. For fractures with greater than 3.0 cm of shortening, skeletal traction may be used before spica casting to obtain adequate length. If the shortening is unacceptable at 6 weeks following the injury, the decision must be made as to whether osteoclasis and distraction with external fixation are preferable to a later limb length equalization procedure. Most authors recommend early external fixation.
- *Osteonecrosis.* Proximal femoral osteonecrosis may result with the antegrade placement of an intramedullary nail due to the precarious vascular supply. This is of particular concern when the proximal femoral physis is not yet closed because the major vascular supply to the femoral head is derived from the lateral ascending cervical artery that crosses the capsule at the level of the trochanteric notch. Radiographic changes may be seen as late as 15 months after antegrade intramedullary nailing.

47. PEDIATRIC KNEE

OVERVIEW

- The knee is a ginglymoid (hinge) joint consisting of three articulations: patellofemoral, tibiofemoral, and tibiofibular.
- Under normal cyclical loading, the knee may experience up to five times the individual's body weight per step.
- The normal range of motion is from 10 degrees of extension to 140 degrees of flexion with 8 to 12 degrees of rotation through the flexion-extension arc.
- The dynamic and static stability of the knee is conferred mainly by soft tissues (ligaments, muscles, tendons, menisci) in addition to the bony articulations.
- Because ligaments in the immature skeleton are more resistant to tensile stresses than are physeal plates, trauma leads to physeal separations and avulsions not seen in the skeletally mature patient.
- Three physeal plates with secondary ossification centers are found.
- Appearance of ossification centers is as follows:
  - Distal femur: 39th fetal week
  - Proximal tibia: birth
  - Tibial tubercle: 7 to 9 years
- Physeal closure occurs as follows:
  - Distal femur: 16 to 19 years
  - Proximal tibia: 16 to 19 years
  - Tibial tubercle: 15 to 17 years
- The patella is a sesamoid bone, with its own ossification center, which appears between the ages of 3 to 5 years.
- The tibial spine is the site of insertion for the anterior cruciate ligament (ACL).
- Two-thirds of the longitudinal growth of the lower extremity is provided by the distal femoral (9 mm/year) and proximal tibial (6 mm/year) physes.

DISTAL FEMORAL FRACTURES

Epidemiology

- The most commonly interrupted physis is around the knee.
- One percent to 6% of all epiphyseal injuries.
- Majority (two-thirds) occur in adolescents.

Anatomy

- The distal femoral epiphysis is the largest and fastest growing physis in the body (9 mm/year).
- No inherent protection of the physis exists; ligamentous and tendinous structures insert on the epiphysis.
- The sciatic nerve divides at the level of the distal femur.
- The popliteal artery gives off the superior geniculate branches to the knee just posterior to the femoral metaphysis.

Mechanism of Injury

- Direct trauma to the distal femur: uncommon but may occur from vehicular trauma, falling onto a flexed knee, or during athletic activity, such as a lateral blow to the knee with a planted cleated foot in football. In infants, this injury must be suspected of occurring as a result of child abuse.
- Indirect injury: varus/valgus; hyperextension/hyperflexion; usually results in simultaneous compression to one aspect of the physis with distraction to another and with the epiphysis separating from the metaphysis due to tension. Most typically, the physeal fracture exits the metaphysis on the compression side, resulting in a Salter-Harris type II fracture (Fig. 47.1).
- Birth injury: breech presentation.
- Minimal trauma: in conditions that cause generalized weakening of the growth plate (osteomyelitis, leukemia, myelodysplasia).

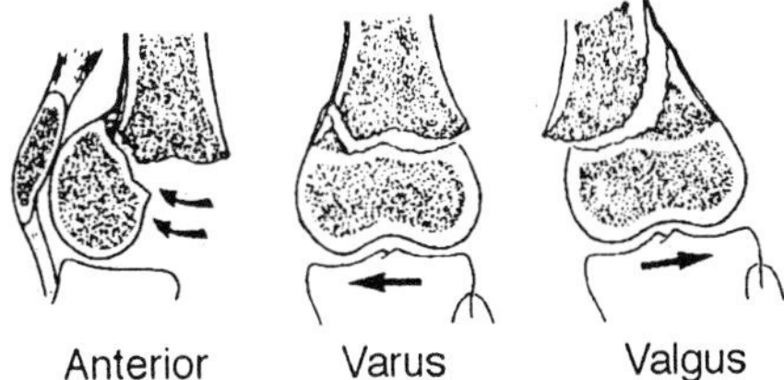

FIG. 47.1. Salter-Harris type II fractures of the distal femur. (From Ogden JA. *Skeletal injury in the child,* 2nd ed. Philadelphia: W.B. Saunders, 1990:725, with permission.)

Clinical Evaluation

- The patient typically presents unable to bear weight on the affected lower extremity, although nondisplaced physeal injuries from low energy mechanisms (e.g., athletic injury) may ambulate with an antalgic gait.
- Older children and adolescents may relate a history of hearing or feeling a "pop"; with associated knee effusion and soft-tissue swelling, this may be confused with a ligamentous injury.
- The knee is typically in flexion due to hamstring spasm.
- Gross shortening or angular deformity varies with potential compromise of neurovascular status due to traction injuries or laceration. A complete neurovascular assessment is thus critical.
- Point tenderness may be elicited over the physis; this is usually performed by palpation of the distal femur at the level of the superior pole of the patella and adductor tubercle.

Radiographic Evaluation

- Anteroposterior, lateral, and oblique views should be obtained. Radiographs of the contralateral lower extremity may be obtained for comparison.
- Stress views may be taken to diagnose nondisplaced separations in which the clinical examination is highly suggestive of physeal injury. The physeal line should be 3 to 5 mm thick until adolescence.
- Salter-Harris type III injuries usually have vertically oriented epiphyseal components that occur in the sagittal plane and are thus best appreciated on anteroposterior views.
- Tomograms or computed tomography may be useful for assessing articular involvement or aiding in fracture definition.
- In infants, separation of the distal femoral physis may be difficult unless gross displacement is present because only the center of the epiphysis is ossified at birth. This should be in line with the anatomic axis of the femur on both anteroposterior and lateral views. Magnetic resonance imaging, ultrasound, or arthrography may aid in the diagnosis of distal femoral injury in these patients.
- Arteriography of the lower extremity should be pursued if vascular injury is suspected.

SALTER-HARRIS CLASSIFICATION

Type I: Seen in newborns and adolescents; diagnosis easily missed; physeal widening may be demonstrated on stress radiographs.

Type II: Most common injury of the distal femoral physis; displacement usually medial or lateral with metaphyseal fragment on compression side.

Type III: Intraarticular fracture exiting the epiphysis.

Type IV: Intraarticular fracture exiting the metaphysis; high incidence of growth inhibition with bar formation; rare injury.

Type V: Physeal crush injury; difficult diagnosis that is often made retrospectively after growth arrest; narrowing of physis possible.

CLASSFICATION BY DISPLACEMENT

Anterior: Results from hyperextension injury; high incidence of neurovascular injury from proximal metaphyseal spike driven posteriorly.
Posterior: Rare injury caused by knee hyperflexion.
Medial: Valgus force most common; usually Salter-Harris type II.
Lateral: Varus force.

Treatment

Nonoperative Treatment

- Nonoperative treatment is indicated for nondisplaced fractures.
- Tense effusions may be addressed with sterile aspiration for symptomatic relief.
- The lower extremity should be immobilized in a long-leg cast or hip spica cast with 15 to 20 degrees of knee flexion; close follow-up with serial radiographs is required to prevent displacement.
- Isometric exercises should be instituted as soon as symptoms permit; straight leg raises are usually possible 1 week after injury.
- Crutch ambulation with toe-touch weight bearing may be instituted at 3 to 6 weeks postinjury.
- The cast may be discontinued between 4 to 8 weeks, depending on the patient's age and healing status. A removable posterior splint and active range-of-motion exercises are instituted at this time.
- Athletic involvement should be restricted until knee range of motion is optimized, symptoms have resolved, and sufficient quadriceps strength has been regained.

Operative Treatment

- Closed reduction under general anesthesia may be performed for displaced fractures in which a stable result can be obtained. Sufficient traction should be applied during manipulation to minimize grinding of physeal cartilage. The position of immobilization varies with the direction of displacement as follows:
  - Medial/lateral: immobilize in 15 to 20 degrees of knee flexion.
  - Anterior: immobilize first at 90 degrees, then decrease with time.
  - Posterior: immobilize in extension.
- Indications for open reduction and internal fixation include the following:
  - Irreducible Salter-Harris type II with interposed soft tissue: cannulated 4.0- or 6.5-mm screw fixation used to secure the metaphyseal spike.
  - Unstable reduction: smooth percutaneous wires or pins used.
  - Salter-Harris type III and IV: joint congruity must be restored.
- To minimize residual deformity and growth disturbance, the following guidelines should be observed for internal fixation:
  - Avoid crossing physis, if possible.
  - If physis must be crossed, use smooth pins as perpendicular as possible to the physis.
  - Remove fixation as soon as possible.
- Postoperatively, the patient is maintained in a long-leg cast in 10 degrees of knee flexion. The patient may be ambulatory with crutches in 1 to 2 days; this should be non–weight bearing with regard to the operated extremity. At 1 week, the patient may begin straight leg raises.
- If at 4 weeks evidence of osseous healing is demonstrated radiographically, the cast may be discontinued and a posterior splint may be placed for protection. The patient may be advanced to partial weight bearing with active range-of-motion exercises.
- The patient typically resumes a normal, active lifestyle between 4 and 6 months following injury.

Complications

Acute

- *Popliteal artery injury (<2%).* This is associated with hyperextension injuries in which a traction injury may be sustained or with direct laceration from the sharp metaphyseal spike.

A cool pulseless foot that persists despite reduction should include an angiography in the work-up to rule out laceration.
Vascular impingement that resolves after reduction should be observed for 48 to 72 hours to rule out an intimal tear and thrombosis.

- *Peroneal nerve palsy (3%).* This is caused by traction injury during fracture or reduction. Persistent peroneal palsy over 3 to 6 months should be evaluated by electromyography with possible exploration when indicated.
- *Recurrent displacement.* Fractures with questionable stability following closed reduction should receive operative fixation (either percutaneous pins or internal fixation) to prevent late or recurrent displacement. Anterior and posterior displacements are particularly unstable.

Late

- *Knee instability.* In up to 40% of patients, knee instability may be present, indicating concomitant ligamentous compromise that was not appreciated at the time of index presentation. The patient may be treated with rehabilitation for lower extremity strengthening or may require operative treatment.
- *Angular deformity (19%).* This may be due to initial physeal injury (Salter-Harris types I and II), asymmetric physeal closure (bar formation, Salter-Harris types III and IV), or unrecognized physeal injury (Salter-Harris type V). Observation, physeal bar excision (<30% of physis, <2 years of remaining growth), hemiepiphysiodesis, epiphyseolysis, or wedge osteotomy may be indicated.
- *Leg length discrepancy (24%).* This is usually clinically insignificant if <2 years of growth remain; otherwise, the discrepancy tends to progress at the rate of 1 cm per year.
  Discrepancy <2.5 cm at skeletal maturity usually is of no functional or cosmetic significance.
  A discrepancy between 2.5 to 5 cm may be treated with contralateral epiphysiodesis (femoral or tibial) or femoral shortening.
  A discrepancy of >5 cm may be an indication for femoral lengthening combined with epiphysiodesis of the contralateral distal femur or proximal tibia.
- *Knee stiffness (16%).* This may be due to adhesions, and it involves capsular or muscular contractures. It is usually related to duration of immobilization; therefore, early discontinuation of the cast with active range of motion is desirable.

PROXIMAL TIBIAL FRACTURES

Epidemiology

- Less than 1% of all physeal injuries.
- Average age of occurrence of 14 years.
- Most in adolescent males.

Anatomy

- The popliteal artery traverses the posterior aspect of the knee and is tethered to the knee capsule by connective tissue septa posterior to the proximal tibia. The vascular supply is derived from the anastomosis of the inferior geniculate arteries (Fig. 47.2).
- The physis is well protected by osseous and soft-tissue structures, which may account for the low incidence of injuries to this structure:
  Lateral: fibula
  Anterior: tibial tubercle
  Medial: medial collateral ligament (inserts into metaphysis)
  Posteromedial: semimembranosus insertion

Mechanism of Injury

- Direct: trauma to the proximal tibia (e.g., motor vehicle bumper, lawnmower accident).
- Indirect: more common; hyperextension, abduction, or hyperflexion from athletic injuries; motor vehicle accidents; falls; or landing from a jump.
- Birth injury: hyperextension during breech delivery.
- Pathologic condition: osteomyelitis of the proximal tibia or myelomeningocele.

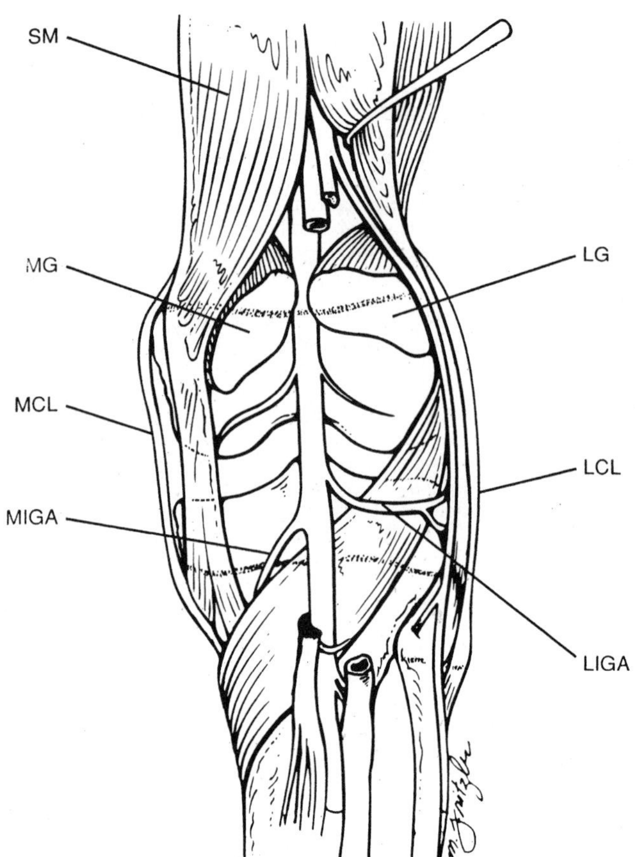

FIG. 47.2. Posterior anatomy of the right popliteal region. Note that the popliteal vessels are protected from bone (especially the tibia) only by the popliteus muscle. The vessels are tethered by the geniculate branches and by the trifurcation. Abbreviations: *LCL*, lateral collateral ligament; *LIGA*, lateral inferior geniculate artery; *MCL*, medial collateral ligament; *MIGA*, medial inferior geniculate artery; *MG* and *LG*, medial and lateral gastrocnemius heads; *SM*, semimembranosus. (From Rockwood CA Jr, Wilkins KE, Beaty JH, eds. *Rockwood and Green's fractures in children*, 4th ed. Vol. 3. Philadelphia: Lippincott-Raven, 1996:1265, with permission.)

Clinical Evaluation

- Patients typically present with an inability to bear weight on the injured extremity. The knee may be tense with hemarthrosis, and extension is limited by hamstring spasm.
- Tenderness is present 1- to 1.5-cm distal to the joint line; variable gross deformity is also present.
- Neurovascular status should be carefully documented to assess for popliteal artery or peroneal nerve compromise. The anterior, superficial posterior, and deep posterior compartments should be palpated for pain or turgor. Patients suspected to have elevated compartment pressures should receive serial neurovascular examinations with measuring of compartment pressures.
- Associated ligamentous injuries should be suspected, although appreciating these injuries secondary to the dramatic presentation of the fracture can be difficult.

Radiographic Evaluation

- Anteroposterior, lateral, and oblique views of the affected knee should be obtained.
- Radiographs of the contralateral knee may be taken for comparison.
- Stress radiographs in coronal and sagittal planes may be obtained, but hyperextension of the knee should be avoided due to potential injury to popliteal structures.
- Most patients with proximal tibial physeal injuries are adolescents in whom the secondary ossicle of the tibial tubercle has appeared. A smooth horizontal radiolucency at the base of the tibial tubercle should not be confused with an epiphyseal fracture.
- Magnetic resonance imaging may aid in identification of soft-tissue interposition in cases in which reduction is difficult or impossible.
- Computed tomography may aid in fracture definition, especially with Salter-Harris type III or IV fractures.
- Arteriography may be indicated in patients in whom vascular compromise (popliteal) is suspected.

SALTER-HARRIS CLASSIFICATION

Type I: Transphyseal injury; diagnosis often missed; may require stress or comparison views.

Type II: Transphyseal injury exiting the metaphysis; one-third are nondisplaced; those that displace usually do so medially into valgus.

Type III: Intraarticular fracture of the lateral plateau; more common than the medial; fracture line exits the physis.

Type IV: Intraarticular fracture of the medial or lateral plateau; fracture line exits the metaphysis.

Type V: Crush injury; retrospective diagnosis after growth arrest.

CLASSIFICATION BY DISPLACEMENT

Medial: Abduction force.

Posterior: Hyperextension force; increased incidence of popliteal artery injury.

Tibial tubercle and fibula prevent anterior and lateral displacements, respectively.

Treatment

Nonoperative Treatment

- Nondisplaced fractures may be treated with a long-leg cast with the knee flexed to 30 degrees. The patient should be followed closely with serial radiographs to avoid displacement.
- Displaced fractures may be addressed with gentle closed reduction with limited varus and hyperextension stress to minimize traction to the peroneal nerve and popliteal vasculature, respectively. The patient is placed in a long-leg cast in flexion (typically 30 to 60 degrees, depending on the position of stability).
- The cast may be discontinued between 4 to 6 weeks postinjury. If the patient is symptomatically improved and if radiographic evidence of healing is documented, active range-of-motion and quadriceps strengthening exercises should be initiated.

Operative Treatment

- Displaced Salter type I or II fractures in which stable reduction cannot be maintained may be addressed with percutaneous smooth pins across the physis (type I) or parallel to the physis (metaphysis, type II).
- Open reduction and internal fixation are indicated for displaced Salter-Harris types III and IV to restore articular congruity. This may be achieved with pin or screw fixation parallel to the physis; articular congruity is the goal.
- Postoperatively, the patient is immobilized in a long-leg cast with the knee flexed to 30 degrees. This is continued for between 6 to 8 weeks at which time the cast may be discontinued with initiation of active range-of-motion exercises.

Complications

Acute

- Recurrent displacement: may occur if closed reduction and casting without operative fixation are performed on an unstable injury.
- Popliteal artery injury: especially in hyperextension injuries; related to the tethering of the popliteal artery to the knee capsule posterior to the proximal tibia. Arteriography may be indicated for cases in which distal pulses do not return after prompt reduction of the injury.
- Peroneal nerve palsy: traction injury due to displacement, either at the time of injury or of attempted closed reduction, especially with a varus moment applied to the injury site.

Late

- Angular deformity: due to initial physeal injury (Salter-Harris types I and II), asymmetric physeal closure (bar formation, Salter-Harris types III and IV), or unrecognized physeal injury (Salter-Harris type V). Observation, physeal bar excision (<30% of physis, <2 years of remaining growth), hemiepiphysiodesis, epiphyseolysis, or wedge osteotomy may be indicated.
- Leg length discrepancy: usually clinically insignificant if <2 years of growth remain; otherwise, discrepancy generally progresses at the rate of 1 cm per year.
  - A discrepancy of <2.5 cm at skeletal maturity usually is of no functional or cosmetic significance.
  - Discrepancies from 2.5 to 5 cm may be treated with contralateral epiphysiodesis (femoral or tibial) or femoral shortening.
  - A discrepancy >5 cm may be an indication for femoral lengthening combined with epiphysiodesis of the contralateral distal femur or proximal tibia.

TIBIAL TUBERCLE FRACTURES

Epidemiology

- Represent 1% to 3% of all physeal injuries.
- Seen most commonly in athletic males from 14 to 16 years of age.
- Important to differentiate from Osgood-Schlatter disease.

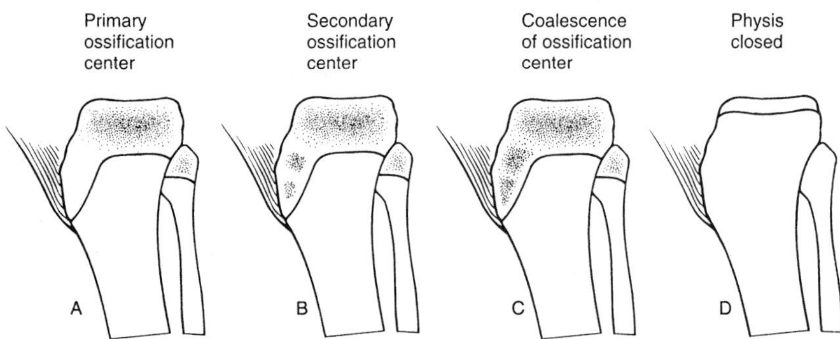

FIG. 47.3. Development of the tibial tubercle. **A.** In the *cartilaginous stage,* no ossification center is present in the cartilaginous anlage of the tibial tubercle. **B.** In the *apophyseal stage,* the secondary ossification center(s) forms in the cartilaginous anlage of the tibial tubercle. **C.** In the *epiphyseal stage,* the primary and secondary ossification centers of the proximal tibial epiphysis have coalesced. **D.** In the *bony stage,* the proximal tibial physis has closed. (From Rockwood CA Jr, Wilkins KE, Beaty JH, eds. *Rockwood and Green's fractures in children,* 4th ed. Vol. 3. Philadelphia: Lippincott-Raven, 1996:1274, with permission.)

Anatomy (Fig. 47.3)

- The tibial tubercle physis, which is continuous with the tibial plateau, is most vulnerable between the ages of 13 and 16 years when it closes from posterior to anterior.
- Because the insertion of the medial retinaculum extends beyond the proximal tibial physis into the metaphysis, limited active extension of the knee is still possible after tibial tubercle fractures, although patella alta and extensor lag are present.

Mechanism of Injury

- The mechanism of injury is typically indirect, usually resulting from a sudden accelerating or decelerating force involving the quadriceps mechanism.
- Predisposing factors include the following:
  - Patella baja;
  - Tight hamstrings;
  - Preexisting Osgood-Schlatter disease;
  - Disorders with physeal anomalies.

Clinical Evaluation

- Patients typically present with a limited ability to extend the knee, as well as an extensor lag.
- Swelling and tenderness over the tibial tubercle are typically present, often with a palpable defect.
- Hemarthrosis is variable.
- Patella alta may be observed if severe displacement has occurred.

Radiographic Evaluation

- Anteroposterior and lateral views of the knee are sufficient for the diagnosis; a slight internal rotation view best delineates the injury as the tibial tubercle lies just lateral to the tibial axis.
- Patella alta may be noted.

WATSON-JONES CLASSIFICATION

Type I: Small fragment avulsed and displaced proximally.

Type II: Secondary ossification center already coalesced with proximal tibial epiphysis; fracture at this junction.

Type III: Fracture line passing proximally through the tibial epiphysis and into the joint.

OGDEN CLASSIFICATION (FIG. 47.4)

Modification of Watson-Jones (above); subdivides each type into A and B categories to account for degree of displacement and comminution.

Treatment

Nonoperative Treatment

- This is indicated for type IA fractures.
- Treatment consists of manual reduction, followed by immobilization in a long-leg cast with the knee extended and patellar molding.
- The cast is continued for 4 to 6 weeks, at which time the patient may be placed in a posterior splint for an additional 2 weeks. Gentle active range-of-motion exercises and quadriceps strengthening exercises are instituted and advanced as the symptoms abate.

Operative Treatment

- This is indicated for type IB, II, and III fractures.
- A vertical midline approach is used to access the fractured tubercle, which may be addressed with smooth pins (>3 years from skeletal maturity), screws, threaded Steinmann pins, or tension bands.
- Postoperatively, the patient is placed in a long-leg cast in extension with patellar molding for 4 to 6 weeks, at which time the patient may be placed in a posterior splint for an additional 2 weeks.

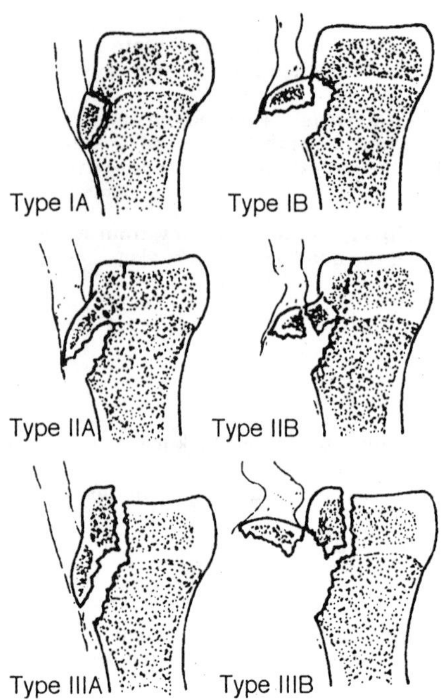

FIG. 47.4. Ogden classification of tibial tuberosity fractures in children. (From Ogden JA. *Skeletal injury in the child,* 2nd ed. Philadelphia: W.B. Saunders, 1990:808, with permission.)

- Gentle active range-of-motion exercises and quadriceps strengthening exercises are instituted and advanced as symptoms subside.

Complications

- *Genu recurvatum.* This is secondary to premature closure of anterior physis and is rare because the injury occurs typically in adolescent patients near skeletal maturity.
- *Possible loss of knee flexion or extension.* Loss of flexion may be related to scarring or postoperative immobilization. The loss of extension may be related to nonanatomic reduction and emphasizes the need for operative fixation of type IB, II, and III fractures.
- *Patella alta.* This may occur if reduction is insufficient.
- *Osteonecrosis of fracture fragment.* This is rare due to soft-tissue attachments.
- *Compartment syndrome.* Although this is rare, it may occur with concomitant tearing of the anterior tibial recurrent vessels that retract to the anterior compartment when torn.

TIBIAL SPINE (INTERCONDYLAR EMINENCE) FRACTURES

Epidemiology

- Relatively rare injury: 3 per 100,000 children per year.
- Most commonly due to a fall from a bicycle (50%).

Anatomy

- Two tibial spines, anterior and posterior, exist. The ACL spans from the medial aspect of the lateral femoral condyle to the anterior tibial spine.
- Because ligaments are more resistant to tensile stresses in the immature skeleton than are physeal cartilage or cancellous bone, forces that would lead to an ACL tear in an adult cause avulsion of the incompletely ossified tibial spine in the child.

Mechanism of Injury

- Indirect trauma: rotatory, hyperextension, valgus forces.
- Direct trauma: extremely rare; secondary to multiple trauma with significant knee injury.

Clinical Evaluation

- Patients typically present with a reluctance to bear weight on the affected extremity.
- A hemarthrosis is typically present with a painful range of motion and a variable bony block to full extension.
- Ligamentous testing, especially of the medial and lateral collateral ligaments, should be performed to rule out associated injuries.

Radiographic Evaluation

- Anteroposterior and lateral views should be obtained. The anteroposterior view should be scrutinized for osseous fragments within the tibiofemoral articulation; these may be difficult to appreciate because only a thin ossified sleeve may be avulsed.
- Taking an anteroposterior radiograph to account for the 5 degrees of posterior slope of the proximal tibia may aid in visualization of the avulsed fragment.
- Stress views may be useful for identification of associated ligamentous or physeal disruptions.

MEYERS AND MCKEEVER CLASSIFICATION (FIG. 47.5)

Type I: minimal or no displacement of fragment
Type II: angular elevation of anterior portion with intact posterior hinge
Type III: complete displacement with or without rotation (15%)
Type IV: comminuted (5%)

Types I and II account for 80% of tibial spine fractures.

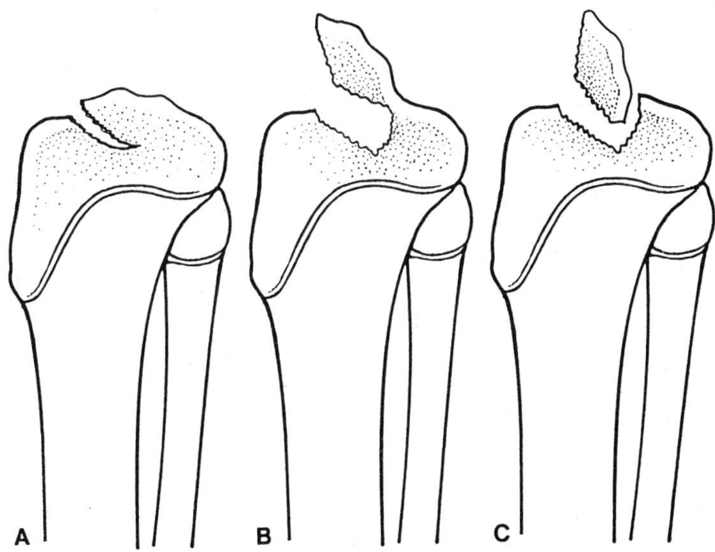

FIG. 47.5. Classification of tibial spine fractures. **A.** Type I—minimal displacement. **B.** Type II—hinged posteriorly. **C.** Type III—complete separation. (From Meyers MH, McKeever FM. Fracture of the intercondylar eminence of the tibia. *J Bone Joint Surg Am* 1959;41A:209–222, with permission.)

Treatment

Nonoperative Treatment

- This is indicated for type I and II fractures of the tibial spine.
- The knee should be immobilized in extension with up to 20 degrees of flexion; the fat pad may contact the spine in extension and thus may help with reduction.
- In 4 to 6 weeks, the cast should be removed with initiation of active range of motion and quadriceps and hamstrings strengthening.

Operative Treatment

- This is indicated with type III and IV fractures of the tibial spine because of uniformly poor results with nonoperative management.
- Debridement of the fracture site is recommended, followed by fixation using sutures, pins, or screws.
- Postoperatively, the patient is placed in a long-leg cast with the knee in slight (10 to 20 degrees) flexion. In 4 to 6 weeks, the cast should be removed, followed by initiation of active range of motion and quadriceps and hamstrings strengthening.

Complications

- Loss of extension: present in up to 60% of cases; loss is no greater than 10 degrees. This is typically clinically insignificant. May represent a bony block to extension caused by malunion of a type III fracture.
- Knee instability: may persist with type III or IV fractures accompanied by collateral ligament injuries and/or physeal fractures.

PATELLA FRACTURES

Epidemiology

Very rare in children; only 1% of all patella fractures are seen in patients under 16 years of age.

Anatomy

- The patella is the largest sesamoid in the body. Its two functions are to protect intra-articular structures and to increase the mechanical advantage of the quadriceps.
- Forces generated by the quadriceps in children are not as high as adults due to a smaller muscle mass and shorter moment arm.
- The blood supply to the patella derives from the anastomotic ring formed by the superior and inferior geniculate arteries. An additional supply through the distal pole is from the fat pad.
- The ossification center appears between 3 and 5 years. Ossification then proceeds peripherally and is complete between 10 to 13 years of age.
- This fracture must be differentiated from the bipartite patella (present in up to 6% of patients), which is located superolaterally.

Mechanism of Injury

- Direct: most common; trauma to the patella secondary to falls or motor vehicle accidents.
- Indirect: sudden accelerating or decelerating force on quadriceps.
- Marginal fracture: usually medial due to patellar subluxation or dislocation laterally.
- Predisposing factors: previous trauma to the knee extensor mechanism; spasticity or contracture of the extensor mechanism (e.g., secondary to cerebral palsy or arthrogryposis).

Clinical Evaluation

- Patients typically present with refusal to bear weight on the affected extremity.
- Swelling, tenderness, and hemarthrosis are present, often with limited or absent active extension of the knee.
- Patella alta may be present with avulsion or sleeve fractures, and a palpable osseous defect may be appreciated.
- An apprehension test may be positive; this may indicate the presence of a spontaneously reduced patellar dislocation that resulted in a marginal fracture.

Radiographic Evaluation

- Anteroposterior, lateral, and patellar (sunrise) views of the knee should be obtained.
- Transverse fracture patterns are most often appreciated on lateral views of the knee. The extent of displacement may be better appreciated on a stress view with the knee flexed to 30 degrees (greater flexion may not be tolerated by the patient).
- Longitudinally oriented and marginal fractures may be best recognized on anteroposterior or sunrise views.
- Stellate fractures and bipartite patella are best seen on anteroposterior radiographs. Comparison views of the opposite patella may aid in delineating a bipartite patella.

CLASSIFICATION BASED ON PATTERN (FIG. 47.6)

Transverse: complete versus incomplete.
Marginal fractures: generally result from lateral subluxation or dislocation of the patella.
Sleeve fracture: unique to immature skeleton; consists of extensive sleeve of cartilage pulled from osseous patella with or without an osseous fragment from the pole.
Stellate: generally from direct trauma in the older child.
Longitudinal
Avulsion

Treatment

Nonoperative Treatment

- Indicated for nondisplaced fractures.
- Consists of a well-molded cylinder cast with the knee in extension.
- Progressive weight bearing permitted as tolerated. Cast generally discontinued at 4 to 6 weeks.

Operative Treatment

- Displaced (>4-mm diastasis or >3-mm articular step-off): treat with loops, tension band, sutures, or screws; retinaculum must also be repaired.
- Sleeve fracture: ensure careful reduction of involved pole and cartilaginous sleeve with fixation and retinacular repair; if this is missed, the result will be an elongated patella with extensor lag and quadriceps weakness.
- Following operation: patient maintained in a well-molded cylinder cast for 4 to 6 weeks.
- Quadriceps strengthening and active range-of-motion exercises instituted as soon as possible.

Complications

- Quadriceps weakness: compromised quadriceps function secondary to missed diagnosis or inadequate treatment; occurs with functional elongation of the extensor mechanism and loss of mechanical advantage.
- Patella alta: due to functional elongation of the extensor mechanism; associated with quadriceps atrophy and weakness.

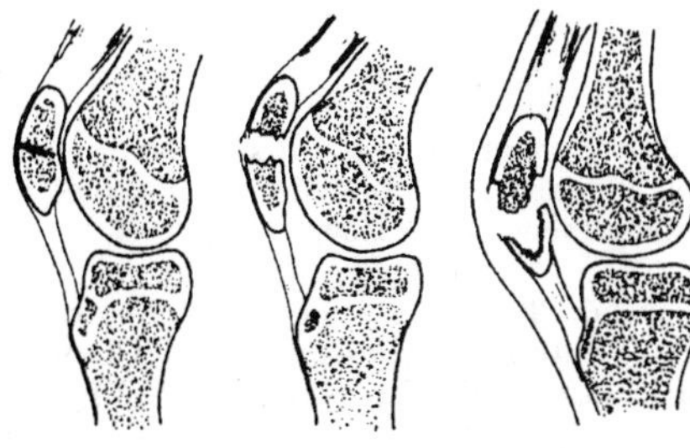

FIG. 47.6. Patellar fractures in children. (From Ogden JA. *Skeletal injury in the child,* 2nd ed. Philadelphia: W.B. Saunders, 1990:761, with permission.)

- Posttraumatic osteoarthritis: degenerative changes secondary to chondral damage at the time of injury.

KNEE DISLOCATION

Epidemiology
Extremely infrequent in skeletally immature individuals because physeal injuries to the distal femur or proximal tibia are more likely to result.

Anatomy
- Typically occurs with major ligamentous disruptions about the knee.
- Associated with major disruptions of soft tissue and damage to neurovascular structures; vascular repair must take place within the first 6 to 8 hours to avoid permanent damage.
- Linked to other knee injuries, including tibial spine fractures, osteochondral injuries, and meniscal tears.

Mechanism of Injury
Most occur as a result of multiple trauma from motor vehicle accidents or falls from heights.

Clinical Evaluation
- Patients almost always present with gross knee distortion. Immediate reduction should be undertaken without waiting for radiographs to be taken in the displaced position. Of paramount importance is the arterial supply; secondary consideration is given to neurologic status.
- The extent of ligamentous injury is related to the degree of displacement, with injury occurring with displacement greater than 10% to 25% of the resting length of the ligament. Gross instability may be realized after reduction.
- A careful neurovascular examination is critical both pre- and postreduction because the popliteal artery is at risk during traumatic dislocations of the knee due to the bowstring effect across the popliteal fossa secondary to proximal and distal tethering. Peroneal nerve injuries are also common, mostly in the form of traction neurapraxias.

Radiographic Evaluation
- Anteroposterior and lateral views are sufficient to establish the diagnosis; the most common direction is anterior.
- Radiographs should be scrutinized for associated injuries to the tibial spine, distal femoral physis, or proximal tibial physis. Stress views may be obtained to detect collateral ligament injury.
- Controversy remains as to whether all patients should receive arteriograms. Some authorities state that if pulses are present both pre- and postreduction, arteriography is not indicated. The patient must be monitored for 48 to 72 hours postreduction because a late thrombus may develop as a result of intimal damage.

DESCRIPTIVE CLASSIFICATION
Based on displacement of the proximal tibia in relation to the distal femur. Also should include open versus closed, reducible versus irreducible. May be classified as occult, indicating a knee dislocation with spontaneous reduction.

- Anterior: forceful knee hyperextension beyond –30 degrees; most common; associated with posterior cruciate ligament (PCL) ± anterior cruciate ligament (ACL) tear; increasing incidence of popliteal artery disruption with increasing degree of hyperextension.

- Posterior: posteriorly directed force against proximal tibia of flexed knee; "dashboard" injury. Accompanied by ACL/PCL disruption and popliteal artery compromise with increasing proximal tibial displacement.
- Lateral: valgus force; medial supporting structures disrupted, often with tears of both cruciate ligaments.
- Medial: varus force; lateral and posterolateral structures disrupted.
- Rotational: varus/valgus with rotatory component; usually results in buttonholing of femoral condyle through the capsule.

Treatment

- Treatment is based on prompt recognition and treatment of the knee dislocation with recognition of vascular injury; operative intervention is used as needed.
- No large series have been reported, but early ligamentous repair is indicated for young patients.
- Closed reduction and splinting, followed by 6 weeks of immobilization in a long-leg cast, are recommended.

Complications

- *Vascular compromise.* Unrecognized and untreated vascular compromise to the leg, usually in the form of an unrecognized intimal injury with late thrombosis and ischemia, represents the most serious and potentially devastating complication from a knee dislocation. Careful serial evaluation of neurovascular status is essential up to 48 to 72 hours postinjury, followed by aggressive use of arteriography as indicated.
- *Peroneal nerve injury.* This usually represents traction neurapraxias that resolve. Electromyography may be indicated if resolution does not occur within 3 to 6 months.

48. PEDIATRIC TIBIA AND FIBULA

EPIDEMIOLOGY

- Tibia fractures represent the third most common pediatric fractures after femoral and forearm fractures.
- They represent 15% of pediatric fractures.
- The average age of occurrence is 8 years.
- Thirty percent are associated with ipsilateral fibular fractures.
- The incidence of boys to girls is 2:1.
- Tibia fractures are the second most commonly fractured bone in abused children; 26% of abused children with fractures will have tibial fractures.

ANATOMY

- The anteromedial aspect of the tibia is subcutaneous with no overlying musculature for protection.
- Three consistent ossification centers form the tibia:
  - Diaphyseal: ossifies at 7 weeks of gestation.
  - Proximal: ossification center appears just after birth; closure occurs at the age of 16 years.
  - Distal: ossification center appears in the second year of life, and closure occurs at age 15.
- In addition, the medial malleolus and tibial tubercle may present as separate ossification centers; they should not be confused with a fracture.
- The fibular ossification centers are as follows:
  - Diaphyseal: ossifies at 8 weeks of gestation.
  - Distal: ossification center appears at the age of 2 years; closure found at the age of 16 years.
  - Proximal: ossification center appears at age 4 years and closure between the ages of 16 to 18 years.

MECHANISM OF INJURY

- Fifty percent of pediatric tibial fractures are due to pedestrian–motor vehicle accidents.
- Twenty-two percent are caused by indirect rotational forces.
- Seventeen percent are caused by falls.
- Eleven percent are due to motor vehicle accidents.
- Children aged 1 to 4 years are susceptible to bicycle-spoke trauma, whereas children aged 4 to 14 most often sustain tibial fractures during athletic or motor vehicle accidents.

CLINICAL EVALUATION

- A full pediatric trauma protocol must be observed, because >60% of tibial fractures are associated with motor vehicle or pedestrian–motor vehicle trauma.
- Patients typically present with the inability to bear weight on the injured lower extremity and pain, variable gross deformity, and painful range of motion of the knee or ankle.
- A careful neurovascular examination, with assessment of both the dorsalis pedis and posterior tibial artery pulses, is essential.
- Palpation of the anterior, lateral, and posterior (deep and superficial) muscle compartments should be performed to evaluate for possible compartment syndrome. When suspected, compartment pressure measurement should be undertaken, and emergent fasciotomies should be performed in the case of compartment syndrome.
- Field dressings/splints should be removed to expose the entire leg in order to assess soft-tissue compromise and to rule out open fracture.

RADIOGRAPHIC EVALUATION

- Anteroposterior and lateral views of the tibia and knee should be obtained. Anteroposterior, lateral, and mortise views of the ankle should be obtained to rule out con-

comitant ankle injury Comparison radiographs of the uninjured contralateral extremity are rarely necessary.
- Technetium-99m bone scans may be obtained to rule out an occult fracture in the appropriate clinical setting.

CLASSIFICATION
Descriptive based on location.

PROXIMAL TIBIAL METAPHYSEAL FRACTURES

Epidemiology
- Uncommon, representing <5% of pediatric fractures and only 11% of pediatric tibial fractures.
- Peak incidence occurs at 3 to 6 years of age.

Anatomy
The proximal tibial physis is generally structurally weaker than the metaphyseal region; this accounts for the lower incidence of fractures in the tibial metaphysis.

Mechanism of Injury
- The most common mechanism is force applied to the lateral aspect of the extended knee that causes the cortex of the medial metaphysis to fail in tension, generally as nondisplaced greenstick fractures of the medial cortex.
- The fibula usually does not fracture, although plastic deformation may occur.

Clinical Evaluation
- The patient typically presents with pain, swelling, and tenderness in the region of the fracture. Motion of the knee is painful, and the child usually refuses to ambulate.
- Because the medial cortex most commonly fails, valgus deformity is typically present.

Radiographic Evaluation
Anteroposterior and lateral views of the tibia should be obtained, as well as appropriate views of the knee and ankle to rule out associated injuries.

DESCRIPTIVE CLASSIFICATION
- Open versus closed
- Angulation
- Displacement
- Pattern—transverse, oblique, spiral, greenstick, plastic deformation, torus
- Degree of comminution

Treatment

Nonoperative Treatment
- Nondisplaced fractures may be treated with a long-leg cast with 10-degree knee flexion.
- Displaced fractures should undergo closed reduction under general anesthesia, followed by application of a long-leg cast with the knee in full extension and a varus moment placed on the cast to prevent valgus collapse.
- The cast should be maintained for 6 to 8 weeks with serial radiographs to rule out displacement.
- Normal activities may be resumed when normal knee and ankle motions are restored and the fracture site is nontender.

Operative Treatment (Fig. 48.1)
- Fractures that cannot be reduced by closed means should undergo open reduction with removal of interposed soft tissue.

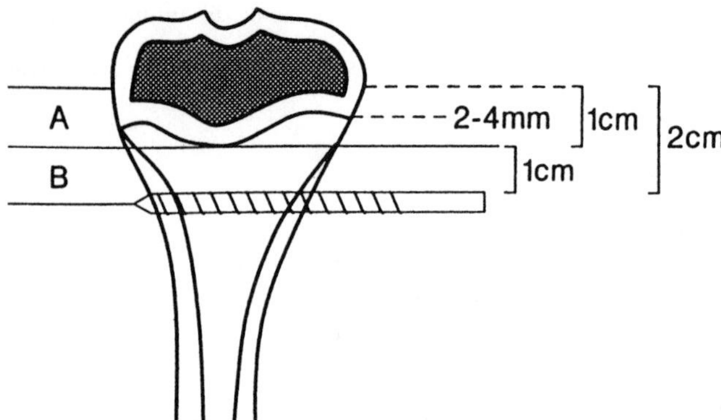

FIG. 48.1. Safe drilling zone. **A.** The area occupied by the physis is about 1 cm proximal because of its undulations. **B.** The safe drilling zone is at least 1 cm distally from the physis. (From Alonso JE. The initial management of the injured child: musculoskeletal injuries. In: MacEwen GD, Kassar J, Heinrich SDH, eds. *Pediatric fractures: a practical approach to assessment and treatment.* Baltimore: Williams & Wilkins, 1993, with permission.)

- The pes anserinus insertion should be repaired with restoration of tension as indicated.
- A long-leg cast with the knee in full extension should be placed and should be maintained for 6 to 8 weeks postoperatively with serial radiographs to monitor healing.
- Open fractures or grossly contaminated fractures with associated vascular compromise may be treated with debridement of compromised tissues and external fixation, particularly in older children. Regional or free flaps or skin grafting may be required for skin closure.

Complications

- Progressive valgus angulation: may be due to a combination of factors, including disruption of the lateral physis at the time of injury, exuberant medial callus formation that results in fracture overgrowth, entrapment of periosteum at the medial fracture site with consequent stimulation of the physis, or concomitant pes anserinus injury that results in a loss of the inhibitory tethering effect on the physis, allowing overgrowth. The deformity is most prominent within 1 year of fracture occurrence; younger patients may experience spontaneous correction with remodeling, although older patients may require hemiepiphysiodesis or corrective osteotomy.
- Premature proximal tibial physeal closure: may occur with unrecognized crush (Salter V) injury to the proximal tibial physis, resulting in growth arrest. This most commonly affects the anterior physis, resulting in a consequent recurvatum deformity of the affected knee.

DIAPHYSEAL FRACTURES OF THE TIBIA

Epidemiology

- Thirty-nine percent of pediatric tibial fractures occur in the middle third.
- Approximately 30% of pediatric diaphyseal fractures are associated with a fracture of the fibula. Occasionally, this occurs in the form of plastic deformation, producing valgus misalignment of the tibia.
- Isolated fractures of the fibular shaft are rare; they occur due to direct trauma to the lateral aspect of the leg.

Anatomy

- The nutrient artery arises from the posterior tibial artery, entering the posterolateral cortex distal to the origination of the soleus muscle at the oblique line of the tibia. Once the vessel enters the intramedullary canal, it gives off three ascending branches and one descending branch. These give rise to the endosteal vascular tree, which anastomoses with periosteal vessels arising from the anterior tibial artery.
- The anterior tibial artery is particularly vulnerable to injury as it passes through a hiatus in the interosseus membrane.
- The peroneal artery has an anterior communicating branch to the dorsalis pedis artery. It may therefore be occluded despite the presence of an intact dorsalis pedis pulse.
- The distal third is supplied by periosteal anastomoses around the ankle where branches enter the tibia through ligamentous attachments.
- The fibula is responsible for 6% to 17% of weight-bearing load. The common peroneal nerve courses around the neck of the fibula, which is nearly subcutaneous in this region; it is therefore especially vulnerable to direct blows or traction injuries at this level.

Mechanism of Injury

- Direct: occurs mostly in the form of vehicular trauma or pedestrian–motor vehicle accidents.
- Indirect: most a result of torsional injuries in younger children. Spiral and oblique fractures occur as the body mass rotates on a planted foot. The fibula prevents significant shortening when intact, but the fracture frequently falls into varus.

Clinical Evaluation

- The patient typically presents with pain, swelling, and tenderness in the region of the fracture. Motion of the knee is painful, and the child usually refuses to ambulate.
- Children with stress fractures of the tibia may complain of pain on weight bearing that is partially relieved by rest.

Radiographic Evaluation

- Standard anteroposterior and lateral views of the leg should be obtained. Radiographs of the ipsilateral ankle and knee should be viewed to rule out associated injuries.
- Comparison views of the uninjured contralateral leg may be taken in cases in which the diagnosis is unclear.
- Technetium-99m bone scans may rule out an occult fracture.

DESCRIPTIVE CLASSIFICATION

- Angulation
- Displacement
- Open versus closed
- Pattern—transverse, oblique, spiral, greenstick, plastic deformation, torus
- Degree of comminution

Treatment

Nonoperative Treatment

- Most pediatric fractures of the tibia and fibula are uncomplicated; they may be treated by simple manipulation and casting, especially when non- or minimally displaced. However, isolated tibial diaphyseal fractures tend to fall into varus angulation, whereas fractures of the tibia and fibula tend to fall into valgus angulation with shortening and recurvatum.
- Displaced fractures may be initially treated with closed reduction and casting under general anesthesia.

    In children, an acceptable reduction includes 50% apposition of the fracture ends, <1 cm of shortening, and <5 to 10 degrees of angulation in the sagittal and coronal planes.

A long-leg cast is applied with the ankle slightly plantar flexed (20 degrees for distal and middle third fractures, 10 degrees for proximal third fractures) to prevent posterior angulation of the fracture in the initial 2 to 3 weeks. The knee is flexed to 45 degrees to provide rotational control and to prevent weight bearing.

The fracture alignment must be serially monitored, particularly during the initial 3 weeks when atrophy and diminished swelling may result in fracture subsidence and loss of reduction. Some patients require remanipulation with cast application under general anesthesia 2 to 3 weeks after initial casting.

The cast may require wedging (opening or closing wedge) to provide correction of an angulatory deformity.

Time to healing varies according to patient age as follows:

Neonates—2 to 3 weeks;
Juveniles—4 to 6 weeks;
Adolescents—8 to 12 weeks.

Operative Treatment

- Operative management of tibial fractures is typically required in <5% of cases.
- Indications for operative management include open fractures, fractures in which a stable reduction is unable to be achieved or maintained, fractures with associated vascular injury, fractures associated with compartment syndrome, severely comminuted fractures, associated femoral fracture (floating knee), fractures in patients with spasticity syndromes (cerebral palsy, head injury), patients with bleeding diatheses (hemophilia), or patients with multisystem injuries.
- Open fractures or grossly contaminated fractures with associated vascular compromise may be treated with debridement of compromised tissues and external fixation, particularly in older children. Severe degloving injuries may require the use of flexible intramedullary nails for fracture stabilization. Regional or free flaps or skin grafting may be required for skin closure.
- Other methods of operative fixation include percutaneous pins, plates and screws, or intramedullary nails (particularly in older children).
- Postoperatively, a long-leg cast is placed with the knee in 45 degrees of flexion to allow rotational control. The cast is maintained for 4 to 16 weeks, depending on the status of healing, as evidenced by serial radiographs and the healing of associated injuries.

Complications

- *Compartment syndrome.* In pediatric tibial fractures, compartment syndrome is most common after severe injuries in which the interosseous membrane surrounding the anterior compartment is disrupted. Elevated compartment pressures of >30 mm Hg or within 30 mm Hg of the diastolic blood pressure should receive emergent fasciotomies of all four compartments of the leg to avoid neurologic and ischemic sequelae.
- *Angular deformity.* Correction of deformity varies by age and gender.
  Girls <8 years and boys <10 years often experience significant remodeling.
  Girls from 9 to 12 years of age and boys between 11 and 12 years can correct up to 50% of angulation.
  In children older than 13 years of age, <25% angular correction is expected.
  Posterior and valgus angulation tend to correct the least with remodeling.
- *Malrotation.* Rotational deformity of the tibia does not correct with remodeling; it is poorly tolerated, often resulting in malpositioning of the foot with the development of associated ankle and foot problems. Supramalleolar osteotomy may be required for rotational correction.
- *Premature proximal tibial physeal closure.* This may occur with unrecognized crush (Salter V) injury to the proximal tibial physis that results in growth arrest. It most commonly affects the anterior physis, resulting in a consequent recurvatum deformity of the affected knee.
- *Delayed union and nonunion.* This is uncommon in children but may occur as a result of infection, the use of external fixation, or from inadequate immobilization.

Fibulectomy, bone grafting, reamed intramedullary nailing (adolescents), or plate fixation with bone grafting have all been described as methods for the treatment of tibial nonunions in the pediatric population.

FRACTURES OF THE DISTAL TIBIAL METAPHYSIS

Epidemiology

- Fractures of the distal third of the tibia comprise approximately 50% of pediatric tibial fractures.
- Most occur in patients younger than 14 years of age, with the peak range of incidence in children between the ages of 2 and 8 years.

Anatomy

Distally, the tibia flares out as the cortical diaphyseal bone changes to cancellous metaphyseal bone overlying the articular surface. This is similar to the tibial plateau in that primarily cancellous bone is found within a thin cortical shell.

Mechanism of Injury

- Indirect: axial load resulting from a jump or a fall from a height.
- Direct: trauma to the lower leg; for example, "bicycle-spoke" injuries in which a child's foot is thrust forcibly between the spokes of a turning bicycle wheel, resulting in severe crush to the distal leg, ankle, and foot with variable soft-tissue injuries.

Clinical Evaluation

- Patients typically present as unable to ambulate, or they are ambulatory only with severe pain.
- Although swelling may occur with variable abrasions or lacerations, the foot, ankle, and leg typically appear relatively normal without gross deformity.
- The entire foot, ankle, and leg should be exposed to evaluate the extent of soft-tissue injury and to assess for possible open fracture.
- A careful neurovascular examination is important, and the presence of compartment syndrome must be ruled out.
- In cases of bicycle-spoke injuries, palpation of all bony structures of the foot and ankle should be undertaken, as well as assessment of ligamentous integrity and stability.

Radiographic Evaluation

- Anteroposterior and lateral views of the leg should be obtained. Appropriate views of the ankle and knee should be taken to rule out associated injuries; views of the foot are used when indicated.
- Fractures of the distal metaphysis typically represent greenstick injuries with anterior cortical impaction, posterior cortical disruption, and tearing of the overlying periosteum, often resulting in a recurvatum pattern of injury.
- In cases of severe torsional injuries with impaction or distraction forces, a spiral fracture may result.
- Computed tomography is usually unnecessary, but it may aid in fracture definition in cases of comminution or complex fractures.

DESCRIPTIVE CLASSIFICATION

- Angulation
- Displacement
- Open versus closed
- Pattern—transverse, oblique, spiral, greenstick, plastic deformation, torus
- Degree of comminution
- Associated injuries: knee, ankle, foot

Treatment

Nonoperative Treatment

- Nondisplaced, minimally displaced, torus, or greenstick fractures should be treated with manipulation and long-leg casting under general anesthesia.

- In cases of recurvatum deformity of the tibial fracture, the foot should be placed in slight plantarflexion (10 degrees) to prevent angulation into recurvatum.
- After 3 to 4 weeks of plaster immobilization, the long-leg cast is discontinued and is changed to a short-leg walking cast with the ankle in the neutral position if the fracture demonstrates radiographic evidence of healing.
- The current recommendation is that a child with a bicycle-spoke injury should be admitted for observation because the extent of soft-tissue compromise may not be evident initially.
  - A long-leg splint should be applied and the lower extremity should be aggressively elevated for 24 hours, with serial examination of the soft-tissue envelope over the subsequent 48 hours.
  - If no open fracture exists and soft-tissue compromise is minimal, a long-leg cast may be placed before discharge as described previously.

Operative Treatment

- Surgical intervention is warranted for cases of open fracture or for cases in which stable reduction is not possible by closed means.
- Unstable distal tibial fractures can typically be managed with closed reduction and percutaneous pinning using Steinmann pins or Kirschner wire fixation. Rarely, a comminuted fracture may require open reduction and internal fixation using pins or plates and screws. Postoperatively, the patient is immobilized in a long-leg cast. The fracture should be monitored with serial radiographs to assess healing. At 3 to 4 weeks the pins may be removed and the cast may be replaced either with a long-leg cast or by a short-leg walking cast, if clinically allowable.
- Open fractures may require external fixation to allow for management of the wound. Devitalized tissue should be debrided as necrosis becomes apparent. Aspiration of large hematomas should be undertaken to avoid plane formation and the compromise of overlying skin. Skin grafts or flaps (regional or free) may be necessary for wound closure.

Complications

- *Recurvatum.* Inadequate reduction or fracture subsidence may result in a recurvatum deformity at the fracture site. Younger patients tend to tolerate this better because remodeling typically renders the deformity clinically insignificant. Older patients may require supramalleolar osteotomy for severe recurvatum deformity that compromises ankle function and gait.
- *Premature distal tibial physeal closure.* This may occur with unrecognized crush (Salter V) injury to the distal tibial physis resulting in growth arrest.

TODDLER FRACTURE

Epidemiology

- Most occur in children younger than 2.5 years of age.
- Average age of incidence is 27 months.
- Tend to occur in males more than females and in the right leg more than the left leg.

Anatomy

The distal epiphysis appears at approximately 2 years of age; thus, physeal injuries of the distal tibia may not be readily apparent and must be suspected.

Mechanism of Injury

- The classic description of the mechanism of a toddler fracture is external rotation of the foot with the knee in fixed position, producing a spiral fracture of the tibia with or without concomitant fibular fracture.
- This injury has also been reported as a result of a fall.

Clinical Evaluation

- Patients typically present as irritable and nonambulatory or with an acute limp.
- The examination of a child refusing to ambulate without readily identifiable causes should include a careful history with attention to temporal progression of symptoms

and signs (e.g., fever) and a systematic evaluation of the hip, thigh, knee, leg, ankle, and foot with attention to points of tenderness, swelling, or ecchymosis. This should be followed by radiographic evaluation and appropriate laboratory analysis if the diagnosis remains in doubt.
- In the case of a toddler fracture, pain and variable swelling occurs with palpation of the tibia. This is usually appreciated over the anteromedial aspect of the tibia where its subcutaneous nature allows minimal soft-tissue protection.

Radiographic Evaluation
- Anteroposterior and lateral views of the leg should be obtained.
- An internal oblique radiograph of the leg may help to demonstrate a nondisplaced spiral fracture.
- Occasionally, an incomplete fracture may not be appreciated on presentation radiographs; however, it may become radiographically evident 7 to 10 days after the injury as periosteal new bone formation occurs.
- Technetium-99m bone scans may aid in the diagnosis of a toddler fracture by visualization of diffusely increased uptake throughout the tibia. This may be differentiated from infection, which tends to produce a localized area of increased uptake.

CLASSIFICATION
A toddler fracture is, by definition, a spiral fracture of the tibia in the appropriate age group. Further characterization of the fracture may include angular deformity, displacement, or shortening.

Treatment
- A long-leg cast for 2 to 3 weeks, followed by conversion to a short-leg walking cast for an additional 2 to 3 weeks, is usually sufficient.
- Manipulation is generally not necessary because angulation and displacement are usually minimal and are within acceptable limits.

Complications
Complications of toddler fractures are rare due to the low energy nature of the injury, the age of the patient, and the rapid and complete healing that typically accompanies this fracture pattern. Rotational deformity, on rare occasions, may result in clinically insignificant rotational deformity of the tibia as the fracture slides minimally along the spiral configuration. This is usually unnoticed by the patient, but it may be appreciated on comparison examination of the lower limbs.

STRESS FRACTURES

Epidemiology
- Most tibial stress fractures occur in the proximal third.
- The peak incidence of tibial stress fractures in children is between the ages of 10 and 15 years.
- Most fibular stress fractures occur in the distal third.
- The peak incidence of fibular stress fractures in children is between the ages of 2 and 8 years.

Anatomy
- An acute fracture occurs when the force applied to a bone exceeds the bone's capacity to withstand it. A stress fracture occurs when a bone is subjected to forces and repeated trauma with a strain that is less than what would have produced an acute fracture.
- With microtrauma, osteoclastic tunnel formation increases to remodel microcracks. New bone formation results in the production of immature woven bone that lacks the strength of the mature bone it replaced, predisposing the area to fracture with continued trauma.

Mechanism of Injury

- Stress fractures in older children and adolescents tend to occur as a result of athletic participation.
- Distal fibular stress fractures have been referred to as the "ice skater's fracture" because of the repeated skating motion that results in a characteristic fibular fracture approximately 4 cm proximal to the lateral malleolus.

Clinical Evaluation

- The patient typically presents with an antalgic gait that is relieved by rest, although younger patients may refuse to ambulate.
- The pain is usually described as insidious in onset, worse with activity, and improving at night.
- Swelling is generally not present, although the patient may complain of a vague ache over the site of fracture with tenderness that is reproduced with palpation.
- Knee and ankle range of motion are full and painless.
- Occasionally, the patient's symptoms and signs may be bilateral.
- Muscle sprains, infection, and osseous sarcoma must be ruled out. Exercised-induced compartment syndrome overlying the tibia may have a similar clinical presentation.

Radiographic Evaluation

- Anteroposterior and lateral views of the leg should be obtained to rule out acute fracture or other injuries, although stress fractures are typically not evident on standard radiographs for 10 to 14 days after initial onset of symptoms.
- Radiographic evidence of fracture repair may be visualized as periosteal new bone formation, endosteal radiodensity, or the presence of an "eggshell" callus at the site of fracture.
- Technetium-99m bone scan reveals a localized area of increased tracer uptake at the site of fracture; it may be performed within 1 to 2 days of injury.
- Computed tomography rarely demonstrates the fracture line, although it may delineate increased marrow density, endosteal/periosteal new bone formation, and soft-tissue edema.
- Magnetic resonance imaging may demonstrate a localized band of very low signal intensity continuous with the cortex.

CLASSIFICATION

Stress fractures may be classified as complete versus incomplete or acute versus chronic or recurrent but rarely are displaced or angulated.

Treatment

- The treatment of a child presenting with a tibial or fibular stress fracture begins with activity modification.
- The child may be placed in a long-leg (tibia) or short-leg (fibular) walking cast, initially non–weight bearing, with a gradual increase in activity level. The cast should be maintained for 4 to 6 weeks until the fracture site is nontender and radiographic evidence of healing is seen.
- Nonunion may be addressed with open excision of the nonunion site, followed by iliac crest bone grafting or electrical stimulation.

Complications

- Recurrent stress fractures: may be the result of overzealous training regimens or ice skating. Activity modification must be emphasized to prevent recurrence.
- Nonunion: rare, occurring most commonly in the middle third of the tibia. As described above, it may be addressed with open curettage of the nonunion with bone grafting and/or electrical stimulation.

49. PEDIATRIC ANKLE

EPIDEMIOLOGY

- Ankle injuries account for 25% to 38% of all physeal injuries, second only in frequency to distal radial physeal injuries.
- Fifty-eight percent of ankle physeal injuries occur during athletic participation.
- They represent between 10% and 40% of all physeal injuries.
- Tibial physeal fractures are most common from 8 to 15 years of age.
- Fibular physeal injuries are most common from 8 to 14 years of age.
- Ligamentous injuries are rare in children because, relative to bone, their ligaments are stronger.
- After ages 15 to 16, an adult fracture pattern is seen.
- Some 25,000 lawnmower injuries occur each year, with over 20% involving children.

ANATOMY

- The ankle is a modified hinge joint stabilized by medial and lateral ligamentous complexes. All ligaments attach distal to the physes of the tibia and fibula; this information is important in the pathoanatomy of pediatric ankle fracture patterns.
- The distal tibial ossific nucleus appears between the ages of 2 and 3 years; it fuses with the shaft at about the age of 15 years in girls and 17 in boys. Over an 18-month period, the lateral portion of the distal tibial physis remains open while the medial part has closed.
- The distal fibular ossific nucleus appears at the age of 2 years and unites with the shaft at age 20. Secondary ossification centers occur, often bilaterally; they may be confused with a fracture of either the medial or lateral malleolus.

MECHANISM OF INJURY

- Direct: trauma to the ankle from a fall, motor vehicle accident, or pedestrian–motor vehicle accident.
- Indirect: axial force transmission through the forefoot and hindfoot or rotational force of the body on a planted foot; may occur in falls or, more commonly, in athletic participation.

CLINICAL EVALUATION

- Patients with severely displaced fractures typically present with severe pain, gross deformity, and an inability to ambulate.
- Physical examination may demonstrate tenderness, swelling, and ecchymosis.
- Ligamentous instability may be present; however, it is usually difficult to elicit on presentation due to pain and swelling from the acute injury.
- Neurovascular examination, with documentation of dorsalis pedis and posterior tibial pulses, capillary refill, sensation to light touch and pinprick, and motor testing, is essential.
- Dressings and splints placed in the field should be removed and soft-tissue damage should be assessed, paying attention to skin lacerations that may indicate open fracture and to fracture blisters that may compromise wound healing.
- The ipsilateral foot, leg, and knee should be examined for concomitant injury.

RADIOGRAPHIC EVALUATION

- Anteroposterior, lateral, and mortise views of the ankle should be obtained. Tenderness of the proximal fibula warrants appropriate views of the leg.
- Clinical examination will dictate the need for obtaining views of the knee and foot.
- Stress views may be taken to determine possible ligamentous instability.
- The presence of secondary ossification centers (a medial os subtibiale in 20% of patients or a lateral os subfibulare in 1% of patients) should not be confused with fracture, although tenderness may indicate injury.

- A Tillaux fragment represents an osseous fragment from the lateral tibia that has been avulsed during injury.
- Computed tomography is often helpful for evaluation of complex intraarticular fracture patterns, such as the juvenile Tillaux or triplane fracture.
- Magnetic resonance imaging has been used to delineate osteochondral injuries in association with ankle fractures.

DIAS AND TACHDJIAN CLASSIFICATION (FIG. 49.1)

- Lauge-Hansen principles correlate with the Salter-Harris classification.
- Typology is simplified by noting the direction of physeal displacement, Salter-Harris type, and location of the metaphyseal fragment.
- Classification aids in determining the proper maneuver for closed reduction.

Supination-External Rotation (SER)

Stage I: Salter-Harris II fracture of the distal tibia with the metaphyseal fragment located posterolaterally; a long spiral fracture of the distal tibia starting laterally at the physis.

Stage II: As external rotation force continues, a spiral fracture of the fibula occurs beginning medially and extending posterosuperiorly; differs from an adult SER injury.

Pronation-Eversion-External Rotation

- Fifteen percent to 20% of pediatric ankle fractures.
- Marked valgus deformity.
- Tibial and fibular fractures simultaneous.
- Salter-Harris type II fracture of the distal tibial physis most commonly seen, but type I also occurs; metaphyseal fragment located laterally.
- Short oblique distal fibular fracture 4 to 7 cm proximal to the tip.

Supination-Plantar Flexion

- Most commonly Salter-Harris type II fracture of the distal tibial physis with the metaphyseal fragment posterior; type I Salter-Harris fracture is rare.
- Fibula fracture: rare.

Supination-Inversion

This is the most common mechanism of fracture, with the highest incidence of complications.

Stage I: Salter-Harris I or II of the distal fibular physis most common; pain noted along physis when x-rays are negative. This is the most common pediatric ankle fracture.

Stage II: Salter-Harris III or IV of the medial tibial physis as the talus wedges into the medial tibial articular surface; rarely a type I or II fracture; occasionally an open injury associated with a talus fracture. These are intraarticular fractures that exhibit the highest rate of growth disturbance (i.e., physeal bar formation).

Axial Compression (Fig. 49.2)

- Salter-Harris type V injury to distal tibia.
- Rare injury with poor prognosis secondary to physeal growth arrest.
- Diagnosis often delayed until premature physeal closure is found with a leg length discrepancy.

Juvenile Tillaux Fractures (Fig. 49.3)

- Salter-Harris type III fracture of the anterolateral tibial epiphysis; occurs in 2.9% of ankle fractures.
- External rotation force causes the anterior tibiofibular ligament to avulse the fragment.
- Occurs in children between the ages of 12 to 14 years when the central and medial portions of the distal tibial physis have already fused; 18-month window where lateral physis remains open.
- Computed tomography helps to distinguish from triplane fractures.

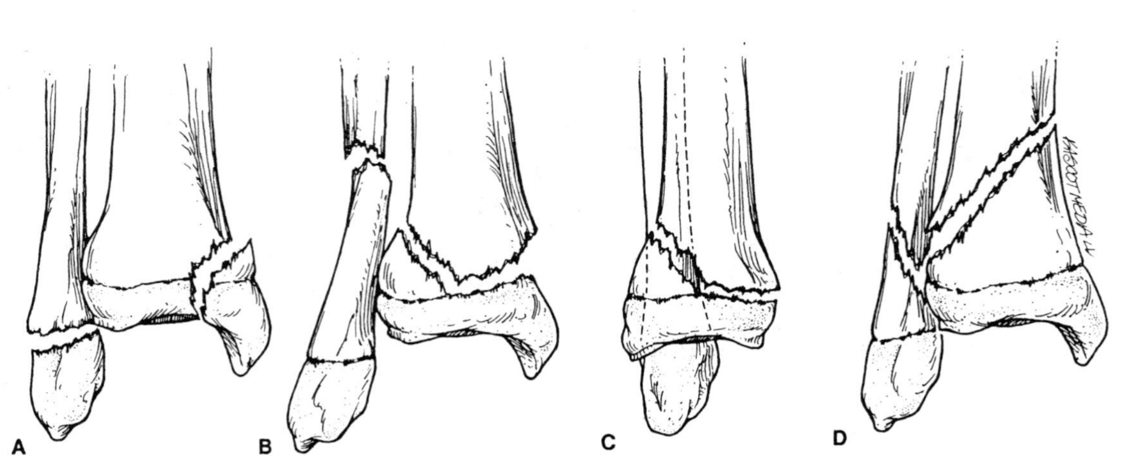

FIG. 49.1. Diaz-Tachdjian classification of physeal injuries of the distal tibia and fibula. (From Rockwood CA Jr, Wilkins KE, Beaty JH, eds. *Rockwood and Green's fractures in children*, 4th ed. Vol. 3. Philadelphia: Lippincott-Raven, 1996:1384, with permission.)

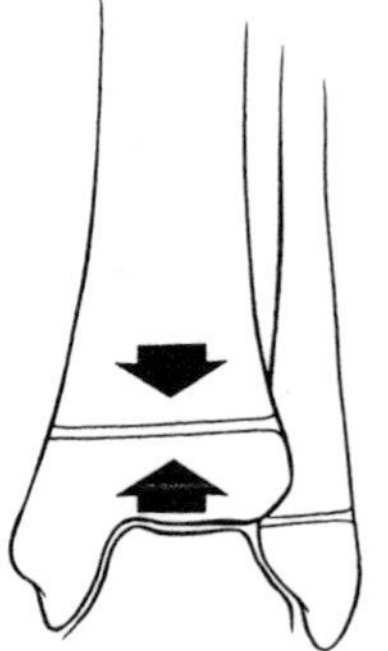

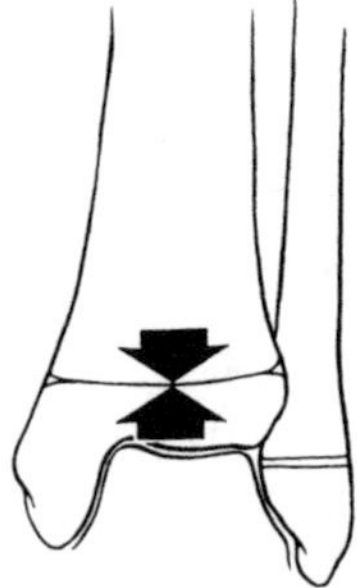

FIG. 49.2. Compression-type injury of the tibial physis. Early physeal arrest can cause leg length discrepancy. (From Rockwood CA Jr, Wilkins KE, Beaty JH, eds. *Rockwood and Green's fractures in children*, 4th ed. Vol. 3. Philadelphia: Lippincott-Raven, 1996: 1401, with permission.)

Triplane Fractures (Fig. 49.4)

- Occur in three planes: transverse, coronal, and sagittal.
- Explained by fusion of the tibial physis from central to anteromedial to posteromedial and finally to lateral.
- Peak age incidence from 13 to 15 years of age in males and 12 to 14 in females.
- Mechanism thought to be external rotation of the foot and ankle.
- Fibular fracture possible; usually oblique from anteroinferior to posterosuperior 4 to 6 cm proximal to the tip.
- Computed tomography is invaluable in preoperative assessment.
- Two- and three-part types have been described:
  - Two-part fractures are either medial, where the coronal fragment is posteromedial, or lateral, where the coronal fragment is posterolateral.
  - Three-part fractures consist of an anterolateral fragment that mimics the juvenile Tillaux fracture (Salter-Harris type III), the remainder of the physis with a posterolateral spike of the tibial metaphysis, and the remainder of the distal tibial metaphysis.

TREATMENT

Lateral Malleolar (Distal Fibula) Fracture

Salter-Harris Type I or II

Closed reduction and casting with a short-leg walking cast for 4 to 6 weeks.

Salter-Harris Type III or IV

- Closed reduction and percutaneous pinning with Kirschner wire fixation followed by placement of a short-leg cast.
- Open reduction with fixation using a Kirschner wire perpendicular to the physis possibly required for interposed periosteum.

Medial Malleolar (Distal Tibia) Fracture

Salter-Harris Type I or II

- Closed reduction is the treatment of choice; it is usually attainable unless soft-tissue interposition prevents reduction.
- In children <10 years of age, some residual angulation is acceptable because remodeling occurs.
- Open reduction may be necessary for interposed periosteum, followed by placement of a transmetaphyseal compression screw or Kirschner wire parallel and proximal to the physis. A long-leg cast for 3 weeks, followed by a short-leg walking cast for 3 weeks, is used.

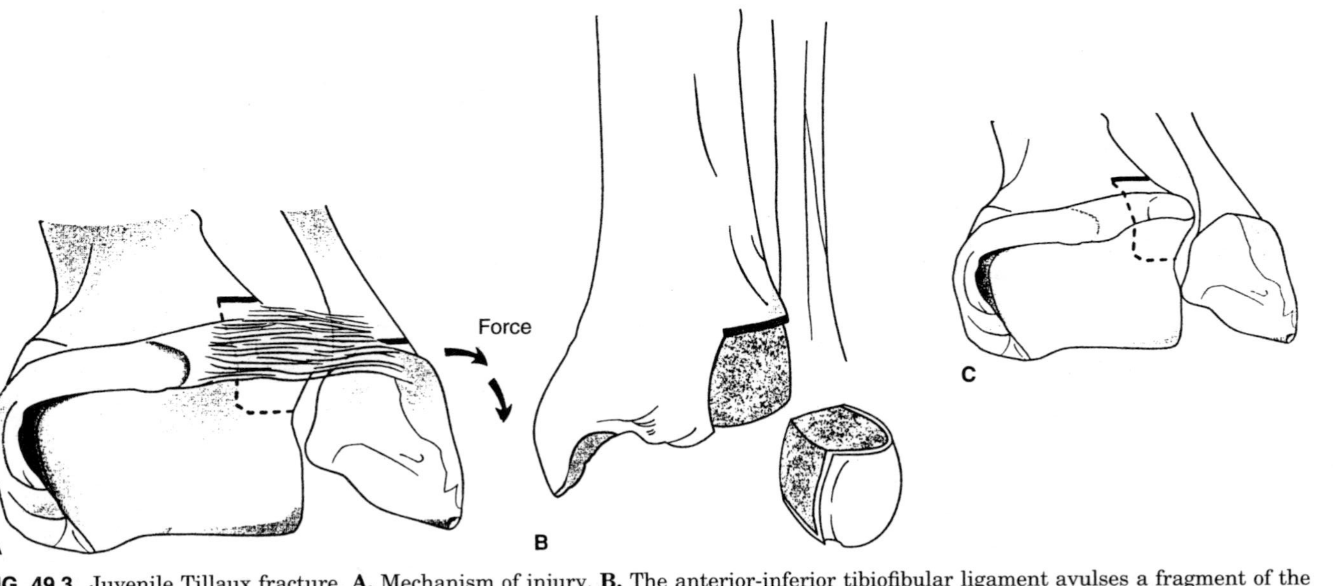

FIG. 49.3. Juvenile Tillaux fracture. **A.** Mechanism of injury. **B.** The anterior-inferior tibiofibular ligament avulses a fragment of the lateral epiphysis, **C.** corresponding to the portion of the physis that is still open. (From Rockwood CA Jr, Wilkins KE, Beaty JH, eds. *Rockwood and Green's fractures in children*, 4th ed. Vol. 3. Philadelphia: Lippincott-Raven, 1996:1407, with permission.)

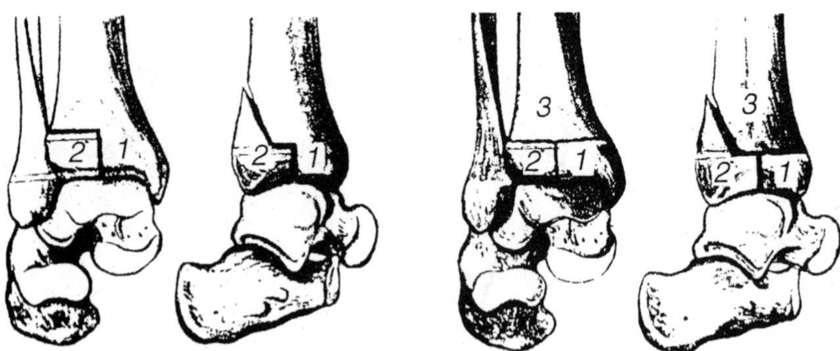

FIG. 49.4. The triplane fracture. (From Tachdjian MO. *Pediatric orthopaedics*, 2nd ed. Philadelphia: W.B. Saunders, 1990:3324, with permission.)

Salter-Harris Type III or IV

- Anatomic reduction is essential.
- Intraarticular displacement of >2 mm is unacceptable; open reduction and internal fixation are indicated.
- Open reduction and internal fixation may be performed through an anteromedial approach with cancellous screw(s) placed parallel below and/or above the physis.
- Postoperative immobilization consists of short-leg casting for 6 weeks.

Juvenile-Tillaux Fracture

- Closed reduction may be achieved via gentle distraction accompanied by internal rotation of the foot and direct pressure over the anterolateral tibia; this may be maintained in a short- or long-leg cast depending on the rotational stability. The patient is non–weight bearing for the initial 3 weeks, followed by a short-leg walking cast for an additional 3 weeks.
- Unstable injuries may require percutaneous pinning with Kirschner wire fixation.
- Displacement of >2 mm is unacceptable; it warrants open reduction and internal fixation with Kirschner wire fixation.
- Open reduction and internal fixation may be achieved via an anterolateral approach with cancellous screw fixation.
- Computed tomography may be used to assess reduction.

Triplane Fracture

- Nondisplaced fractures may be treated in a long-leg cast with the knee flexed to 30 degrees for 3 to 4 weeks, followed by an additional 3 weeks in a short-leg walking cast.
- Articular displacement of >2 mm warrants operative fixation, either by closed reduction and percutaneous pinning or by open reduction and internal fixation using a combination of cancellous screws or Kirschner wires for fixation.
- Computed tomography may be used to assess the adequacy of reduction.
- Postoperative immobilization consists of a short- or long-leg cast (depending on stability of fixation) for 3 to 4 weeks, followed by a short-leg walking cast for an additional 3 weeks.

COMPLICATIONS

- Angular deformity: may occur secondary to premature physeal arrest, especially after Salter-Harris type III and IV injuries.

Varus deformity is most common in supination-inversion injuries with premature arrest of the medial tibial physis.

Valgus deformity is seen with distal fibular physeal arrest and may be due to poor reduction or interposed soft tissue.

Rotational deformities may occur with inadequately reduced triplane fractures; extraarticular rotational deformities may be addressed with derotational osteotomies, but intraarticular fractures cannot.

- Leg length discrepancy: complicates up to 10% to 30% of cases and is dependent on the age of the patient. Discrepancy of 2 to 5 cm may be treated by epiphysiodesis of the opposite extremity, although skeletally mature individuals may require osteotomy.
- Posttraumatic arthritis: may occur as a result of inadequate reduction of the articular surface in Salter-Harris type III and IV fractures.

50. PEDIATRIC FOOT

TALUS

Epidemiology

- Extremely rare in children.
- Most represent fractures through the talar neck.

Anatomy

- The ossification center of the talus appears at 8 months *in utero*.
- The body of the talus is covered superiorly by the trochlear articular surface through which the body weight is transmitted. The anterior aspect is wider than the posterior aspect, which confers intrinsic stability to the ankle.
- Arterial supply to the talus is from two main sources:
  - Artery to the tarsal canal: arises from the posterior tibial artery 1 cm proximal to the origin of the medial and lateral plantar arteries. Gives off a deltoid branch immediately after its origin that anastomoses with branches from the dorsalis pedis over the talar neck.
  - Artery of the tarsal sinus: originates from the anastomotic loop, the perforating peroneal, and lateral tarsal branches of the dorsalis pedis artery.
- An os trigonum is present in up to 50% of normal feet. It arises from a separate ossification center just posterior to the lateral tubercle of the posterior talar process.

Mechanism of Injury

- Forced dorsiflexion of the ankle from a motor vehicle accident or fall represents the main mechanism of injury in children. This typically results in a fracture of the talar neck, which is extraarticular.
- Isolated fractures of the talar dome and body have been described but are extremely rare.

Clinical Evaluation

- Patients typically present with extreme pain on weight bearing on the affected extremity.
- Range of motion is typically painful; it may elicit crepitus.
- Diffuse swelling of the hindfoot may be present as may tenderness to palpation of the talus and subtalar joint.
- A neurovascular examination should be performed.

Radiographic Evaluation

- Standard anteroposterior, mortise, and lateral radiographs of the ankle should be obtained in addition to anteroposterior, lateral, and oblique views of the foot.
- A canale view provides an optimum view of the neck; with the ankle in maximum equinus, the foot is placed on a cassette and pronated 15 degrees and the x-ray tube is directed cephalad 15 degrees from the vertical.

DESCRIPTIVE CLASSIFICATION

Location: most talar fractures in children occur through the talar neck
Angulation
Displacement
Dislocation: subtalar, talonavicular or ankle joints
Pattern: presence of comminution

HAWKINS CLASSIFICATION OF TALAR NECK FRACTURES

Type I: nondisplaced
Type II: associated subtalar subluxation or dislocation

Type III: associated subtalar and ankle dislocation
Type IV: type III with associated talonavicular subluxation or dislocation

Treatment

Nonoperative Treatment
Nondisplaced fractures may be managed in a long-leg cast with the knee flexed to 30 degrees to prevent weight bearing. This is maintained for 6 to 8 weeks with serial radiographs to assess healing status. The patient may then be advanced to weight bearing in a short-leg walking cast for an additional 2 to 3 weeks.

Operative Treatment
- Indicated for displaced fractures (defined as >5-mm displacement or >5-degree malalignment on the anteroposterior radiograph).
- Minimally displaced fractures (type II) often treated successfully with closed reduction and plantarflexion of the forefoot with hindfoot eversion or inversion, depending on the displacement. A short-leg cast is then placed for 6 to 8 weeks; may require plantarflexion of the foot to maintain reduction. If it cannot be maintained by simple positioning, operative fixation is indicated.
- Displaced fractures usually amenable to internal fixation using a posterior approach; 4.0-mm cannulated screws introduced from a posterior to anterior direction to avoid dissection around the precarious talar neck.
- May be reduced and held with Kirschner wire fixation.
- Postoperatively, patient is maintained in a short-leg cast for 6 to 8 weeks with removal of pins at 3 to 4 weeks.

Complications

Osteonecrosis: may occur with disruption or thrombosis of the tenuous vascular supply to the talus. Related to initial degree of displacement and angulation and theoretically to time until reduction. Tends to occur within 6 months of injury. Hawkins sign represents subchondral osteopenia in the vascularized non–weight bearing talus at 6 to 8 weeks; although this tends to indicate talar viability, the presence of this sign does not rule out osteonecrosis.

- Type I fractures: 0 to 27% incidence of osteonecrosis reported
- Type II fractures: 42% incidence
- Type III and IV fractures: >90% incidence

CALCANEUS

Epidemiology

- Rare injury typically involving older children (>9 years) and adolescents.
- Most are extraarticular, involving the apophysis or tuberosity.
- Thirty-three percent associated with other injuries, including lumbar vertebral and ipsilateral lower extremity injuries.

Anatomy

- The primary ossification center appears at 7 months *in utero*; a secondary ossification center appears at the age of 10 years and fuses by age 16.
- Calcaneal fracture patterns in children differ from those of adults. This is primarily due to the following three reasons:
  - The lateral process, which is responsible for calcaneal impaction resulting in joint depression injury in adults, is diminutive in the immature calcaneus.
  - The posterior facet is parallel to the ground rather than inclined as in adults.
  - In children, the calcaneus is comprised of a ossific nucleus surrounded by cartilage.

These are responsible for the dissipation of the injurious forces that produce classic fracture patterns in adults.

Mechanism of Injury

- Almost all calcaneal fractures occur as a result of a fall or a jump from a height.
- Open fractures may result from lawnmower injuries.

Clinical Evaluation

- Patients typically present unable to walk due to hindfoot pain.
- On physical examination pain, swelling, and tenderness can usually be appreciated at the site of injury.
- Examination of the ipsilateral lower extremity and lumbar spine is essential because associated injuries are common.
- A careful neurovascular examination should be performed.

Radiographic Evaluation

- Dorsal-plantar, lateral, axial, and lateral oblique views should be obtained for the evaluation of pediatric calcaneal fractures.
- The Bohler tuber joint angle is represented by the supplement (180-degree measured angle) of two lines: a line from the highest point of the anterior process to the highest point of the posterior articular surface and a line drawn between the same point on the posterior articular surface and the most superior point of the tuberosity. Normally, this angle is between 25 and 40 degrees; flattening of this angle indicates collapse of the posterior facet.
- Technetium-99m bone scanning may be used in cases in which calcaneal fracture is suspected but is not appreciated on standard radiographs.
- Computed tomography may aid in fracture definition, particularly in intraarticular fractures, in which preoperative planning may be facilitated by three-dimensional characterization of fragments.

SCHMIDT AND WEINER CLASSIFICATION (FIG. 50.1)

Type I:
  A. Fracture of the tuberosity or apophysis
  B. Fracture of the sustentaculum
  C. Fracture of the anterior process
  D. Fracture of the anterior inferolateral process
  E. Avulsion fracture of the body

Type II: Fracture of the posterior and/or superior parts of the tuberosity

Type III: Fracture of the body not involving the subtalar joint

Type IV: Nondisplaced or minimally displaced fracture through the subtalar joint

Type V: Displaced fracture through the subtalar joint
  A. Tongue type
  B. Joint depression type

Type VI: Either unclassified (Rasmussen and Schantz) or serious soft-tissue injury, bone loss, and loss of the insertions of the Achilles tendon.

Treatment

Nonoperative Treatment

- Cast immobilization is recommended for pediatric patients with extraarticular fractures and nondisplaced intraarticular fractures of the calcaneus. Weight bearing is restricted for 6 weeks, although some authors have suggested that in the case of truly nondisplaced fractures in a very young child, weight bearing may be permitted with cast immobilization.
- Mild degrees of joint incongruity tend to remodel well; however, severe joint depression is an indication for operative management.

Operative Treatment

- Operative treatment is indicated for displaced articular fractures, particularly in older children and adolescents.

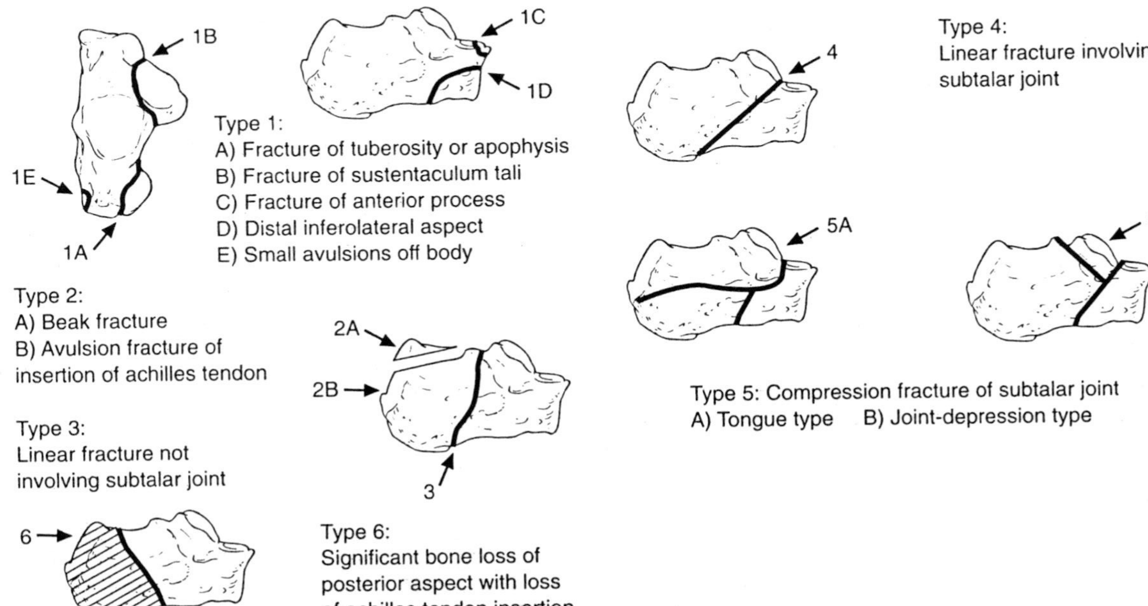

FIG. 50.1. Classification used to evaluate calcaneal fracture patterns in children. **A.** Extraarticular fractures. **B.** Intra-articular fractures. **C.** Type VI injury with significant bone loss, soft-tissue injury, and loss of insertion of Achilles tendon. (From Schmidt TL, Weiner DS. Calcaneus fractures in children: an evaluation of the nature of injury in 56 children. *Clin Orthop* 1982;171:150, with permission.)

- Displaced fractures of the anterior process of the calcaneus represent relative indications for open reduction and internal fixation because up to 30% may result in nonunion.
- Anatomic reconstitution of the articular surface is imperative, followed by compression screw technique for operative fixation.

Complications

- *Posttraumatic osteoarthritis.* This may result due to residual or unrecognized articular incongruity. Although younger children remodel very well, this difficulty emphasizes the need for anatomic reduction and reconstruction of the articular surface in older children and adolescents.
- *Heel widening.* This is not as significant a problem in children as it is in adults because the mechanisms of injury tend not to be as high energy (i.e., falls from lower heights with less explosive impact to the calcaneus) and remodeling can partially restore architectural integrity.
- *Nonunion.* This complication is rare; it most commonly involves displaced anterior process fractures treated nonoperatively with cast immobilization. This is likely due to the attachment of the bifurcate ligament, which tends to produce a displacing force on the anterior fragment with motions of plantarflexion and inversion of the foot.

TARSOMETATARSAL (LISFRANC) INJURIES

Epidemiology

- Extremely uncommon in children.
- Tend to occur in older children and adolescents (>10 years of age).

Anatomy

- The base of the second metatarsal is the "keystone" of an arch that is interconnected by tough plantar ligaments.
- The plantar ligaments generally are much tougher than the dorsal ligamentous complex.
- The ligamentous connection between the first and second metatarsal bases is weak relative to those between the second through fifth metatarsal bases.

Mechanism of Injury

- Direct: secondary to a heavy object impacting the foot dorsum and causing plantar displacement of the metatarsal with compromise of the intermetatarsal ligaments.
- Indirect: more common; due to violent abduction, forced plantarflexion, or twisting of the forefoot.
  - Abduction: tends to fracture the recessed base of the second metatarsal and to cause lateral displacement of the forefoot, variably producing a "nutcracker" fracture of the cuboid.
  - Plantarflexion: often accompanied by fractures of the metatarsal shafts as the axial load is transmitted proximally.
  - Twisting: may result in purely ligamentous injuries.

Clinical Evaluation

- Patients typically present with swelling over the dorsum of the foot with either an inability to ambulate or with painful ambulation.
- Deformity is variable because spontaneous reduction of the ligamentous injury is common.
- Tenderness over the tarsometatarsal joint can usually be elicited; this may be exacerbated by maneuvers that stress the tarsometatarsal articulation.

Radiographic Evaluation

- Anteroposterior, lateral, and oblique views of the foot should be obtained.
- The anteroposterior radiograph should elucidate the following:
  - The medial border of the second metatarsal should be co-linear with the medial border of the middle cuneiform on the anteroposterior view.

A fracture of the base of the second metatarsal should alert the examiner to the likelihood of a tarsometatarsal dislocation because often the dislocation will have spontaneously reduced.
The combination of a fracture at the base of the second metatarsal and a cuboid fracture indicates that severe ligamentous injury has occurred, as well as dislocation of the tarsometatarsal joint.
Greater than 2 to 3 mm of diastasis between the first and second metatarsal bases indicates ligamentous compromise.

- The lateral radiograph should elucidate the following:
  Dorsal displacement of the metatarsals is indicative of ligamentous compromise.
  Plantar displacement of the medial cuneiform relative to the fifth metatarsal on a weight-bearing lateral view may indicate subtle ligamentous injury.
- The oblique radiograph should elucidate the medial border of the fourth metatarsal, which should be co-linear with the medial border of the cuboid.

QUENU AND KUSS CLASSIFICATION (FIG. 50.2)

Type A: incongruity of the entire tarsometatarsal joint
Type B: partial instability, either medial or lateral
Type C: divergent partial or total instability

Treatment

Nonoperative Treatment

- Minimally displaced tarsometatarsal dislocations (<2 to 3 mm) may be managed with elevation and a compressive dressing until the swelling subsides. This is followed by short-leg casting for 2 to 4 weeks until symptomatic improvement occurs. The patient may then be placed in a hard-soled shoe or cast boot until ambulation is well tolerated.
- Displaced dislocations often respond well to closed reduction under general anesthesia.
  This is typically accomplished with the patient prone, finger-traps on the toes, and 10 pounds of traction.
  If the reduction is determined to be stable, a short-leg cast is placed for 4 weeks, followed by a hard-soled shoe or cast boot until ambulation is well tolerated.

Operative Treatment

- Surgical management is indicated with displaced dislocations in which a reduction cannot be achieved or maintained.
- Closed reduction may be attempted as described above, followed by the placement of percutaneous Kirschner wires to maintain the reduction.
- In the rare case in which a closed reduction cannot be obtained, open reduction using a dorsal incision may be performed. Kirschner wires are used to maintain reduction; these are typically left protruding from the skin to facilitate removal.
- A short-leg cast is placed postoperatively; this is maintained for 4 weeks, at which time the wires and cast may be discontinued and the patient can be placed in a hard-soled shoe or cast boot until ambulation is well tolerated.

Complications

- Persistent pain: may result due to unrecognized or untreated injuries to the tarsometatarsal joint as a result of ligamentous compromise and residual instability.
- Angular deformity: may result despite treatment; emphasizes the need for reduction and immobilization by surgical intervention if indicated.

METATARSALS

Epidemiology

- Very common injuries in children; true incidence of injury is unknown.
- Metatarsals involved in only 2% of stress fractures in children; in adults, metatarsals involved in 14% of stress fractures.

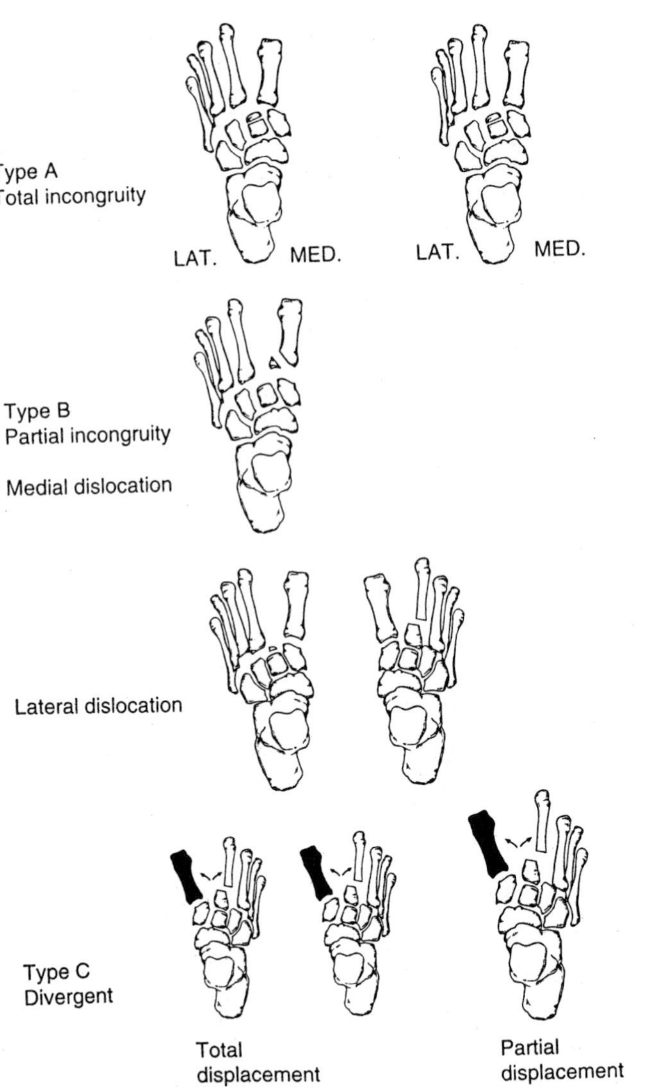

FIG. 50.2. Quenu and Kuss classification of tarsometatarsal injuries. (From Hardcastle PH, Reschauer R, Kitscha-Lissberg E, et al. Injuries to the tarsometatarsal joint. Incidence, classification, and treatment. *J Bone Joint Surg Br* 1982; 64B:349, with permission.)

Anatomy

- Ossification of the metatarsals is apparent by 2 months *in utero*.
- The metatarsals are interconnected by tough intermetatarsal ligaments at their bases.
- The configuration of the metatarsals in coronal section forms an arch, with the second metatarsal representing the "keystone" of the arch.

- Fractures through the metatarsal neck occur most frequently due to their relatively small diameter.
- Fractures at the base of the fifth metatarsal must be differentiated from an apophyseal growth center or an os vesalianum, a sesamoid proximal to the insertion of the peroneus brevis. The apophysis is not present before the age of 8 years; it usually unites to the shaft by the age of 12 in girls and of 15 in boys.

Mechanism of Injury

- Direct: trauma to the foot dorsum, mainly from heavy falling objects.
- Indirect: more common; results from axial loading with force transmission through the plantarflexed ankle or by torsional forces as the forefoot is violently twisted.
- Avulsion at the base of the fifth metatarsal: occurs as a result of tension at the insertion of the peroneus brevis muscle, the tendinous portion of the abductor digiti minimi, or the insertion of the tough lateral cord of the plantar aponeurosis.
- "Bunk-bed" fracture: fracture of the proximal first metatarsal caused by jumping from a bunk bed with impact on the plantarflexed foot.
- Stress fractures: occur with repetitive loading, such as long-distance running.

Clinical Evaluation

- Patients typically present with swelling, pain, and ecchymosis; they may be unable to ambulate on the affected foot.
- Minimally displaced fractures may present with minimal swelling and tenderness to palpation.
- A careful neurovascular examination should be performed.
- The presence of compartment syndrome of the foot should be ruled out in cases of dramatic swelling, pain, venous congestion in the toes, or a history of a crush mechanism of injury. The interossei and short plantar muscles are contained in closed fascial compartments.

Radiographic Evaluation

- Anteroposterior, lateral, and oblique views of the foot should be obtained.
- Bone scans may be useful for identifying occult fractures in the appropriate clinical setting or stress fractures with plain radiographs that are apparently negative.
- With conventional radiographs of the foot, exposures sufficient for penetration of the tarsal bones typically result in overpenetration of the metatarsal bones and phalanges; therefore, when injuries to the forefoot are suspected, optimal exposure of this region may require underpenetration of the hindfoot.

DESCRIPTIVE CLASSIFICATION

- Location: metatarsal number, proximal, midshaft, distal
- Pattern: spiral, transverse, oblique
- Angulation
- Displacement
- Degree of comminution
- Articular involvement

Treatment

Nonoperative Treatment

- Most fractures of the metatarsals may be treated initially with splinting, followed by a short-leg walking cast once swelling subsides. If severe swelling is present, the ankle should be splinted in slight equinus to prevent neurovascular compromise at the ankle. Care must be taken to ensure that circumferential dressings are not constrictive at the ankle, causing further congestion and possible neurovascular compromise.
- Alternatively, in cases of truly nondisplaced fractures with no or minimal swelling, a cast may be placed initially. This is typically maintained for 3 to 6 weeks until radiographic evidence of union.

- Fractures at the base of the fifth metatarsal may be treated with a short-leg walking cast for 3 to 6 weeks until radiographic evidence of union. True Jones fractures (occurring at the metaphyseal-diaphyseal junction) have questionable rates of healing. For these, open reduction and intramedullary screw fixation should be considered controversial.
- Stress fractures of the metatarsals may be treated with a short-leg walking cast for 2 weeks, at which time it may be discontinued if tenderness has subsided and walking is painless. Pain from excessive metatarsophalangeal motion may be minimized by the use of a metatarsal bar sunk into the sole of the shoe.

Operative Treatment
- If a compartment syndrome is identified, all nine fascial compartments of the foot should be released.
- Unstable fractures may require percutaneous pinning with Kirschner wires for fixation, particularly with fractures of the first and fifth metatarsals. Considerable lateral displacement and dorsal angulation may be accepted in younger patients because remodeling will occur.
- Open reduction and pinning are indicated in fractures in which reduction is unable to be achieved or maintained. The standard technique includes dorsal exposure, Kirschner wire placement in the distal fragment, fracture reduction, and intramedullary introduction of the wire in a retrograde fashion to achieve operative fixation.
- Postoperatively, the patient should be placed in a short-leg non–weight bearing cast for 3 weeks, at which time the pins are removed and the patient is changed to a walking cast for an additional 2 to 4 weeks.

Complications
- Malunion: typically does not result in functional disability because remodeling may achieve partial correction. Severe malunion resulting in disability may be treated with osteotomy and operative pinning.
- Compartment syndrome: an uncommon but devastating complication that may result in fibrosis of the interossei and an intrinsic minus foot with claw toes. Clinical suspicion must be high in the appropriate clinical setting, workup should be aggressive, and treatment must be expedient because the compartments of the foot are small in volume and are bounded by tight fascial structures.

PHALANGES

Epidemiology
Uncommon; true incidence unknown due to underreporting.

Anatomy
- Ossification of the phalanges ranges from 3 months *in utero* for the distal phalanges of the lesser toes, 4 months *in utero* for the proximal phalanges, 6 months *in utero* for the middle phalanges, and up to the age of 3 years for the secondary ossification centers.

Mechanism of Injury
- Direct trauma accounts for nearly all the injuries; force transmission is typically on the dorsal aspect from heavy falling objects or is axial when an unyielding structure is kicked.
- Indirect mechanisms are uncommon; rotational forces from twisting are responsible for most of these.

Clinical Evaluation
- Patients typically present ambulatory but display guarding of the affected forefoot.
- Ecchymosis, swelling, and tenderness to palpation may be appreciated.
- A neurovascular examination, with documentation of digital sensation on the medial and lateral aspects of the toe and an assessment of capillary refill, is important.
- The entire toe should be exposed and examined for open fracture or puncture wounds.

Radiographic Evaluation

- Anteroposterior, lateral, and oblique films of the foot should be obtained.
- The diagnosis is usually made from the anteroposterior or oblique films; lateral radiographs of lesser toe phalanges are usually of limited value.
- Contralateral views may be taken for comparison.

DESCRIPTIVE CLASSIFICATION

- Location: toe number, proximal, middle, distal
- Pattern: spiral, transverse, oblique
- Angulation
- Displacement
- Degree of comminution
- Articular involvement

Treatment

Nonoperative Treatment

- Nonoperative treatment is indicated for almost all pediatric phalangeal fractures unless severe articular incongruity or an unstable displaced fracture of the first proximal phalanx is present.
- Reduction maneuvers are rarely necessary; severe angulation or displacement often may be addressed by simple longitudinal traction.
- External immobilization typically consists of simple buddy taping with gauze between the toes to prevent maceration; a rigid-soled orthosis may provide additional comfort by limiting forefoot motion. This is maintained until symptomatic relief, typically between 2 and 4 weeks.
- Kicking and running sports should be limited for an additional 2 to 3 weeks to ensure complete healing.

Operative Treatment

- Surgical management is indicated for cases in which a reduction is unable to be achieved or maintained, particularly for displaced or angulated fractures of the first proximal phalanx.
- Relative indications include rotational displacement that cannot be corrected by closed means and severe angular deformities that, if uncorrected, would lead to cock-up toe deformities or to an abducted fifth toe.
- Reduction is maintained via retrograde intramedullary Kirschner wire fixation. Nailbed injuries should be repaired. Open reduction may be necessary to remove interposed soft tissues or to achieve adequate articular congruity.
- Postoperative immobilization consists of a rigid-soled orthosis or splint. The pins are typically removed at 3 weeks.

Complications

Malunion: uncommonly is functionally significant; this is usually a result of fractures of the first proximal phalanx that may result in varus or valgus deformity. Cock-up toe deformities and fifth toe abduction may result in cosmetically undesirable results and poor shoe fitting or irritation.

SUBJECT INDEX

SUBJECT INDEX

Note: Page numbers followed by an *f* indicates figures; page numbers followed by a *t* indicate tables.

R

T